# THE MANAGEMENT OF WORKING CAPITAL IN HOSPITALS

Robert W. Broyles, Ph.D.
University of Ottawa

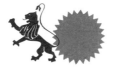

AN ASPEN PUBLICATION
Aspen Systems Corporation
Rockville, Maryland
London
1981

Library of Congress Cataloging in Publication Data

Broyles, Robert
The management of working capital in hospitals.

Includes index.
1. Hospitals—Finance.   2. Working capital.
3. Hospitals—United States—Finance.
4. Hospitals—Canada—Finance.   I. Title [DNLM:
1. Financial management.   2. Economics, Hospital.
WX 157 B885m]
RA971.3.B76        362.1'1'0681        80-26802
ISBN: 0-89443-335-0

Library of Congress Catalog Card Number: 80-26802
ISBN: 0-89443-335-0

*Printed in the United States of America*

1  2  3  4  5

# Table of Contents

Preface ..................................................... xi

PART 1    — INTRODUCTION ............................. 1

Chapter 1    — Introduction to Working Capital Management ...... 3

    1.1 — The Basic Problem ......................... 3
    1.2 — The Objective of Management .............. 4
    1.3 — A Definition of Working Capital Management .. 5
    1.4 — Relationship between Working Capital
            Management and Internal Control ........... 5
    1.5 — The Value of Working Capital Management .... 7
    1.6 — Two Approaches in Financing Care .......... 10

Chapter 2    — Financing Hospital Care in the U.S. .............. 13

    2.1 — Introduction ............................... 13
    2.2 — Source of Revenue ........................ 14
    2.3 — Blue Cross .............................. 14
        2.3.1 — The Benefit Package .................... 14
        2.3.2 — Allowable Costs ...................... 15
        2.3.3 — Financing Hospital Costs ............... 18
        2.3.4 — Methods of Payment ................... 18
    2.4 — The Commercial Insurance Industry .......... 19
        2.4.1 — The Benefit Structure .................. 20
        2.4.2 — Financing Care under Commercial Insurance 21
        2.4.3 — Methods of Payment ................... 22
    2.5 — Medicare ................................ 22
        2.5.1 — Benefit Structure ...................... 23

2.5.2 — Financing Medicare Benefits . . . . . . . . . . . . .    24
2.5.3 — Allowable Costs . . . . . . . . . . . . . . . . . . . . . .    25
2.5.4 — Amount and Receipt of Medicare Payments .    26
2.6 — Medicaid . . . . . . . . . . . . . . . . . . . . . . . . . . . . . .    29

**Chapter 3    — Financing Hospital Care In Canada** . . . . . . . . . . . . . .    **33**

3.1 — Introduction . . . . . . . . . . . . . . . . . . . . . . . . . . . .    33
3.2 — Benefit Structure and Sources of Revenue . . . . . .    34
3.2.1 — Inpatient Benefits . . . . . . . . . . . . . . . . . . . . .    34
3.2.2 — Outpatient Benefits . . . . . . . . . . . . . . . . . . . .    34
3.2.3 — Other Sources of Revenue . . . . . . . . . . . . . .    37
3.3 — Allowable costs . . . . . . . . . . . . . . . . . . . . . . . . .    38
3.4 — Financing Mechanism . . . . . . . . . . . . . . . . . . . . .    40
3.4.1 — The Federal Contribution . . . . . . . . . . . . . . .    41
3.4.2 — The Provincial Contribution . . . . . . . . . . . . .    44
3.5 — Methods of Payment . . . . . . . . . . . . . . . . . . . . . .    45
3.6 — Summary and Implications for Working Capital
          Management . . . . . . . . . . . . . . . . . . . . . . . . . . .    45

**Chapter 4    — Introduction to Matrix Algebra** . . . . . . . . . . . . . . . . . .    **49**

4.1 — Introduction . . . . . . . . . . . . . . . . . . . . . . . . . . . .    49
4.2 — A General Description . . . . . . . . . . . . . . . . . . . . .    50
4.3 — Matrix Addition . . . . . . . . . . . . . . . . . . . . . . . . .    52
4.4 — Matrix Subtraction . . . . . . . . . . . . . . . . . . . . . . .    52
4.5 — Matrix Multiplication . . . . . . . . . . . . . . . . . . . . .    53
4.6 — The Determinant and Inverse of a Matrix . . . . . . .    59

**PART II    — WORKING CAPITAL MANAGEMENT** . . . . . . . . . . .    **67**

**Chapter 5    — Fundamentals of Working Capital Management** . . . . .    **69**

5.1 — Definitions . . . . . . . . . . . . . . . . . . . . . . . . . . . . .    69
5.2 — The Importance of Working Capital Management    70
5.3 — Working Capital Needs . . . . . . . . . . . . . . . . . . . . .    72
5.3.1 — A Cash Flow Approach . . . . . . . . . . . . . . . .    72
5.3.2 — Working Capital Needs and Financial
            Statements . . . . . . . . . . . . . . . . . . . . . . . . .    81
5.4 — Financing Working Capital . . . . . . . . . . . . . . . . .    97
5.4.1 — Nature of Working Capital . . . . . . . . . . . . . .    98
5.4.2 — Sources of Funding . . . . . . . . . . . . . . . . . . .    99

5.4.3 — Financing Temporary Working Capital
Needs . . . . . . . . . . . . . . . . . . . . . . . . . . . . .   104
5.4.4 — Choice of Short-Term Finance . . . . . . . . . . . .   106
Appendix 5-1 . . . . . . . . . . . . . . . . . . . . . . . . . . . . . .   108

**Chapter 6    — Management of Accounts Receivable . . . . . . . . . . . . . .   111**

6.1 — Introduction . . . . . . . . . . . . . . . . . . . . . . . . . . . . .   111
6.2 — Characteristics of Accounts Receivable . . . . . . . .   112
6.3 — The Cost of Accounts Receivable: The General
Case . . . . . . . . . . . . . . . . . . . . . . . . . . . . . . . . . .   113
6.3.1 — Opportunity Costs . . . . . . . . . . . . . . . . . . . . . .   113
6.3.2 — Routine Credit and Collection Costs . . . . . . .   114
6.3.3 — Delinquency Costs . . . . . . . . . . . . . . . . . . . .   114
6.4 — Advantages of Trade Credit . . . . . . . . . . . . . . . . .   115
6.5 — Management and Control of Accounts
Receivable . . . . . . . . . . . . . . . . . . . . . . . . . . . . .   116
6.5.1 — The Preadmission Phase . . . . . . . . . . . . . . . . .   116
6.5.2 — The Admission Phase . . . . . . . . . . . . . . . . . . .   118
6.5.3 — The Production Phase . . . . . . . . . . . . . . . . . . .   118
6.5.4 — The Discharge Phase . . . . . . . . . . . . . . . . . . . .   119
6.5.5 — The Post-Discharge Phase . . . . . . . . . . . . . . .   120
6.5.6 — Evaluation of Accounts Receivable
Management . . . . . . . . . . . . . . . . . . . . . . .   120
6.6 — Estimation of Cash Receipts . . . . . . . . . . . . . . . .   125
6.6.1 — Institutional Sources . . . . . . . . . . . . . . . . . . .   125
6.6.2 — Noninstitutional Sources . . . . . . . . . . . . . . . . .   131
Appendix 6-1 . . . . . . . . . . . . . . . . . . . . . . . . . . . . . .   149

**Chapter 7    — Management of Cash . . . . . . . . . . . . . . . . . . . . . . . . . . .   151**

7.1 — The Functions of Money . . . . . . . . . . . . . . . . . . .   151
7.1.1 — Unit of Value . . . . . . . . . . . . . . . . . . . . . . . . . .   152
7.1.2 — Medium of Exchange . . . . . . . . . . . . . . . . . . .   152
7.1.3 — Standard of Deferred Payments . . . . . . . . . . .   152
7.1.4 — Store of Value . . . . . . . . . . . . . . . . . . . . . . . . .   153
7.2 — The Composition and Importance of Cash . . . . . .   154
7.2.1 — The Composition of Cash . . . . . . . . . . . . . . . .   154
7.2.2 — The Importance of Cash . . . . . . . . . . . . . . . . .   154
7.3 — The Management and Control of Cash . . . . . . . . .   155
7.3.1 — General Guidelines . . . . . . . . . . . . . . . . . . . . .   155
7.3.2 — An Internal Control System . . . . . . . . . . . . . .   156

7.3.3 — Evaluation of the Control System ......... 161
7.4 — The Cash Balance Decision .................. 165
7.4.1 — Motives for Holding Cash ............... 165
7.4.2 — The Costs of Holding Cash ............. 166
7.5 — Elements of the Cash Balance Decision ........ 166
7.5.1 — The Nature of Cash Flows .............. 167
7.5.2 — The Minimum Cash Balance ............. 169
7.6 — The Cash Balance under Conditions of Certainty 170
7.7 — Optimum Cash Balance and Uncertainty ....... 172
7.7.1 — Expected Short-Cost Function ............ 173
7.7.2 — Expected Long-Cost Function ........... 176
7.7.3 — The Optimum Cash Balance ............. 178

Chapter 8   — Management of Marketable Securities ............. 187

8.1 — Investment Alternatives .................... 188
8.1.1 — Government Treasury Bills.............. 188
8.1.2 — Certificates of Deposit ................. 188
8.1.3 — Bonds............................... 189
8.1.4 — Stocks ............................. 190
8.2 — The Evaluation of Bonds ................... 191
8.3 — The Process of Stock Selection .............. 195
8.3.1 — Historical Analysis .................... 196
8.3.2 — The Forecasting Phase ................. 200
8.3.3 — The Analysis Phase.................... 202
8.4 — A Management Model: The Case of a Single
        Security ................................ 206
8.4.1 — The Basic Model ...................... 206
8.4.2 — An Illustration ....................... 212
8.5 — The Portfolio Problem .................... 221
8.5.1 — Reduction of Risk ..................... 221
8.5.2 — Marketability and Liquidity ............. 222
8.5.3 — Maturity ............................ 223
8.5.4 — An Investment Strategy ................ 223

Chapter 9   — Inventory Management ......................... 227

9.1 — The Importance of Inventories and Inventory
        Management Functions ................... 228
9.1.1 — The Importance of Inventories ........... 228
9.1.2 — Inventory Management Functions ........ 229
9.2 — The ABC Classification System ............. 230

9.3 — The Control of Inventory ..................... 232
9.4 — Costs of Inventory ........................ 236
   9.4.1 — Ordering Costs ........................ 236
   9.4.2 — Carrying Costs ........................ 237
   9.4.3 — Long-Costs .......................... 239
   9.4.4 — Short-Costs .......................... 240
9.5 — Inventory Management: Certanty ............. 241
9.6 — Inventory Management: Uncertainty ........... 245
   9.6.1 — The EOQ and Reorder Point: Uncertainty ... 246
   9.6.2 — The Reorder Point: A Mathematical
          Expectation Model .................. 252

**PART III    — INTERNAL CONTROL** ........................ **255**

**Chapter 10 — Cost Analysis** ................................... **257**

10.1 — Managerial Uses of Cost Analysis ........... 257
   10.1.1 — Planning Operational Activity ........... 258
   10.1.2 — Controlling Operational Activity ......... 259
10.2 — Necessary Prerequisites ................... 260
   10.2.1 — Organization Chart and Chart of Accounts . 260
   10.2.2 — Classification of Cost Centers .......... 260
   10.2.3 — Accurate Accounting System ........... 261
   10.2.4 — Information System ................... 261
10.3 — Methods of Apportionment ................. 262
   10.3.1 — Direct Apportionment .................. 263
   10.3.2 — Step-Down Method .................... 267
   10.3.3 — Double Distribution Method ............. 274
   10.3.4 — A Comparison of the Methods .......... 282
   10.3.5 — Alternate Organizational Structures ....... 283
   10.3.6 — Alternate Methods of Cost Analysis ...... 283
   10.3.7 — Computer Applications ................. 284

**Chapter 11 — Introduction to Budgeting** ...................... **285**

11.1 — The Importance of Budgeting ............... 285
11.2 — Budgeting and the Functions of Management .. 286
   11.2.1 — Planning ........................... 286
   11.2.2 — Control ............................ 286
   11.2.3 — Coordination ........................ 288
   11.2.4 — Organizing ......................... 288
11.3 — Techniques of Budgeting ................... 289

11.3.1 — The Global Budget .................... 289
11.3.2 — Line Item Budgeting .................. 290
11.3.3 — Responsibility Budgeting .............. 290
11.3.4 — Program Budgeting .................... 291
11.3.5 — Zero-Base Budgeting ................. 296
11.4 — Approaches to the Budgeting Process ........ 306
11.4.1 — Comprehensive and Partial Budgets ....... 307
11.4.2 — Fixed and Flexible Budgets ............ 307

**Chapter 12 — The Budgeting Process** ......................... **311**

12.1 — Introduction ............................... 311
12.2 — The Phases of Budget Preparation ........... 311
12.2.1 — The First Phase ....................... 312
12.2.2 — The Second Phase ..................... 315
12.2.3 — The Third Phase ..................... 316
12.2.4 — The Fourth Phase .................... 317

**Chapter 13 — Traditional Budgeting Techniques** ................. **321**

13.1 — Components of the Budget ................. 321
13.2 — Estimation of Work Load ................. 323
13.2.1 — The Moving Average and the Geometric
Mean ............................ 323
13.2.2 — Exponential Smoothing ................. 328
13.2.3 — Regression Analysis ................... 330
13.3 — Expense Budget ......................... 331
13.3.1 — The Salary and Wage Budget ........... 331
13.3.2 — Supply Expense Budget ............... 337
13.4 — The Revenue Budget ..................... 339
13.4.1 — Standardized Services ................. 342
13.4.2 — Stay-Specific Services ............... 344
13.4.3 — Services Measured by Hours of Use ...... 347
13.4.4 — Merchandising Function ............... 348
13.5 — The Capital Budget ...................... 349
13.6 — Cash Budget ........................... 350
13.6.1 — Cash Receipts Budget ................. 350
13.6.2 — Cash Disbursement Budget ............. 353
13.6.3 — Summary of Cash Receipts and
Disbursements ..................... 354

**Chapter 14 — Traditional Systems of Internal Control and
Reporting** ................................... **357**

14.1 — Basic Principles of Internal Control .......... 357
14.2 — Basic Statistical Reports ................... 360
14.2.1 — Work Performance Reports ............. 360
14.2.2 — Cost Variances: A Summary View ....... 365
14.3 — Reporting Revenues and Expenses .......... 366

**Chapter 15 — Program Budgeting** ........................... **371**

15.1 — Introduction ............................. 371
15.2 — The Program Area ....................... 372
15.3 — The Components of Hospital Care .......... 373
15.4 — An Overview .......................... 375
15.5 — The Operational Budget of the Program Area .. 377
15.5.1 — The Size of the Patient Population ....... 377
15.5.2 — The Expected Diagnostic Mix .......... 377
15.5.3 — Service Requirements of the Program Area 381
15.5.4 — Estimation of Resource Requirements ..... 387
15.6 — Labor and Supply Costs of the Program Area .. 392
15.6.1 — Standard Factor Prices ................ 393
15.6.2 — Labor Costs ......................... 394
15.6.3 — Supply Costs ........................ 397
15.7 — Overhead and Direct Equipment Costs of
Program Areas ........................ 398
15.8 — Full Program Costs ....................... 401
15.9 — Obtaining the Data ....................... 402

**Chapter 16 — Responsibility Budgeting** ........................ **405**

16.1 — Introduction ............................. 405
16.2 — Operational Budget of the Responsibility Center 406
16.3 — Financial Budget of the Responsibility Center .. 410
16.3.1 — Financial Budget for Department $D_3$ ...... 411
16.3.2 — Financial Budget for Departments $D_1$ and
$D_2$ ................................ 415
16.4 — Equipment and Overhead Costs of the
Responsibility Center .................... 416
16.5 — Full Costs of Operation ................... 418
16.6 — Rate Setting ........................... 419
16.6.1 — Direct Costs ......................... 419

16.6.2 — Indirect or Overhead Costs . . . . . . . . . . . . . .    420
16.6.3 — Full Cost Pricing . . . . . . . . . . . . . . . . . . . . . .    421

**Chapter 17 — Controlling the Program Area** . . . . . . . . . . . . . . . . . . . .    **423**

17.1 — Introduction. . . . . . . . . . . . . . . . . . . . . . . . . . . . .    423
17.2 — An Overview of the Reporting System . . . . . . . .    425
17.3 — The Total Cost Variance . . . . . . . . . . . . . . . . . . .    427
17.4 — Diagnostic Mix Variance . . . . . . . . . . . . . . . . . . .    434
17.5 — Service Mix Variance. . . . . . . . . . . . . . . . . . . . . .    437
17.6 — Labor Efficiency Variance . . . . . . . . . . . . . . . . .    439
17.7 — Supply Efficiency Variance . . . . . . . . . . . . . . . .    442
17.8 — Wage Variance . . . . . . . . . . . . . . . . . . . . . . . . . .    444
17.9 — Supply Price Variance . . . . . . . . . . . . . . . . . . . .    446
17.10 — Management Reports . . . . . . . . . . . . . . . . . . . . .    448

**Chapter 18 — Controlling the Responsibility Center** . . . . . . . . . . . . . .    **451**

18.1 — The Total Cost Variance . . . . . . . . . . . . . . . . . .    452
18.2 — Volume Variance . . . . . . . . . . . . . . . . . . . . . . . . .    455
18.3 — Efficiency Variance . . . . . . . . . . . . . . . . . . . . . .    458
18.4 — Price Variance . . . . . . . . . . . . . . . . . . . . . . . . . .    463
18.5 — The Interactive Variance . . . . . . . . . . . . . . . . . .    467
18.6 — Management Reports . . . . . . . . . . . . . . . . . . . . . .    469
18.7 — Productivity Reports . . . . . . . . . . . . . . . . . . . . . .    474

**Chapter 19 — Short-Term Forecasting**. . . . . . . . . . . . . . . . . . . . . . . .    **479**

19.1 — Introduction. . . . . . . . . . . . . . . . . . . . . . . . . . . . .    479
19.2 — Forecasting Techniques . . . . . . . . . . . . . . . . . . . .    480
19.2.1 — Time Series Analysis-Regression Analysis .    481
19.2.2 — Causal Models-Regression Analysis . . . . . .    482
19.2.3 — Simulation . . . . . . . . . . . . . . . . . . . . . . . . .    483

**Index** . . . . . . . . . . . . . . . . . . . . . . . . . . . . . . . . . . . . . . . . . . . . .    **485**

# Preface

The purpose of this text is to familiarize practicing administrators and students of health care administration with the fundamentals of working capital management and the techniques of controlling operational activity, particularly in achieving the goals and objectives of the hospital enterprise.

Accordingly, this book is comprised of three parts. The first phase discusses the financial environment of the institution and examines methods that have been used in the United States and Canada to finance hospital care. As documented in Part I, the two countries have relied, in varying degrees, on prospective and retrospective methods of financing the costs of care. As a result, the techniques of working capital management as developed here accommodate both mechanisms.

Many techniques are expressed in the notation of matrix algebra. Matrix algebra not only simplifies the expression of complex mathematical operations but also provides the basis for developing programs that permit management to use high-speed electronic computers to perform the calculations. Since many readers may not be familiar with this area of mathematics, Chapter 4 is devoted to a discussion of the fundamentals of matrix algebra.

In Part II of this book, Chapter 5 addresses the fundamentals of working capital management; Chapter 6, the principles of managing outstanding receivables; Chapter 7, cash management; Chapter 8, managing the hospital's investment in marketable securities; and Chapter 9, inventory management.

While the retrospective system of financing hospital care predominates in the United States and the prospective mechanism in Canada, elements of these systems are present in both countries. To accommodate both methods of reimbursement, separate models are developed in selected sections of this text.

Since one of the most important aspects of working capital management is the control and evaluation of the hospital's day-to-day functioning, the final section of this volume, Part III, discusses the techniques that may be used in monitoring, evaluating, and controlling the institution's operational activity. In discharging these responsibilities, managers must develop indexes of current activity as well as a standard against which actual operational performance is compared. Data to carry out these functions are obtainable through the application of cost-finding techniques. Cost finding is a method by which management may determine the actual or expected expenditures in operating units that provide direct patient care and thereby earn revenue for the hospital.

Accordingly, Chapter 10 examines cost analysis as a system by which management may derive the data required for such activities as:

1. the prospective development of the hospital's rate structure;
2. the preparation of the revenue budget;
3. the construction of indexes that reflect current operational activity.

Following the discussion of cost finding are chapters on the process and techniques of budgeting. These provide a frame of reference for understanding the budgeting process as well as the techniques that may be used in developing a budget in which expectations concerning desired performance are expressed in real and monetary terms. This section also examines a system of internal reporting and control based on indexes of current operational activity and standards of performance as expressed by the budget. The discussion analyzes exceptions to the budget that facilitate identification of areas that require remedial actions or policies in order to control or realign current operating activity.

The final chapter is a general discussion of various approaches to the development of short-term projections as well as the role of forecasts in managing working capital and in formulating the plans by which the administration expects to achieve the goals of the hospital enterprise.

*Robert W. Broyles*
Ottawa, Ontario
March 1981

# Acknowledgments

The author is indebted to a number of contributors whose suggestions have resulted in a far better product than would have been possible otherwise. Particular gratitude is expressed to Colin Lay, who provided valuable insights and recommendations for an improved presentation. The author also is indebted to George Hamilton and J. A. Kendree of the Canadian Ministry of Health for their helpful comments. In addition, the suggestions and recommendations provided by those who reviewed this manuscript are gratefully acknowledged.

The author also wishes to extend sincere gratitude to Micheline LeBlanc for her dedication and the effort required in the preparation of this text. In addition, the efforts of Mike Brown, Margot Raphael, Eileen Higgins, and Sam Sharkey are gratefully acknowledged. Finally, no endeavor such as this would have been possible without the support and encouragement of my family, Rita and Erin.

Recognizing the contribution of others, the responsibility for any errors or oversights must rest with the author.

# Part I

# Introduction

# Chapter 1

# Introduction to Working Capital Management

## Objectives

After completing this chapter you should be able to:

1. Identify the objectives of the hospital enterprise.
2. Understand the basic components of working capital management.
3. Understand the interrelationship among the components of working capital management.
4. Understand the importance of working capital management to achieving the goals of the hospital enterprise.

## 1.1 THE BASIC PROBLEM

That the costs of medical care in the United States and Canada have risen at unprecedented rates in recent years requires no documentation. In response to this rapid escalation, governmental authorities and other entities responsible for financing health care have intensified efforts to reduce the total costs of providing health services or to abate the rate at which those costs have risen. Since expenditures have increased more rapidly for hospital care than for any other form of medical care, administrators have been subjected to even greater pressure to contain costs and to improve the efficiency of their operations.

In such an economic environment, the problems usually associated with working capital management as well as with monitoring, evaluating, and controlling operational activity have become even more crucial. In recent years, the importance of working capital management as an integral part of operational management has become increasingly recognized. Indeed, it is difficult, if not impossible, to conceive of an operational decision that does not have a financial ramification. Given the increased pressure for economic efficiency and cost

3

containment, the importance of managing the working capital of the hospital and controlling operational activity in an effective and efficient manner cannot be denied.

The purpose of the following discussion is to outline the importance of working capital management and internal control when viewed from the perspective of achieving the goals of the hospital enterprise. However, it is necessary first to specify management goals and to define working capital management.

## 1.2 THE OBJECTIVES OF MANAGEMENT

To identify the basic objectives of management, assume that the supply of hospital services in a given area is not excessive and that the continued existence of the institution is required to provide an adequate level of health services to the population at risk. Under this assumption, it may be argued that management's objective is to ensure the continued existence of the institution so as to provide the services required in meeting the community's health needs. Clearly, then, one management objective is to ensure that total revenues are at least equal to total costs; in turn, that tends to assure the continued existence of the institution. Such an objective, while pragmatic and realistic, fails to reflect the economic realities that confront the administrator. As a result, the definition of management's objective function must be modified and expanded.

Obviously, the goal of ensuring the equality of total revenues and total costs is far too restrictive. The increasing demands for health care, coupled with improvements in medical technology that become embodied in hospital capital, plus the impact of inflation, require that the institution earn revenues in excess of costs so as to maintain the productive capability necessary for providing service. Thus, even though the nonprofit status of the average hospital requires that total revenues only equal total costs, the environment in which such an institution operates dictates that revenues *in excess* of costs must be earned if it is to discharge its service responsibility.

As noted, the rapid escalation in the cost of hospital care has resulted in increased demands for cost containment and economic restraint. Given this economic reality, it also is necessary to reflect the goal of cost containment in specifying the objectives associated with the average short-term hospital.

These considerations suggest that the objectives of management might be modified and expanded as follows. In the case of the hospital, the objective may be defined as preserving its long-run and short-run financial viability as well as its productive capability so as to provide required services to the community at an acceptable level of quality and at minimum costs.

## 1.3 A DEFINITION OF WORKING CAPITAL MANAGEMENT

Working capital is a term commonly employed to represent the current assets of an institution. It includes items that appear in the current asset portion of the balance sheet. As a consequence, the institution's investment in accounts receivable, cash, inventories, and marketable securities represents the lion's share of the current assets held by most acute care hospitals. Since one of the objectives is to provide required services at minimum cost, management must ensure that the use of the hospital's current assets is planned, controlled, and coordinated so as to minimize the cost of operation.

Management also must be concerned with the methods by which working capital assets are financed. Management frequently is confronted with numerous sources of either long-term or short-term financing. Obviously, if services are to be provided at least cost, management must select the funding method that minimizes the expense of financing current assets—an integral component of working capital management. As a consequence, working capital management involves the administration not only of the hospital's current assets but also of the liabilities it frequently incurs when these resources are acquired.

The problem of controlling operational activity will be expressed in both real and financial terms. Because most operational decisions exert an impact on one or more components of working capital, it is imperative to recognize the interrelationship between the operational and financial spheres of activity in the hospital.

## 1.4 RELATIONSHIP BETWEEN WORKING CAPITAL
## MANAGEMENT AND INTERNAL CONTROL

This section examines the relation between working capital management and the process of planning, monitoring, evaluating, and controlling operational activity, as expressed in real or physical terms. In fact, the hospital's operational activity is central to the problem of managing its current assets and liabilities (Figure 1-1). Operational activity is represented by the combination of factor inputs (i.e., land, labor, capital equipment, and consumable supplies) in a production process that results in providing hospital care. Obviously, the provision of patient care during a given time interval generates revenues and expenses from which the net income, or loss, for the period can be determined.

When the hospital is reimbursed retrospectively, the generation of income simultaneously creates an account receivable that represents a sum of money that is owed to the hospital by the patient or a third party payer. In many situations, the generation of revenue is related closely to one of the major components of working capital, namely, the accounts receivable of the institu-

**Figure 1-1** Relationship Between the Components of Working Capital Management

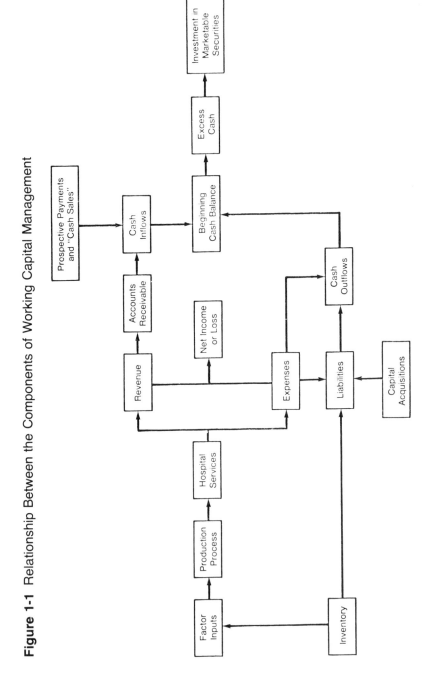

tion. Outstanding receivables also are related closely to the cash inflows of the institution. In this case, the realization of receivables represents a major source of cash to the hospital. In addition to the payments made on outstanding receivables, the hospital can receive cash in the form of a prepayment from a third party or a patient as well as payments that occur more or less simultaneously with the provision of service.

The next consideration involves the hospital's cash disbursements. Unlike cash receipts, a cash disbursement usually terminates a direct market transaction in which the hospital acquires needed goods or services. For example, it is common for the hospital to acquire required resources by issuing either a long-term or a short-term debt instrument. However, the liquidation of the resulting liability ultimately requires a cash disbursement by the hospital. As Figure 1-1 shows, the liabilities of the hospital represent one of the major mechanisms by which current assets are financed.

At this point, it should be noted that the cash available to the institution during a given period is simply the sum of the initial cash balance and the amount of cash received through prospective payments, the realization of outstanding receivables, and cash sales. Cash receipts, cash disbursements, and the cash balance all are major elements of cash management, which is one of the basic components of working capital management.

Closely related to the management of cash is the problem of managing the institution's investment in marketable securities, also a component of working capital management. For example, in a world of certainty, the initial cash balance coupled with cash receipts represent the amount of cash available. Subtracting cash disbursements from available cash yields a sum of money that may be invested in marketable securities that earn interest income for the institution. As a result, the management of cash and the institution's investment in marketable securities are closely interrelated activities that belong to the domain of working capital management.

Finally, it is important to recognize that consumable supplies, when held in inventory, are regarded as a current asset of the institution. As a result, the process of acquiring and holding an adequate supply of inventory represents one of the most important problems of working capital management.

## 1.5 THE VALUE OF WORKING CAPITAL MANAGEMENT

As an example of the value of working capital management in achieving the goal of providing required services at minimum cost, consider the problem of managing the current assets of the hospital. To begin such a discussion, the output of the hospital during some specified period of time may be defined as the provision of diagnostic, therapeutic, and support services required in the medical management of a given number of patients. Obviously, these services require the use of labor, capital equipment, and consumable supplies.

Recognizing that cash is the universal vehicle by which such resources are acquired, it is clear that cash management plays an integral role in the process by which required services are provided to the patient population. On the one hand, frequent cash shortages may jeopardize the hospital's ability to acquire the resources it needs to provide service. Moreover, should the hospital encounter frequent cash shortages, it incurs financial costs, which may take the form of a deteriorating credit rating or interest charges that must be paid to obtain a short-term loan. Consequently, frequent cash shortages may result in disruptions in the process by which care is provided as well as give rise to additional financial costs. On the other hand, idle cash earns nothing for the hospital. Indeed, during periods of inflation, excess funds that remain in idle cash balances earn a negative return—an opportunity cost that is equal to the rate of return that could have been earned by investing the funds in an interest-bearing security.

Thus, if management is to achieve the goal of providing required services at minimum costs, these considerations suggest that neither "too little" nor "too much" cash should be on hand at any given time. Techniques such as cash forecasting, cash budgeting, and probability models of cash management can provide the administrator with the information and the frame of reference with which to reach decisions concerning the desired cash balance.

As noted, the hospital's cash receipts depend on the rate at which outstanding receivables are converted into cash. As a result, patient care depends, by indirection, on the effectiveness with which accounts receivable are managed. The management of these receivables is a purely financial area of activity and, as such, can be managed at least cost. As will be seen later, one of the primary objectives in managing outstanding receivables is to accelerate the rate at which these accounts are transformed into cash. When applied appropriately, the techniques of working capital management are of considerable value in achieving this goal.

Closely related to receivables and the cash balance are decisions concerning the hospital's investment in interest-earning securities. To avoid both the opportunity costs described earlier and the reduction in the purchasing power of cash that results from increases in factor prices, management must ensure that excess funds are invested in an alternative that earns income for the hospital. Competent decisions concerning the level and composition of the hospital's investment in marketable securities can improve the institution's financial position significantly. Techniques of working capital management such as present value analysis, internal rates of return, and the intrinsic value approach to evaluating investment alternatives can be of real value when reaching decisions concerning the hospital portfolio.

As mentioned, patient service requires the use of consumable supplies and, if disruptions in the process of providing care are to be avoided, management must maintain an adequate inventory. When the hospital acquires and possesses inventory, it incurs costs; and if they are to be minimized, considerable time and effort must be devoted to inventory management. Of considerable value in coping with inventory management problems are the financial techniques of economic order quantity, buffer or safety stocks, and probability models. As will be seen, the appropriate application of these techniques can provide the information and the basis on which management can reach inventory decisions that minimize the cost of holding adequate stocks of consumable supplies.

One of the primary goals of management is to ensure the financial viability of the hospital, which implies that, in the long run, revenues must be equal to or greater than total costs of operation. Since the amount of reimbursement from governmental authorities and other third party payers frequently is related to the costs of providing care, management must determine accurately the full cost of producing those services that earn revenue for the hospital. Thus, management must allocate the costs of operating the departments or cost centers that offer general support to the departments that provide services that earn revenue for the hospital. Once the costs of providing support services have been allocated, management may use the resulting data to establish or revise the hospital's rate structure. Given that the major part of revenue is derived through the provision of patient services, the rate structure must reflect both the direct and indirect costs of operation as well as the costs of capital if management is to ensure the equality between total revenues and total expenditures. The method frequently used to derive the data for the development of such a rate structure is the technique of cost finding or cost analysis.

Cost-finding techniques, when coupled with standards of performance, also are of value to the administrator when monitoring, controlling, and evaluating current operations. At the heart of any system by which internal operations are controlled and evaluated is a standard that expresses the institution's desired or expected performance. As such, the standard constitutes the basis against which actual performance may be compared, monitored, and controlled. Such comparisons are of value in identifying areas of hospital operations in which actual performance has deviated from the desired or expected performance. On the basis of this information, management may take corrective action to realign the results of actual operational activity with the desired standard of performance.

The standard against which actual operational activity is compared usually is expressed by the hospital budget. When coupled with indicators of actual performance, the budget plays a central role in the process by which operational activity is monitored, evaluated, and controlled. As will be discussed in more detail later, the operating budget of the hospital is composed of a revenue budget and an expense budget. The expense budget usually is an expression of the costs management expects to incur in providing service. Once the expense budget for each department has been developed, management may use cost-finding techniques to estimate the full expense of providing services for which the hospital earns revenue. Management then is in a position to determine the rate structure that is expected to prevail during the budget period, which provides the basis for the development of the revenue budget.

The components of the operating budget represent the standard against which actual costs and revenues can be compared. A comparison of actual costs with expected costs may identify areas of operational activity in which management must take corrective action so as to achieve its goal of containing costs. Similarly, a comparison of actual costs with expected revenues provides management with the information it requires when assessing the extent to which the goal of maintaining equality between total revenues and expenses is being achieved. As a result, cost finding and budgeting are techniques that may be used productively in monitoring, evaluating, and controlling current performance as well as in assuring that total revenues are equal to or greater than total costs.

This section has emphasized working capital management rather than accounting. The difference between accounting and the financial management of working capital is critical and must be clear to avoid misunderstanding in the remaining chapters.

Accounting may be defined as the art of recording, summarizing, reporting, and interpreting financial information concerning the economic enterprise. The earlier definition suggested that working capital management focuses on the problem of financing required resources at least cost as well as ensuring that these resources were used efficiently and effectively once they had been acquired. These considerations suggest that working capital management and accounting are closely related but are separate functions that must be performed efficiently and accurately if the objectives of the health care enterprise are to be achieved. As described previously, working capital management may be viewed as the application of a set of tools and techniques in a decision-making process that uses the information generated by the accounting system. The accounting system performs a basic informational function that provides much of the data required when applying those tools and techniques. Working capital management, then, is the use of accounting information to improve the operational and financial activities of the institution.

## 1.6 TWO APPROACHES IN FINANCING CARE

That competent working capital management is conducive to the efficient operation of a hospital should be clear from this discussion. The application of the tools and techniques of working capital management depends to a significant extent on the financial environment of the hospital. For example, the relative importance and management of such assets as cash and accounts receivable depend on the method used to finance the costs of hospital care. Essentially two approaches to the problem of financing the costs of hospital care can be identified:

1. Used extensively in the United States, the first is characterized as retrospective in that payment normally is received after service has been provided.
2. Predominant in Canada, the second is regarded as a prospective system since payment usually is received before service is provided.

Since an understanding of when and how to apply the tools and techniques of working capital management depends on the external financial environment, the next two chapters describe the methods by which hospital care is financed in the United States and Canada.

# Chapter 2

# Financing Hospital Care in the U.S.

## Objectives

After completing this chapter, you should be able to:

1. Identify the major third party payers in the United States.
2. Describe the basic benefit packages offered by third party payers.
3. Describe the costs recoverable from Blue Cross and Medicare.
4. Describe the methods used by third parties to finance the costs of hospital care.
5. Describe methods of paying hospitals in the United States.

## 2.1 INTRODUCTION

One of the most important factors that influences the management of working capital is the method by which hospital costs are financed. As mentioned, essentially two methods are used in the United States to finance hospital care—retrospective and prospective payment. In the first technique, public or private payers reimburse the health care institution for services provided previously and payers assume financial responsibility for the costs actually incurred by the hospital. Under prospective reimbursement, the amounts or rates are determined prior to the current period. The hospital is paid that predetermined amount or rate regardless of costs actually incurred during the current period. In contrast to the Canadian system in which prospective reimbursement usually results in the hospital's receiving cash before it provides service, the hospital in the United States that is reimbursed prospectively usually receives cash on a concurrent basis.

## 2.2 SOURCES OF REVENUE

The average hospital in the United States relies on third party payers as its major source of revenue and cash. A third party payer may be defined as any agent, other than the patient, who agrees to assume the financial responsibility for the hospital bill of the individual receiving care. The primary third party payers are Blue Cross, Blue Shield, commercial insurance companies, Medicare, Medicaid, and workmen's compensation, each of which represent a major source of revenue and cash to the hospital. Management can depend on these third party payers to make payments, which usually are known with certainty, within a given system of reimbursement and within a reasonably constant period of time. As a consequence, the third party payer plays a central role in financing hospital activity as well as in assuring the financial viability and solvency of the average hospital. In describing the financial environment of the hospital in the United States, the benefit structure, methods of financing costs, and methods of making payments to the institution are considered for each of the third parties. Moreover, since the amount of the reimbursement received from Medicare and most Blue Cross plans usually is determined on a cost or cost-plus basis, it is necessary to discuss expenditures that are recognized as allowable costs that may be recovered from these third party payers.

## 2.3 BLUE CROSS

Blue Cross is composed of 80 separate and autonomous plans that operate in the United States, Canada, Puerto Rico, and Jamaica. In general, these are non-profit organizations that are committed to a public service orientation evidenced by their adherence to the goal of covering the costs of hospital care from the day of admission to the day of discharge. However, it is not possible to infer that Blue Cross covers all hospital charges. Some Blue Cross contracts limit the extent of insured benefits while others contain deductibles and coinsurance clauses. A deductible is a fixed amount that must be paid by the patient before the insurance carrier, in this case Blue Cross, assumes financial responsibility for the care used by the insured individual. The coinsurance feature provides that, in addition to the deductible, the insured patient is required to pay a percentage (usually 20 to 25 percent) of the remaining amount. As a consequence, the coverage offered by Blue Cross is not completely comprehensive since the patient usually is required to assume financial responsibility for a portion of the hospital bill.

### 2.3.1 The Benefit Package

Since there are a large number of independent plans and each offers several policy options, Blue Cross offers no single or uniform set of insured benefits.

Even though it is not possible to examine all of the benefit packages offered by each of the local plans, it is possible to describe the range of insured inpatient and outpatient benefits available under Blue Cross.

When describing the range of Blue Cross inpatient benefits, it is convenient to divide the hospital's services into essentially two components: (1) stay-specific services (which may be defined as those that depend only on the number of days of care), and (2) ancillary services.

The number of days of stay-specific care insured by Blue Cross varies from plan to plan. In general, Blue Cross contracts insure no less than 30 days of care for conditions requiring hospitalization and no more than 365 days per hospital episode. However, most contracts contain a clause that permits a new benefit period to begin 90 days after the first set of insured days has been exhausted. Most Blue Cross contracts also insure the inpatient use of a wide range of ancillary services such as delivery room, operating room, and treatment room, laboratory examinations, oxygen therapy, physical therapy, hydrotherapy, casts, drugs, intravenous solutions, anesthesia, and electroencephalographs.

As a supplement to these inpatient benefits, several Blue Cross plans offer contracts that include hospital care for patients presenting specific diseases or conditions. These benefits usually are limited to a specified number of insured days of care by patients presenting such conditions as impacted teeth, tuberculosis, alcoholism and drug addiction, dental problems requiring extractions, and mental or nervous disorders. In most Blue Cross plans, ambulance service as well as blood and blood products usually are excluded as insured benefits.

As for outpatient benefits, most contracts include emergency treatment of accidental injuries if care is sought within 24 to 72 hours. Outpatient services in the benefit package usually are similar to the insured ancillary services just described.

## 2.3.2 Allowable Costs

Since Blue Cross usually pays the hospital on a cost or cost-plus basis, the issue of allowable and excluded costs is of considerable importance to the hospital when recovering the expenditures incurred when providing care to the insured members. Even though most Blue Cross plans include the costs of diagnostic, therapeutic, and support services, other cost components are the subject of continuing negotiations between hospital and Blue Cross authorities; the results of these discussions are by no means uniform, so the composition and magnitude of allowable costs vary from plan to plan.

One primary area of concern involves the extent to which Blue Cross recognizes the costs of operating teaching and research programs. Since most plans will reimburse the hospital for the direct and indirect costs of providing service to their members, approval of teaching and research activities hinge on the extent to which they contribute to the patient's care. Obviously, the resources expended on teaching and research activities depend on the size and function of the hospital. As an example, a small, short-term hospital probably will spend very little on teaching and research while a large university hospital may devote a relatively large proportion of its resources to these activities. Most Blue Cross plans recognize the net expense of operating approved teaching and research programs as an allowable cost. Here, the term net expense refers to the difference between the total cost of carrying out the teaching and research and the sum of any grants, donations, scholarships, or other monies received and intended for use in these areas.

In the opinion of the author, teaching and research programs that are consistent with the goal of providing required service at an acceptable level of quality should be regarded as patient-related areas of activity. Since teaching and research play a central role in the process by which medical care is delivered, the costs of operating those programs that contribute to the attainment of the institution's goals should be recognized as an allowable expenditure.

A second area of concern involves the treatment of depreciation charges as an allowable cost. Even though most third parties recognize depreciation as a recoverable expense, the calculation of these charges is a matter of continuing debate. The depreciation base (i.e., the amount that is depreciated), the method of calculating the charges, and the life expectancy of capital equipment are subjects of negotiation and persistent concern to hospital administrators.

Regarding the depreciation base, most third party payers contend that these charges should be computed using historical rather than replacement costs, predicated on the notion that historical costs are objectively verifiable while replacement costs are based on projections or estimates of future conditions. On the other hand, most hospital administrators argue that, because of inflation and improvements in medical technology, the cost of capital equipment has increased dramatically in recent years. As a consequence, the costs of replacing plant and equipment usually exceed the historical costs being used to determine the amount or the rate of hospital reimbursement. The hospital industry contends that reimbursement on historical rather than replacement costs has limited the ability of many institutions to finance capital acquisitions with internally generated funds.

In fact, it seems quite legitimate to argue that the increased reliance on external debt as a mechanism of financing the replacement or expansion of the hospital's capital complement is, in part, a result of using historical costs to determine the depreciation expense recoverable from Blue Cross and other third party payers. Without adequate reserves that might be generated by using replacement costs to determine depreciation charges, it would appear that hospitals' debt burden will continue to increase. However, such increases cannot be sustained indefinitely and it is likely that the debate over the depreciation base will intensify.

During periods in which the costs of capital increase, the method of calculating depreciation also exerts an impact on the ability of the hospital to replace or expand its capital complement. Accelerated depreciation techniques (e.g., sum-of-years-digit or declining balance methods) return the costs of capital to the hospital more rapidly than the straight-line method. During periods of inflation, hospitals must recover the cost of capital equipment as quickly as possible so that they can either invest the funds, and thereby offset a part or all of the increase in capital costs, or use the funds immediately to acquire equipment. It is in this regard that accelerated depreciation is preferred to the straight-line method of determining these charges.

Even though most Blue Cross plans recognize the direct and indirect costs of providing patient care to their membership, certain expenses have been excluded from the formula by which the magnitude of payments to the hospital are determined. Although policy varies from plan to plan, the costs usually excluded are:

1. bad debt expense
2. cost of providing service to charity patients
3. allowances and discounts

The exclusion of bad debt expenses from the formula is perhaps one of the most questionable policies of Blue Cross. It usually is contended that hospital services provided to the insured membership are purchased in accordance with a contractual arrangement that eliminates the possibility of bad debts arising directly from the hospital-Blue Cross relationship. Such an argument, however, tends to ignore the presence of the deductibles and coinsurance clauses in most Blue Cross contracts. As is well known, the patient usually assumes the responsibility for paying deductible and coinsurance charges. These bills are costly to collect and may result in bad debts. Thus, there is a legitimate basis for arguing that a portion of the hospital's bad debt expense should be regarded as an allowable cost by Blue Cross.

Administrators are concerned because Blue Cross excludes costs of service provided to charity patients. The basic difference between charity care and an outstanding receivable that must be written off as a bad debt involves the ability of the patient to pay. A bad debt usually arises when management decides that an individual has the financial resources to pay for service but for some reason is unwilling to make the payment. On the other hand, providing free service frequently is related to the hospital's inability to deny care to individuals who either are uninsured or are financially unable to pay. In both cases, real costs are incurred and must be financed if the continued existence of the institution is to be assured. Thus, if the hospital is to preserve its financial viability and its ability to provide service to the enrolled membership, it would seem to be in the interests of Blue Cross authorities to recognize a portion of free or charity care expenses as an allowable cost.

A comment concerning the exclusion of discounts and allowances is appropriate. In accounting for hospital revenues, discounts and allowances are recorded as reductions in revenue rather than as expenses. This is because the hospital agrees to provide service at a discount or at a price less than its full established rates. Usually these reductions are extended as a courtesy to hospital employees, staff physicians, or indigent patients. Since the hospital offers these rate reductions voluntarily, there is no reason to believe that they should be included as an allowable cost by Blue Cross or any other third party payer.

### 2.3.3 Financing Hospital Costs

As noted earlier, the costs of the care frequently are financed jointly by Blue Cross and the insured patient. The financial liability of Blue Cross usually is limited to a specified number of days of hospital care. However, in the absence of additional coverage, patients usually are responsible for charges when they use care in excess of the maximum benefits offered under the Blue Cross contract. Many Blue Cross contracts also contain deductibles and coinsurance clauses that force the patient to share in the financial risks of disease or injury and the subsequent use of hospital care. Recognizing that the patient frequently is required to finance a portion of the institution's bill, the following discussion focuses on how Blue Cross finances its share of hospital costs or charges.

In any form of health insurance, the population at risk contributes to a common pool out of which the costs of health and hospital care are financed. In the case of Blue Cross, the periodic payment of premiums by insured individuals or their employers is the dominant method by which the common pool is funded. The amount of cash flowing into the pool depends not only on the number of subscribers but also on the premiums charged by Blue Cross. The author simply observes that the membership of Blue Cross has grown in both absolute and relative terms since 1958, when enrollment declined briefly, while the increase in premiums has been commensurate with the rise in hospital costs.

### 2.3.4 Methods of Payment

The process by which the hospital receives reimbursement for services to an insured member begins with a submission of the subscriber's bill to Blue Cross. Blue Cross processes the statement and usually pays the hospital within a given period that has been agreed upon previously. Most Blue Cross plans reimburse the hospital on a cost or cost-plus basis while a far smaller proportion determines the amount on the basis of hospital charges. Since management usually knows the basis for determining the amount of reimbursement, the amount of cash that will be received also is known with relative certainty but the timing of the receipts may be more problematical.

In an attempt to contain costs, several Blue Cross plans have either proposed or experimented with prospective reimbursement as a method of paying hospitals. As proposed or implemented in the United States, under prospective reimbursement amounts or rates of pay are established at the beginning of the reporting period. In turn, the hospital is paid the established rate or amount irrespective of costs actually incurred during the period. The units of analysis that represent the basis for the prospective reimbursement include the hospital budget, the departmental budget, days of care, the case, the hospital stay, and specific services.

As is obvious, prospective reimbursement tends to shift the risk of increasing costs from the third party payer to the hospital. Proponents of prospective reimbursement argue that, by determining the amount or rate of pay in advance of the coming period, management is forced to plan, monitor, evaluate, and control operational activity so as to ensure that actual expenditures are not in excess of the established rate or amount of reimbursement. Moreover, in the event that actual expenditures are less than the established reimbursement, the hospital is allowed to retain a portion of the surplus. As a consequence, it is possible to argue that the potential losses or surpluses induce management to improve efficiency and to contain cost.

However, prospective reimbursement, as implemented in the United States and in Canada, tends to ignore the physician's role in controlling cost. In this regard, the cost of hospital care depends not only on the efficiency with which resources are used in providing service but also on the quantity and composition of care. However, the volume of service depends more on the admitting and prescribing pattern of the physician than on the discretionary actions of management. As a consequence, unless physician behavior is given explicit recognition, any scheme designed to control costs is likely to fail.

## 2.4 THE COMMERCIAL INSURANCE INDUSTRY

After Blue Cross, a second major source of hospital revenue is the commercial insurance company. Unlike Blue Cross, the commercial insurance company is operated to earn a profit. As a result, most companies offer benefit packages that limit their financial liability to definite dollar indemnities that are paid when certain accommodations and certain services are used by the insured person. Given the large number of commercial insurance companies, it is not possible to provide a detailed description of the benefit packages and the reimbursement methods associated with each of these third party payers. As a result, the following discussion provides only a general profile of the commercial insurance industry.

## 2.4.1 The Benefit Structure

The range of benefits offered by the commercial insurance industry includes hospital, maternity, surgical, obstetrical, and inhospital medical care. Most companies also offer outpatient coverage but these benefits usually are limited to group policies or are offered in conjunction with major medical policies that cover these as well as many other types of health care expenses.

With regard to inpatient hospital benefits, most policies cover room and board charges on an indemnity basis that provides for reimbursement up to the specified daily maximum for a given and limited number of days. For example, an insurance company may agree to pay up to $100 per day for a maximum of 10 days. Such a benefit limits the liability of the insurance company for room and board charges to $1,000 ($100 per day $\times$ 10 days).

Most commercial insurance companies also provide an allowance for ancillary services. Usually, such benefits are stated as a multiple of the maximum daily payment for room and board charges. For example, suppose that a policy entitles the insured to a maximum daily payment of $100. If the policy also provides an additional allowance of four times the maximum daily payment for ancillary services, the insured patient is entitled to a maximum of $400 (4 $\times$ $100) that may be used to defray the costs of these services during the hospital stay. It is less common for insurance companies to express ancillary benefits in terms of specified dollar limits for each procedure. Most companies have abandoned this approach in favor of the unallocated blanket allowance that may be used to defray the costs of required ancillary services.

As mentioned, many companies also offer outpatient benefits that cover a portion of the charges when diagnostic x-ray and laboratory services and emergency treatment are involved. These benefits may be expressed in terms of the number of uses of each service in a list of services to which the individual is entitled. The policy also may express the outpatient benefits as an overall dollar limit that may apply to each illness or accident, to a 12-month period, or to both, and may be used to pay the costs of outpatient care.

This set of inpatient and outpatient benefits may be regarded as basic coverage. In addition, many companies offer major medical or catastrophic insurance. When the basic coverage is incorporated with a major medical policy and surgical insurance in a single package, the resulting coverage is called comprehensive.

The major characteristics of catastrophic insurance are (1) its broad coverage of most types of medical and hospital expenses; (2) the absence of internal limits; and (3) a high overall maximum limit that may apply to each illness or injury, to a calendar or benefit year, or to the lifetime of the policyholder. Major medical policies are not limited to hospital-based care; rather, the dollar indemnity may be used to pay for hospital care, nursing service, physician service, prescribed medication, and so on.

Another distinguishing characteristic of major medical policies is their deductible and coinsurance clauses. The deductible amount depends on whether the policy is a group or individual contract and may apply to each illness or injury separately or to the calendar or benefit year. It should be recognized that major medical policies usually are intended to supplement basic coverage. As such, they become effective only after the benefits in the basic package have been exhausted and the insured has satisfied an additional deductible clause. In most cases, the deductible in the catastrophic policy must be paid after the expiration of the basic coverage and before the provisions of the major medical contract become effective. The deductible in catastrophic coverage is regarded as a "corridor" that connects the basic coverage with the major medical policy.

## 2.4.2 Financing Care Under Commercial Insurance

As in the case of Blue Cross, the costs of the care used by the commercially insured patient are financed jointly by the insurance company and the insured individual. The first consideration involves the components of the hospital bill that must be financed by the patient; the second covers the methods by which the insurance industry finances the indemnity benefits.

As might be surmised from the earlier discussion, the indemnity benefits offered by the commercial insurance company usually are in effect throughout the lifetime of the policy and rarely cover the total charges incurred by the patient. Thus, even though premium payments are stabilized by the set of fixed benefits, the patient is forced to assume the financial responsibility for a portion of the hospital bill as well as any increases in the costs of care that may occur during the lifetime of the policy.

The fact that the maximum benefits offered by the commercial company rarely cover all of the hospital's charges is a reflection of the belief that the insured patient should share in the financial risks of disease or injury. This belief also is reflected by the deductible and coinsurance clauses found in many commercial policies. For example, suppose that a policy guarantees the insured 100 days of hospital care per year or per episode of hospitalization or contains a deductible and a coinsurance clause. In this case, the patient assumes the financial responsibility for all costs that exceed the indemnity benefits of the policy or all relevant deductible and coinsurance charges.

These observations suggest that when services are provided to an individual covered by a commercial insurance company, a portion of the hospital bill is the patient's financial responsibility. Such accounts frequently are costly to collect and occasionally it is necessary to write them off as bad debts. Here, as in the case of Blue Cross, one of the major problems confronting management is controlling the length of time required to convert the charges that are the responsibility of the patient into cash. In addition, since not all patients will pay their outstanding accounts in full, management also faces the problem of controlling the portion of these receivables that must be written off as bad debts.

### 2.4.3  Methods of Payment

There essentially are two methods by which a hospital can obtain payment for services insured under a commercial policy. First, the hospital can seek payment for the *entire* bill from the insured patient. This process is initiated by the hospital's submitting a bill to the patient who, in turn, submits a claim to the insurance carrier. After processing the claim, the carrier forwards a check to the patient, who may use the funds to reimburse the hospital. However, it is not uncommon for the patient to divert insurance payments to personal uses, which may imply that the hospital bill will go unpaid. This process is time consuming and results in undue delays in receiving payment. Even worse, this method of collection may result in writing off the total amount as a bad debt.

In the second method, rather than rely on the insured to remit insurance payments to the institution, management should require the patient to execute an assignment that authorizes the carrier to pay benefits directly to the hospital. When an assignment of this sort is initiated, management reduces the time required to convert outstanding receivables into cash. This practice also increases the value of the outstanding receivables for which management is certain of receiving payment and this, of course, may reduce the accounts receivable that must be written off as bad debts.

### 2.5  MEDICARE

On July 1, 1966, Titles XVIII and XIX of the Social Security Act became effective. Known more generally as Medicare and Medicaid, these amendments to the Social Security Act ushered in an area in which governmental authorities have played an increasingly important role in financing the costs of health and hospital care to identifiable segments of the American population.

Medicare is a federally sponsored program designed to pay for health services used by persons aged 65 and over. Part A of the Medicare legislation is insurance for hospital care and related services while Part B, which is called Supplementary Medical Insurance, is designed to help pay for physician care. Since the primary objective here is to describe the financial environment of the hospital, only the provisions pertaining to Part A of Title XVIII are addressed in this section.

## 2.5.1 Benefit Structure

Part A of Title XVIII helps finance the costs of care provided in a hospital, in a skilled nursing facility after a stay in an approved hospital, or in the home after a stay in either a hospital or skilled nursing facility. The benefit structure of Medicare Part A is governed by the notion of a benefit period. A benefit period is said to begin when a beneficiary is registered as an inpatient in a hospital and ends when the individual has not been in a hospital or a skilled nursing facility for a period of 60 consecutive days.

Hospital benefits under Medicare Part A include the occupancy of a semiprivate room and all meals for up to 90 days during a benefit period. Each Medicare recipient also is entitled to a "lifetime" reserve that is limited to 60 days of care. Thus, if the Medicare beneficiary requires more than 90 days of hospital care during a given benefit period, the person may use a portion of the "lifetime" reserve. Inpatient hospital benefits also include the use of drugs, laboratory tests, regular nursing care, operating room, x-ray, and other radiological services as well as other appliances provided by the hospital. Outpatient benefits included in the legislation are:

1. laboratory and other diagnostic services
2. x-ray and other radiological services
3. medical supplies
4. emergency room services

As noted, Medicare Part A also helps finance the cost of care of qualified recipients in skilled nursing facilities. The recipient must satisfy the following conditions:

1. the patient must have been in a participating or qualified hospital for three days in a row prior to admission to the skilled nursing facility
2. the patient must be admitted to the skilled nursing facility within 14 days of discharge from the hospital
3. the patient must be admitted to the skilled nursing facility for the same condition that precipitated the hospital stay
4. existing medical conditions must require continuing care
5. a physician must determine that the patient requires extended care and must order that care.

Once these conditions have been satisfied, the recipient is entitled to 100 days of care in the skilled nursing facility for each benefit period. The benefits include occupancy of a semiprivate room and all meals as well as the use of drugs furnished by the facility; regular nursing care; physical, speech, and occupational therapy; medical supplies, and medical social services.

Part A of Title XVIII also entitles the Medicare recipient to the use of certain services provided by a participating home health agency. Among these services are:

1. the use of part-time nursing care
2. the services of part-time home aides
3. medical social work
4. medical supplies provided by the agency
5. physical, occupational, and speech therapy
6. the use of medical appliances

The legislation authorizes up to 100 visits by a nurse therapist or any other person providing these services during the year following the most recent discharge from a participating hospital or skilled nursing facility. The conditions that must be satisfied before the recipient is entitled to the home health benefits are similar to those in a skilled nursing facility.

As might be inferred from this discussion, one of the objectives of Part A is to match the use of care with the medical needs of the patient. In addition, by providing a mechanism by which the patient is transferred from the hospital to a skilled nursing facility and from a skilled nursing facility to home care, Part A is intended to induce the substitution of less costly care for relatively expensive service. These provisions represent an attempt to contain hospital care costs which, in turn, have increased the importance of less expensive alternatives such as outpatient services, care in skilled nursing facilities, in the patient's home, and so on.

## 2.5.2 Financing Medicare Benefits

The costs of care under Part A are financed jointly by the recipient and the federal government. The federal share of Medicare costs is financed primarily by a special percentage assessment added to the payroll deductions of employees and by the contribution of employers and the self-employed. Any program deficits are financed by the federal government's general funds.

The recipient's contribution to the cost of benefits under Part A assumes the form of specified deductibles and coinsurance charges. With regard to hospital services, the patient pays a fixed deductible for the first 60 days of the hospital stay. The coinsurance provisions then require the patient to pay a fixed amount per day from the 61st to the 90th day of hospitalization. Medicare pays all other covered charges and the deductible is paid only once during the benefit period even though the patient may be hospitalized several times. The coinsurance provisions for care in a skilled nursing facility require the patient to pay a fixed dollar charge per day from the 21st to the 100th day.

The deductible and the coinsurance charges have been increased since Medicare came into effect, reflecting changes in the average costs of care. This implies that Medicare recipients have been asked to bear a portion of the increased costs of hospital care and related services. When viewed from the perspective of managing the accounts receivable and cash assets of institutions that provide a large volume of service to Medicare recipients, the increases in the deductible and coinsurance charges have tended to increase the value of outstanding receivables as well as to lengthen the average time required to convert these receivables into cash.

### 2.5.3 Allowable Costs

Medicare reimburses the hospital on a reasonable cost basis and, like Blue Cross, its basic principle is to pay no more than the cost of care provided. Thus, expenses that may be recovered from Medicare are similar to costs that Blue Cross recognizes as allowable expenditures.

In addition to the direct and indirect costs of providing diagnostic, therapeutic, and support services to hospitalized beneficiaries, Medicare recognizes "net" interest charges on hospital loans related to patient care. Here, the term "net" interest refers to the difference between interest expense and interest income except for the investment income earned on restricted and unrestricted gifts as well as donations that are not commingled with other funds. Furthermore, even though depreciation funding is not required by Medicare, it is encouraged by the provision that interest earned on such funds need not be deducted from interest expenses when determining allowable costs.

Like Blue Cross, Medicare recognizes a portion of net costs associated with the educational activities of the hospital. In this case, the term "net" expense refers to the salaries, stipends, and other costs less any grants, donations, tuition, or other resources that have been received to support the educational programs. Only expenditures associated with educational activities that contribute to providing care to beneficiaries are approved by the Social Security Administration as allowable costs.

As for the costs of conducting research, the institution is allowed to include the expenses associated with surveys and studies that are related to administrative and program needs. On the other hand, research costs that are not directly related to patient care are not regarded as an allowable expenditure. Medicare's basic position is that federally and privately sponsored grants are sufficient to support most research.

Bad debts, courtesy discounts, and the costs of providing charity care are not generally recognized as allowable costs by Medicare, as noted earlier. Rather, these items are considered to be reductions in revenue and, as such, are not allowable costs. The sole exception to this principle involves the coinsurance and deductible provisions mentioned earlier. If Medicare beneficiaries fail to pay the deductible or coinsurance charges, the hospital may recover any outstanding amounts from the Medicaid program after exhausting the usual methods of obtaining payment.

## 2.5.4 Amount and Receipt of Medicare Payments

Since Blue Cross acts as the principal financial intermediary for Medicare, the process of obtaining payments for service to Medicare beneficiaries is similar to that for Blue Cross. That is, the process is initiated by submitting the hospital bill for review to the financial intermediary; the intermediary processes the bill, then makes a payment to the hospital within a period agreed upon previously.

Of considerable importance to some hospitals is the voluntary prepayment plan in which interim payments are based on expected or projected costs. Under this system, at the beginning of each year the hospital estimates the amount of reimbursement for the coming period. The projected reimbursement is divided by the number of weeks in the reporting period and the resulting amount is paid to the hospital in the form of Periodic Interim Payments (P.I.P.) on a weekly basis. The rate or amount of reimbursement may be revised on a quarterly basis. However, once revisions have been approved, the reimbursement remains constant irrespective of costs incurred by the hospital. As a consequence, a portion of the risks associated with inflation is shifted from Medicare to the hospital.

Medicare uses a method slightly different from Blue Cross's in determining the amount of the hospital's reimbursement. As mentioned, Medicare payments are based on the cost of providing care to beneficiaries. The departmental method, also called the ratio of charges to charges technique, and the combination method are used to determine the amount of reimbursement to the hospital. These methods are described next.

### 2.5.4.1 The Departmental Method

Under the departmental method, the ratio of beneficiary charges to total patient charges is used to determine the proportion of total departmental expenditures that represent the costs of providing care to Medicare beneficiaries. For each department responsible for providing these services, a ratio similar to

$$r = \frac{C}{TC}$$

is calculated. Here, $C$ represents charges assessed for the use of the departmental services by Medicare patients and $TC$ those for the use of these services by all patients treated in the hospital. Hence, the ratio $r$ is simply the proportion of total departmental charges attributable to Medicare beneficiaries. Multiplying the ratio of charges to charges by the costs associated with the corresponding department yields the total cost of providing departmental services to Medicare beneficiaries. Summing over all departmental units yields the total cost of providing hospital care to beneficiaries for whom Medicare assumes financial responsibility. These calculations are illustrated in Table 2-1, where the Medicare contribution to hospital operations is found to be $334,550.

### 2.5.4.2 The Combination Method

The combination method of determining the cost of services to Medicare patients involves essentially two steps. In the first, the cost of routine services (room, board, nursing care, and floor drugs) is determined by the product of the average cost per day and the number of days of care used by Medicare recipients. In the second, the cost of providing ancillary services is found by first calculating the ratio of beneficiary charges to the charges to all patients for these services. The cost of providing ancillary services then is obtained by multiplying the resulting ratio by the total cost of providing care.

Consider first the Medicare share of the costs of providing routine services to beneficiaries. Table 2-1 reveals that the total costs associated with this component of care amounted to $1,850,000. If a total of 18,500 days of care were provided by the institution, the average cost per day is given by

$$\$1,850,000/18,500 \text{ days}$$

or $100 per day. Assuming that beneficiaries used 4,500 days of care, the Medicare share of the costs of providing routine care is given by the product

$$4,500 \text{ days} \times \$100/\text{day}$$

or $450,000.

**Table 2-1** Departmental Method

| Department | Charges to Beneficiaries (C) | ÷ | Total Charges to All Patients (TC) | = | Ratio C/TC (r) | × | Total Allowable Costs (TAC) | = | Cost of Medicare Benefits |
|---|---|---|---|---|---|---|---|---|---|
| Routine services | $220,000 | | $1,760,000 | | .125 | | $1,850,000 | | $231,250 |
| X-ray | 10,000 | | 50,000 | | .200 | | 65,000 | | 13,000 |
| Laboratory | 30,000 | | 60,000 | | .500 | | 80,000 | | 40,000 |
| Pharmacy | 15,000 | | 40,000 | | .375 | | 60,000 | | 22,500 |
| Operating room | 10,000 | | 100,000 | | .100 | | 110,000 | | 11,000 |
| Other | 20,000 | | 50,000 | | .400 | | 42,000 | | 16,800 |
| Total | 305,000 | | 2,060,000 | | | | 2,207,000 | | 334,550 |

Consider next the Medicare share of the costs of providing ancillary services. Table 2-1 shows that these expenses may be calculated as follows:

| Component | Charges to Beneficiaries | Charges to All Patients | Costs |
|---|---|---|---|
| X-ray | $10,000 | $50,000 | $65,000 |
| Laboratory | 30,000 | 60,000 | 80,000 |
| Pharmacy | 15,000 | 40,000 | 60,000 |
| Operating room | 10,000 | 100,000 | 110,000 |
| Other | 20,000 | 50,000 | 42,000 |
| Total | 85,000 | 300,000 | 357,000 |

In this case, the ratio of charges to charges is given by

$$r = \frac{\$85,000}{\$300,000}$$

or approximately .283. Given that the costs of providing ancillary services to all patients amounted to $357,000, the amount of reimbursement the hospital receives from Medicare is given by the product (.283) × $357,000 or $101,031. These calculations are summarized in Table 2-2, where the contribution of the Medicare program to hospital operations is found to be $450,000 + $101,031 or $551,031.

As suggested by the data in Tables 2-1 and 2-2, the relative use of service by beneficiaries influences the amount of Medicare reimbursement. As a result, management can increase the reimbursement by either creating or eliminating cost/revenue centers. In Table 2-1, a reimbursement of $16,800 is generated by providing "other" services to Medicare recipients. Suppose that physical therapy and inhalation therapy are subsumed in this category of care. Since Medicare beneficiaries use a high proportion of these services, assume further that management decides to create a cost/revenue center for each of these areas of activity and that the relevant information is as follows:

| | Area of Activity | | | |
|---|---|---|---|---|
| | Combined Category | Physical Therapy | Inhalation Therapy | Other Services |
| Allowable cost | $42,000 | $23,000 | $13,000 | $6,000 |
| Total charges | 50,000 | 9,000 | 25,000 | 16,000 |
| Beneficiary charges | 20,000 | 7,000 | 12,000 | 1,000 |
| Ratio (r) | .40 | .78 | .48 | .06 |
| Reimbursement | 16,800 | 17,940 | 6,240 | 360 |

**Table 2-2** The Combination Method

| Component | | Calculations | | |
|---|---|---|---|---|
| Routine Services: | Total costs | = | $1,850,000 | |
| | Total inpatient days | = | 18,500 | |
| | Average cost/day | = | $100 | |
| | Total beneficiary days | = | 4,500 | |
| | Beneficiary cost for routine services | = | 4,500($100) | = $450,000 |
| Ancillary Services: | Total charges for ancillary services | = | $300,000 | |
| | Total charges to beneficiaries for ancillary services | = | $85,000 | |
| | Ratio of charge to charge | = | .283 | |
| | Total cost of ancillary services | = | $357,000 | |
| | Medicare share of ancillary costs | = .283($357,000) | = | 101,031 |
| Total Medicare share: | | | | 551,031 |

The creation of a cost/revenue center for these two categories of care thus increases Medicare reimbursement from $16,800, as calculated in Table 2-1, to $17,940 + $6,240 + $360 or $24,540. Although this example is overly simplified, it illustrates the need to examine the advantages of creating cost/revenue centers to increase the reimbursement for providing care to Medicare beneficiaries.

## 2.6 MEDICAID

As mentioned, Title XIX of the Social Security Act, more generally known as Medicaid, became effective on July 1, 1966. Medicaid is a program intended to assist in financing the costs of care for medically indigent patients. Here, medical indigency refers to patients who are unable to pay for medical care even though they can finance other normal living expenses.

With regard to the benefit structure, it is important to note that Medicaid is a state-directed program and, as a consequence, definitions of medical indigency as well as the extent and scope of benefits vary from state to state. Some states have minimal benefits while others offer a more comprehensive range of services. However, inpatient, outpatient, physician, and skilled nursing services as well as certain laboratory tests are basic to the Medicaid program.

Hospital charges for Medicaid usually are cost based in a manner similar to Medicare reimbursement. Medicaid claims usually are processed through the state department of health, department of social services, or some other intermediary. In most cases the recipient does not share in financing the costs of care.

In addition to financing the cost of care to Medicaid recipients, states can use funds to pay the deductible and coinsurance charges under Part A of Title XVIII. Usually the institution must exhaust all reasonable means of collecting receivables from the beneficiary before relying on Medicaid for payment.

When viewed from the perspective of the institution, there can be little doubt that the Medicaid program has reduced the magnitude of unmet costs as well as the number and value of receivables that must be written off as uncollectable. Clearly, the payment of hospital charges of the medically indigent as well as the deductibles and coinsurance charges associated with Part A of Title XVIII have improved the financial solvency of hospitals that provide a large volume of care to the poor and the aged.

---

**REFERENCES**

*Governmental Agencies*

Ansley, B. "Non-Profits Should Have Investor Owned Reimbursement Formula." *Hospital Progress,* vol. 57, no. 8, August 1976, pp. 6–12.

Commerce Clearing House, Inc. *Medicare and Medicaid Guide* (Topical Law Reports), 3 vols. Chicago: Commerce Clearing House, Inc., 1974.

Epstein, J. D., and Dennis, B. "Medicare Reimbursement Controversies and Appeals." *Topics in Health Care Financing,* vol. 2, no. 3, Spring 1976.

Hester, J., and Sussman, E. "Medicaid Prepayment: Concept and Implementation." *Milbank Memorial Fund Quarterly,* vol. 52, no. 4, pp. 415–444.

Hitt, D. H. "Reimbursement System Must Recognize Real Costs." *Hospitals,* JAHA, vol. 51, no. 1, January 1, 1977, pp. 47–53.

Myers, R. J. *Medicare.* Bryn Mawr, Pa.: McCahan Foundation, 1970.

Schlag, D. W. "Medicare and the Departmental Method of Reimbursement." *Hospital Progress,* vol. 53, no. 4, April 1972, pp. 56–57.

————— . "Medicare Reimbursement Pitfalls." *Hospital Progress,* vol. 54, no. 1, January 1973, pp. 82–84.

*Blue Cross*

Eilers, R. D. *Regulation of Blue Cross and Blue Shield Plans.* Homewood, Ill.: Richard D. Irwin, Inc., 1963.

Hill, L. A. "Hospitals, Blue Cross Plans Should Examine Mutual Concerns." *Hospitals,* JAHA, vol. 69, no. 18, September 16, 1975, pp. 47–49.

Law, S. A. *Blue Cross: What Went Wrong?* New Haven, Conn.: Yale University Press, 1974.

Lewis, H. L. "A Blue Cross Model: How One Plan Makes 'Em Love Cost Cutting." *Modern Healthcare,* vol. 4, no. 4, October 1975, pp. 37–41.

Prussin, J. A., and Wood, J. C. "Private Third Party Reimbursement." *Topics in Health Care Financing,* vol. 2, no. 1, Fall 1975.

Rogatz, P. "Blue Cross Plans Cannot Separate Financing from Quality and Organization for Care." *Hospital Financial Management,* vol. 27, no. 9, September 1973, pp. 26–35.

*Commercial Insurance Companies*

American Hospital Association. *Manual on Insurance for Hospitals and Related Health Care Facilities.* Chicago: American Hospital Association, 1966.

David, G. "Other Third Party Payers: End Blue Cross Discount." *Modern Healthcare,* vol. 6, no. 1, January 1977, pp. 24–25.

Hetherington, R. W., *et al. Health Insurance Plans: Promise and Performance.* New York: John Wiley & Sons, Inc., 1975.

Marrow, C. K. *Health Care Guidance: Commercial Health Insurance and National Health Policy.* New York: Praeger Publishers, 1976.

*Alternate Reimbursement Methods*

Buck, C. R., Jr. "Point of View: Hospitals Produce What They Are Paid For: Costs and Patient Days." *Health Care Management Review,* vol. 2, no. 4, Fall 1977, pp. 59–65.

Dowling, W. L. "Prospective Reimbursement of Hospitals." *Inquiry,* vol. 11, no. 3, September 1974, pp. 163–180.

Lave, J. R., *et al.* "A Proposal for Incentive Reimbursement for Hospitals." *Medical Care,* vol. 11, no. 2, March/April 1973, pp. 74–89.

McCarthy, C. "Incentive Reimbursement as an Impetus to Cost Containment." *Inquiry,* vol. 12, no. 4, December 1975, pp. 320–329.

Mueller, W. J. "A Perspective on Prospective Reimbursement." *Hospital Financial Management,* vol. 25, no. 1, January 1971, pp. 16–22.

Pauly, M. V. "Efficiency, Incentives and Reimbursement for Health Care." *Inquiry,* vol. 7, no. 4, December 1970, pp. 114–131.

Chapter 3

# Financing Hospital Care
# In Canada

### Objectives

After completing this chapter you should be able to:

1. Describe the insured inpatient and outpatient services in Canada.
2. Describe the other sources of revenue earned by the Canadian hospital.
3. Describe costs that are recoverable by the Canadian hospital.
4. Describe the method of determining the federal contribution to the health programs of the provincial government.
5. Describe the methods employed to finance the provincial share of health costs.
6. Describe the methods used by provincial authorities to pay participating hospitals.

## 3.1 INTRODUCTION

In Canada, the financial environment of the hospital is dominated by a governmentally supported system in which the institution receives a series of prospective payments that usually are made before the service is provided. Since 1956, a more or less fixed and homogeneous set of inpatient services and a more heterogeneous bundle of outpatient services have been financed jointly by the provincial and federal governments. When discussing the insured benefits and methods of making payments to the hospital, it is necessary to focus on the Hospital Insurance and Diagnostic Services Act and the Federal-Provincial Fiscal Arrangements and Established Programs Financing Act of 1977.

The basic inpatient benefit structure offered by all hospitals is specified in the Hospital Insurance and Diagnostic Services Act which, prior to April 1, 1977, also contained the formula used to determine the federal contribution to the various provincial programs. With the passage of the Federal-Provincial Fiscal Arrangements and Established Programs Financing Act on April 1, 1977, however, the responsibility for administering the system of financing health and hospital services shifted from the federal government to provincial governments. Since these two acts have dominated the hospital financial environment, the following discussion considers their provisions in some detail.

## 3.2 BENEFIT STRUCTURE AND SOURCES OF REVENUE

Among the primary objectives of the hospital and diagnostic services program is to ensure that the receipt of service is determined by medical need rather than by economic status or ability to pay. Pursuant to this major goal, the Hospital Insurance and Diagnostic Services Act specifies a set of inpatient benefits to which residents of each province are entitled without direct charges. The exceptions to this rule involve authorized and differential charges that are described below.

### 3.2.1 Inpatient Benefits

Table 3-1 lists and explains the inpatient services that are insured benefits in each province. Several comments concerning this benefit structure are appropriate. As noted above, the insured inpatient is entitled to the set of services listed in this table without additional direct charges. However, when a patient occupies a private or semiprivate room, the individual is responsible for the portion of the rate that is in excess of that for standard ward care. The fee for occupancy of a preferred accommodation is referred to as a differential charge. Several provincial plans have coinsurance provisions that require patients or the third party to pay an authorized charge, usually a fixed charge per day.

### 3.2.2 Outpatient Benefits

With respect to outpatient services, the act guarantees federal participation in financing the use of "any or all" of the services specified above when they are provided on an outpatient basis.

However, each province is allowed to determine which of these services will be incorporated as an insured benefit when used by outpatients. Unlike the set of insured inpatient services, the extent to which outpatient care is insured varies among the provinces and territories.

Table 3-2 summarizes the major outpatient services that are insured benefits in each of the provinces and territories. This table demonstrates that insured benefits are not uniform across provinces. For example, all outpatient services provided by the hospital, including physiotherapy and dietetic counselling serv-

**Table 3-1** Insured Inpatient Benefits

| Insured Benefits | Explanation |
|---|---|
| Accommodations and meals at the standard ward level | Accommodations and meals at the standard or public ward level is an insured service provided in all Canadian hospitals except institutions approved for outpatient services only. |
| Required nursing services | Necessary nursing care is an insured service provided by all hospitals. However, the care provided by a private duty nurse, as defined in the usual way, is not included as an insured service. |
| Laboratory, radiological, and other diagnostic procedures | In addition to the set of diagnostic and monitoring services provided by the hospital, the act specifies that any necessary interpretation of the results of such procedures also is an insured service. |
| Drugs, biologicals, and related preparations | The drugs included as an insured service vary from province to province and only drugs specified in provincial agreements and administered in the hospital are considered to be an insured benefit. |
| Use of special rooms | Included in this benefit are the use of operating rooms, case rooms, and anesthetic facilities, including equipment and supplies. |
| Routine surgical supplies | This benefit includes surgical dressings and other materials required during or following an operation. This benefit does not include prosthetic devices that may be required unless the appliances are used while the individual is a patient in the hospital. |
| Radiotherapy | In hospitals with radiotherapy facilities, the use of these facilities is included as an insured benefit. This includes, for example, the use of equipment and facilities for superficial and deep x-ray therapy as well as cobalt, radium, and other radioactive treatments. |
| Physiotherapy | Even though numerous hospitals have a physiotherapy department or physiotherapy facilities, these facilities are not available in smaller institutions. Where these facilities exist, physiotherapy services are included as an insured benefit. |
| Other services of hospital employees | In addition to the previous factors, the services provided by individuals who have contractual arrangements with the hospital are included as insured benefits. For example, the services of physiotherapists, radiotherapy technicians, occupational therapists, and social workers are insured benefits if such services are incorporated in the provincial plan. Further, the services of interns, residents, or physicians engaged in hospital administration or in the direction of medical departments are included. |
| Other services specified by the province | In addition to the services specified above, the province may decide to include additional ones in the set of insured benefits. As an example of special services, the |

**Table 3-1** continued

| Insured Benefits | Explanation |
|---|---|
| | province may decide to develop specialized programs for the diagnosis and treatment of cancer. For such services to be considered an insured benefit, they must be available to all residents of the province after a proper medical referral. |

ices as well as all outpatient services offered by provincial cancer clinics and diagnostic services at provincial laboratories, are benefits that are insured by the Alberta Health Services Commission. A somewhat less comprehensive approach has been taken by the provincial plans of Saskatchewan, New Brunswick, Manitoba, and Newfoundland. Even less comprehensive is the outpatient coverage offered in the Yukon Territory and the Northwest Territory.

**Table 3-2** Summary of Insured Outpatient Services in Canada, by Province

| Province or Territory | Insured Outpatient Services |
|---|---|
| British Columbia | Emergency services, minor surgical procedures; day care surgical services; outpatient cancer therapy; psychiatric day and night care; day care rehabilitation; narcotic addiction services; physiotherapy; diabetic day care, and dietetic counselling. |
| Alberta | All outpatient procedures provided by the hospital; all diagnostic, physiotherapy, and dietetic counselling services; all outpatient services provided by provincial cancer clinics and laboratories. |
| Saskatchewan | All outpatient services provided by the hospital. |
| Manitoba | All outpatient services except drugs and dressings in certain cases. |
| Ontario | Most outpatient services including physiotherapy, occupational therapy, radiotherapy, and inhalation therapy as well as other hospital services when medically necessary. |
| Quebec | Twenty-four-hour emergency service; minor surgery, including x-ray and laboratory examinations; physiotherapy; radiotherapy; occupational, speech, and audiology therapy; and medical orthoptics. |
| New Brunswick | All approved available services. |
| Nova Scotia | Broad range of essential services, including medically necessary diagnostic and laboratory examinations; radiotherapy for nonmalignant conditions; physiotherapy; |

**Table 3-2** continued

| Province or Territory | Insured Outpatient Services |
|---|---|
| | hemodialysis; emergency diagnostic and treatment services within 48 hours of an accident; minor medical and surgical procedures, and dietary counselling. |
| Prince Edward Island | Basic laboratory and radiological diagnostic procedures; radioactive isotopes; drugs and related preparations for emergency diagnosis and treatment. All other services specified as inpatient services. |
| Newfoundland | Laboratory, radiological, and other diagnostic procedures; radiotherapy and physiotherapy; occupational therapy; outpatient visits; emergency room visits; operating room facilities; drugs, medical, and surgical supplies when provided in the hospital. |
| Yukon Territory | Diagnostic procedures, treatment of injury, illness, or disability excluding normal physician services; day care surgical services. |
| Northwest Territory | Emergency and follow-up treatment of injury; radiological diagnostic procedures; laboratory examinations; minor surgical procedures; physiotherapy and radiotherapy; certain day care surgical procedures. |

## 3.2.3 Other Sources of Revenue

Although most of the institution's revenue is earned by providing insured services to the population covered under the provincial plan, the Canadian hospital also earns income from services that are insured by other third party payers. The hospital earns revenue by providing service to patients who are covered by other governmental agencies such as the municipal, provincial, or federal governments as well as those whose care is financed through the Workmen's Compensation Board. To a lesser extent, the hospital may earn revenues by providing services to insured patients who are not residents of the province in which the institution is located. In such cases, the income from this source consists of direct charges to the patient or to the provincial plan concerned.

The final source of operating revenue involves the portion of hospital charges that represents the financial liability of the patient. The situations in which the patient is responsible for a portion or all of the hospital's charges may be summarized as follows:

1. *Inpatient use*
   a. Authorized charges
   b. Differential charges

     c. Uninsured patient
  2. *Outpatient use*
     a. Authorized charges
     b. Uninsured services
     c. Uninsured patient

With regard to inpatient services, it will be recalled that a differential charge is imposed directly on patients, or their third party payers, for the use of preferred accommodations while the authorized charge represents a deterrent fee that is assessed in several provinces. As was seen earlier, the composition of insured outpatient benefits varies from provincial plan to provincial plan. When these services are not included as an insured benefit under a third party contract, the financial liability resulting from their use rests with the patient. The responsibility for a portion or all of the costs of care for an uninsured patient might be assumed by the individual.

When compared with the provincial plan and other governmental units, the hospital can place far less reliance on actually receiving payment from the patient. This is so for several reasons. First, as in the United States, the unwillingness of Canadian hospitals to pursue vigorous collection procedures or to assess carrying or interest charges on unpaid balances in patients' accounts has placed the institutions at a comparative disadvantage when competing with other creditors for payment. A second factor involves the possibility that the illness for which the patient received service reduces the individual's ability to perform normal economic functions and limits the capability to earn income. The first factor obviously influences the patient's willingness to pay, the second influences the ability to pay. Both tend to reduce the probability that patients will honor their financial liability to the hospital.

Finally, the Canadian hospital may earn nonoperating revenue by selling goods and services to individuals or institutions other than the patient. For example, the hospital may sell dietary services, laundry services, or heat or steam to other health care facilities. In addition, income may be derived through the rental of rooms or other accommodations as well as of land and buildings owned by the hospital to persons or institutions other than patients. In these instances, the income earned is referred to as a "recovery" and the entity responsible for payment frequently is another health care institution such as a local nursing home or another hospital.

## 3.3 ALLOWABLE COSTS

Most provincial plans and other third party payers recognize the direct and indirect expenditures incurred in providing insured services as allowable costs. These cost elements are as follows:

1. *Costs of employment:* This category includes wages, salaries, and employee benefits. With the exception of a few minor items, all employee costs are regarded as shareable by all provincial plans.
2. *Cost of purchased services:* In this category are the costs of services that are primarily substitutes for employment costs.
3. *Consumable supplies:* This category covers the costs of supplies used in the production of service as well as in the maintenance and operation of the hospital.
4. *Occupancy costs:* This category includes costs related to heat, light, power, etc. In addition, most provincial plans recognize depreciation charges on major equipment, nonmovable equipment, and outright purchases of equipment.

When calculating the expenses that constitute the basis for provincial plan payments, the hospital must deduct certain items from recorded costs. These items are regarded as sources of revenue that compensate the hospital for costs incurred in providing uninsured service. Since the hospital will recover these expenses from nonplan sources, most provincial plans require that the institution deduct the items listed in Table 3-3 from recorded costs when determining allowable costs.

It is important to note, however, that the offset revenues recognized by most provincial plans do not usually include such items as gifts, bequests, endowments, chapel receipts, contributed services, or investment income. As a result, these items are not treated as offset revenues and need not be deducted from total recorded expenditures when determining allowable cost.

In addition to the items of offset revenue summarized in Table 3-3, most provincial plans exclude certain items from allowable costs. Table 3-4 lists the major expenditures that must be excluded by the provider in most provinces when calculating allowable costs. Most of these exclusions are self-explanatory but several deserve further comment.

As noted in the table, any amounts expended on land, land inprovements, buildings, built-in equipment, and building service equipment as well as any provision for depreciation on these items are not regarded as allowable costs in most provinces. Most provincial authorities would defend this exclusion by noting that the acquisition of these items was financed primarily through governmental grants. Since governmental agencies provide most of the funding for the construction of the hospital's physical plant, there is no reason to recognize depreciation charges, debt principal, or interest charges related to the acquisition and use of these capital assets.

As indicated, any provision for depreciation on the value of the hospital's physical plant is not recognized as an allowable cost by most provincial authorities. It should be noted, however, that the term "physical plant" usually

**Table 3-3** Major Items of Offset Revenue

| Item | Explanation |
|---|---|
| Differential charges | A portion (usually 50 percent) of the revenue earned by providing preferred accommodations is treated as offset revenue. |
| Accounts receivable | Receivables generated by providing service to patients, such as members of the Royal Canadian Mounted Police or the armed forces, who are entitled to service under any act of Parliament or any other legislation or jurisdiction, usually are deducted from total costs. In addition, amounts owed by other provincial plans or other entities are regarded as offset revenues. |
| Grants | Contributions or National Health Grants intended to finance current operating activity or teaching and research programs usually are deducted from total costs when determining allowable costs. |
| Recoveries | Cash received or income earned by engaging in recovery transactions is treated as offset revenue. |
| Cash discounts | Total recorded costs are reduced by the amount of cash discounts on purchases made by the hospital. This deduction pertains only to institutions using the gross invoice method of recording accounts payable. This deduction is justified on the ground that cash discounts do not involve a cash disbursement by the hospital. |
| Unnecessary services | The earnings from insured services, the use of which is considered to be unnecessary by provincial authorities, must be deducted from total cost when determining allowable costs. |

is defined to exclude furniture and movable and nonmovable equipment designed specifically for use in a hospital. As a consequence, most provinces recognize depreciation charges on these items as allowable costs.

In many provinces, the hospital cannot recover the costs of research from provincial authorities. Thus, gross wages and salaries; the costs of medical, surgical, and pharmaceutical supplies, and any outlays for equipment purchased for the express purpose of conducting research are not recognized as allowable costs in most provinces. This exclusion is justified on the ground that most research in Canada is financed through federal and provincial grants. As a consequence, most provincial authorities would argue that funding provided through such grants is sufficient to finance most hospital-based research.

## 3.4 FINANCING MECHANISM

As mentioned, the costs of hospital care in Canada are financed jointly by federal and provincial governments. In describing how the cost of hospital care

**Table 3-4** Major Cost Exclusions

| Item | Explanation |
|---|---|
| Capital costs | This exclusion refers to amounts expended on land, land improvements, buildings, building equipment, and building service equipment. |
| Capital debts | Amounts expended on payment of capital debts and any interest on such debts usually are excluded from allowable costs. |
| Depreciation | The exclusion covers any provision for depreciation on the value of land, land improvements, and the physical plant of the hospital. |
| Prior debts | This exclusion involves any amounts expended for the payment of debts prior to the enactment of legislation creating governmental responsibility for financing hospital costs. |
| Research costs | This exclusion pertains to any direct and indirect costs incurred in whole or in part for research purposes. |
| Cost of commercial operations | This exclusion refers to the direct and indirect costs incurred in the operation of commercial enterprise such as the hospital gift shop, barber shop, etc. |

is financed, the first consideration is the method of determining the federal contribution to hospital operations and then the various methods employed by provincial governments to pay for their share of hospital costs.

## 3.4.1 The Federal Contribution

The basic thrust of the Federal-Provincial Fiscal Arrangements and Established Programs Financing Act of 1977 was to establish the basis for determining the federal contribution to the hospital insurance programs of the provinces and territories. It is important to note that, apart from altering the formula for determining the amount of the federal contribution, the act did not change any of the other provisions of the Hospital Insurance and Diagnostic Services Act. As a result, the contribution of the federal government under the 1977 act remains conditional on the preservation of the structure of insured benefits guaranteed by the Hospital Insurance and Diagnostic Services Act.

Since April 1, 1977, the new arrangement has constituted the basis for determining the amount of the federal contribution to the provinces and territories to help them provide:

1. hospital services as defined by the Hospital Insurance and Diagnostic Services Act
2. physician services

3. Extended Health Care
4. postsecondary education

Extended Health Care is recognized specifically by the legislation. The major purpose of this provision is to give the provinces flexibility in determining the manner and form in which these services are provided. Depending on local requirements, some provinces may emphasize home care as a low-cost alternative while others may emphasize ambulatory or residential care.

The annual federal contribution to these areas of program activity consists of:

1. a reduction in federal income taxes that enables provinces to increase provincial taxation without a net increase in the total level of taxation
2. a set of cash contributions consisting of
   a. a basic cash contribution
   b. a leveling payment

Of these components, the basic cash contribution is perhaps the most important. This is because this element comprises approximately half of the federal funding of established programs. Given the importance of the basic cash contribution, this component is considered first.

### 3.4.1.1 Basic Cash Contribution

The basic cash contribution is based on the total amount paid by the federal government in support of hospital insurance, medical care, and postsecondary education programs during the fiscal year 1975–1976. The calculation of the basic cash contribution requires the following steps:

1. The basic per capita rate *(PCR)* is obtained by dividing the total federal contribution to these programs during 1975–1976 by the total population in 1975–1976. Thus,

$$PCR = \frac{\text{Total Federal Contributions in 1975--1976}}{\text{Population 1975--1976}}$$

where *PCR* is the per capita rate.

2. The *per capita base* is then derived by multiplying the per capita rate by one-half, to which $7.63 is added. Thus,

$$PCB = \tfrac{1}{2}(PCR) + \$7.63$$

where *PCB* is the per capita base.

3. The basic federal cash contribution *(BCC)* to a given province for any fiscal year is derived by multiplying the per capita base by

a. the population of the province for the fiscal year in question;
b. an escalator adjustment equal to the three-year compound rate of growth in the Gross National Product (GNP) as expressed in current dollars.

Thus, the basic cash contribution to a given province *j* for the fiscal year *t* is given by

$$BCC_{jt} = PCB \times P_{jt} \times \alpha$$

where $P_{jt}$ represents the population of province *j* in time *t* and $\alpha$ represents the three-year compound rate of growth in GNP.

### 3.4.1.2 Leveling Payments

As seen, the national per capita rate, which is based on the total federal contributions during the fiscal year 1975–1976, was employed in calculating the basic cash contribution to a given province. Prior to the Act of 1977, provinces in which the per capita costs of hospital care exceeded the national average received a relatively low percentage of their costs from the federal government; those where these costs were less than the national average received a relatively high percentage. As a consequence, the federal per capita contribution varied from province to province during fiscal 1975–1976.

By implementing the national per capita rate immediately, the Act of 1977 would have exerted an adverse effect on some provinces and a beneficial effect on others. Provinces that received a relatively high per capita federal contribution would have suffered a loss had the national average been used immediately to compute the basic cash contribution; conversely, provinces that received a relatively low per capita payment from the federal government would have experienced a windfall gain. Therefore, a leveling payment was added or subtracted from the federal cash contribution to each province in the following fashion:

1. Provinces that received a per capita federal contribution in excess of the national average in 1975–1976 were to remain somewhat above the national average during the first four years of operation under the new legislation. By the fifth year, after narrowing the gap between the per capita rate in 1975–1976 and the national average by 20 percent per year, these provinces were to be receiving the national average payment.
2. Provinces that received a per capita contribution from the federal government in 1975–1976 that was less than the national average remained somewhat below the national average during the first two years under the new legislation. By the third year, after narrowing the difference between the per capita contribution from the federal government and the per capita contribution in 1975–1976 by one-third each year, these provinces also were receiving the national average payment.

In short, then, provinces gradually moved through a series of leveling payments from the per capita contribution received in the base year to the national average payment in three to five years.

### 3.4.1.3 Reduction in Federal Income Taxes

The reduction in federal income taxes consists of:

1. a transfer of 13.5 personal income tax points* from the federal government to the provincial government
2. a transfer of 1 corporate income tax point from the federal government to the provincial government

The reduction in federal income taxes enables the province to increase the level of provincial taxation in these areas without a *net* increase in its total level of corporate and personal income taxes. Thus, the transfer of tax points from the federal government to the provincial governments simply alters the composition of taxation without a net increase in the total level of corporate or personal income taxes.

## 3.4.2 The Provincial Contribution

Presented in Table 3-5 is a summary of the various methods employed by provincial governments to finance the portion of the costs of hospital care that are not the responsibility of the federal government. In accordance with the legislation enacted in 1977, all provinces rely on general revenues to finance the costs of health and hospital care. In addition, an inspection of the table will reveal that several provinces also employ premium payments as well as direct patient charges as a major source of required funds.

## 3.5 METHODS OF PAYMENT

The amount of the contribution to hospital operations by the provincial plan is determined by the hospital's budget which must be approved by provincial authorities. Once approved, the hospital receives one-twelfth or one-twenty fourth of the annual budget in monthly or semimonthly installments respectively. The purpose of these payments is to finance the operations of the hospital on

---

* From the perspective of the federal government, the value of a tax point is equal to 1 percent of the basic federal taxes generated by a specific tax base such as personal or corporate income. From the perspective of the provincial government, the value of the transferred tax point is equal to the number of transferred points multiplied by the value of a tax point in the province.

**Table 3-5** Provincial Health Care Financing Methods Before 1977 Act

| | Method of Financing | | | |
|---|---|---|---|---|
| | General Revenue | | Premium | Patient Charges |
| Province | In Whole | In Part | | |
| Newfoundland | ★ | | | |
| Prince Edward Island | ★ | | | |
| Nova Scotia | ★ | | | |
| New Brunswick | ★ | | | |
| Quebec | ★ | | | |
| Ontario | | ★ | ★ | |
| Manitoba | ★ | | | |
| Saskatchewan | ★ | | | |
| Alberta | | | ★ | ★ |
| British Columbia | | ★ | | ★ |
| Northwest Territories | | ★ | | ★ |
| Yukon Territory | ★ | | | |

a current basis until the next pay period. Presented in Table 3-6 is a representative sample of the methods employed by the provinces in paying participating hospitals in selected provinces.

Since the preparation of the budget and the resulting periodic disbursement from the provincial plan to the hospital are based on expectations and predictions, each plan allows for periodic or end-of-year adjustments. These adjustments reflect the fact that the actual performance of the hospital is seldom, if ever, in balance with the expected performance as expressed in the budget. The adjustment process, then, is the mechanism by which the hospital might be compensated for justifiable deficits. On the other hand, if actual costs are less than budgeted costs, the hospital may be forced to reimburse all or a portion of the surplus to the provincial plan.

As noted in Table 3-6, the adjustment process usually occurs at year's end after an external audit of the hospital's books has been completed. In seeking additional funds, the hospital usually must prove that the deficits were due to changes in volume, standards of care, or an unusual circumstance that could not be foreseen at the time the budget was prepared. In certain provinces such as Manitoba, a firm budget procedure is in effect and the hospital is responsible for any deficits.

### 3.6 SUMMARY AND IMPLICATIONS FOR WORKING CAPITAL MANAGEMENT

The last two chapters have examined the financial environment in which working capital is managed in Canada and the United States. That hospitals in

**Table 3-6** Methods of Paying Hospitals in Selected Provinces

| Province | Method of Payment | Adjustment Process |
|---|---|---|
| Manitoba | 24 payments per year based on approved annual budget | Hospitals usually are responsible for any unfavorable differences between actual and budgeted cost. On the other hand, they are permitted to retain a small percentage of any surplus. |
| Prince Edward Island | 12 monthly payments based on the approved budget less 50 percent of all differential revenues earned by the hospital; standard ward rates reimbursed by bulk payments | Adjustments during the year are negotiated on the basis of material differences between actual and budgeted rates of activity. Year's end adjustment is negotiated after audit. |
| Newfoundland | 24 payments per year based on approved annual budget | Hospital may request budget review after midyear (June 1); final review and adjustments occur at year's end. |
| British Columbia | 24 payments per year based on approved annual budget | Adjustments made when occupancy rates are markedly different from budgeted standards; adjustments = variation in days × value of one day's supplies. |
| Alberta | 12 monthly payments based on approved annual budget | Adjustment permitted if the hospital can prove a deficit is due to unusual circumstances. |
| Saskatchewan | 24 payments per year based on approved annual budget | Rates are changed if volume or standards of care change; adjustment made at year's end and the hospital may retain surplus if it was a result of efficient operations. |

the two countries depend on third party payers and, to a lesser extent, self-pay patients as a major source of revenue and cash should be clear. Also shown was the fact that the lion's share of the United States hospital's reimbursement is received on a retrospective basis, most of the average Canadian hospital's on a prospective basis.

Despite these differences, the basic techniques of working capital management may be used appropriately in both systems of reimbursement. To illustrate this point, consider the impact of these two systems on the problem of estimating the cash inflows for some specified period.

Under retrospective reimbursement, the hospital's cash inflows depend on the rate at which payments are made on receivables. When estimating these cash inflows, it is convenient to divide the amounts owed to the hospital into essentially two groups. The first group consists of receivables for which a third party payer (e.g., Blue Cross, Medicare, the commercial insurance company, etc.) assumes financial responsibility. For this group, the amount of the payment usually is known with certainty but the timing of subsequent cash receipts is far more problematical. The second group consists of accounts receivable for which the patient assumes financial responsibility. In this case, neither the amount nor the timing of subsequent cash receipts can be known with certainty.

A similar situation arises under prospective reimbursement. As seen above, the cash receipts of such a hospital consist of random and nonrandom components. With regard to the nonrandom component, the timing and the amount of the periodic prepayment is usually known with relative certainty. On the other hand, the random component depends on the rate at which payments are made on receivables. As before, the accounts receivable of such a hospital may be divided into two groups. The first group consists of receivables for which a third party payer (e.g., other provincial plans, commercial insurance companies, Workmen's Compensation Board, etc.) assumes financial responsibility while the second consists of amounts owed to the hospital by self-responsible patients. Factors that give rise to this component are the imposition of direct patient charges as well as the use of uninsured service. As before, management usually is certain of receiving payment in full from the third party payer but is less certain of the timing of these receipts. On the other hand, management is certain of neither the amount nor the timing of cash inflows from patient payments.

These observations suggest that hospitals in Canada and in the United States are faced with similar problems when estimating the cash inflows from payments on receivables. In the case of the third party payer, only the timing of cash receipts is problematical and it will be seen that an application of the principles of mathematical expectation permits an estimation of the magnitude of cash receipts during a given period. When estimating the cash inflows from payments on the receivables for which the patient is responsible, it is necessary to address not only the problem of estimating the timing of these receipts but also the value of the accounts that will be paid in full and the value of those that must be written off as uncollectable. In this regard, an absorbing Markov chain, which is a method of estimating the value of outstanding receivables that will be paid in full or written off as uncollectable, will be found to be a useful management tool. These probability models may be used appropriately in both systems of reimbursement.

Concerning the other components of working capital, administrators in the United States and Canada are faced with similar problems when managing inventories and the institutions' investment in marketable securities as well as when reaching decisions regarding the best method of financing working capital needs. As a consequence, the tools and techniques of working capital management are appropriate to both systems of reimbursement.

At this point it is important to note that the last two chapters provided the basis for subsequent analyses of the tools and techniques of working capital management. In addition, it will be found that many of the techniques discussed in this text may be expressed by using the notation and operations of matrix algebra. Thus, before discussing working capital management and the process of internal control, it is necessary first to review the basic principles of this area of mathematics.

# Chapter 4

# Introduction to Matrix Algebra

## Objectives

After completing this chapter, you should be able to:

1. Use matrices to display information.
2. Perform the operations of
   a. matrix addition.
   b. matrix subtraction.
   c. matrix multiplication.
3. Find the transpose of a matrix.
4. Find the determinant and the inverse of a square matrix.

## 4.1 INTRODUCTION

The notation and operations of matrix algebra are used extensively throughout this book. The reliance on matrix algebra is predicated on two fundamental premises:

1. The operations and notation of matrix algebra greatly simplify the expression of many of the quantitative techniques described in this text.
2. Once the methods of analysis have been expressed in the notation of matrix algebra, management may develop programs that permit the use of high-speed electronic computers to perform required calculations. This reduces the time and energy needed to carry out long and tedious calculations, thus providing management with the time to devote attention to other areas of responsibility.

These two factors are of considerable importance in the discussion of cost finding, the technical aspects of budget preparation, the analysis of cost variances, techniques of projecting cash receipts that emanate from the realization of receivables, the determination of the optimum cash balance, and the identification of the optimum investment strategy. The techniques described here require a rudimentary understanding of the fundamental operations of matrix algebra; therefore, this chapter is devoted to the operations of addition, subtraction, and multiplication as applied to matrices. The inverse of a matrix, which is the matrix algebra counterpart to algebraic division, also is considered. It should be noted that an understanding of matrix algebra requires only a small investment of time that can yield significant dividends. In fact, the prerequisites to an understanding of matrix algebra involve nothing more than an ability to perform the algebraic operations of addition, subtraction, multiplication, and division.

## 4.2 A GENERAL DESCRIPTION

A matrix is a rectangular array or table of numbers that have been arranged in rows and columns. A matrix is a device that is used to organize and present numerical data so that they may be manipulated mathematically with ease. One of the primary advantages of employing matrix notation is that the algebra of matrices provides a means of organizing data and simplifying the expression of a large number of computations.

Consider first the aspect of a matrix as an aid in organizing data. Suppose we are provided with information concerning the number of days of hospital care used by patients of differing ages during the last three years. Suppose further that the information is conveyed in tabular form as in Table 4-1.

These data may be written in matrix notation as follows:

$$\begin{bmatrix} 80,000 & 82,000 & 86,000 \\ 60,000 & 65,000 & 68,000 \\ 50,000 & 56,000 & 62,000 \\ 90,000 & 92,000 & 85,000 \end{bmatrix}$$

**Table 4-1** Use of Service by Age of Patient during the Period 1978–1980

| | Days of Care Utilized by Year | | |
|---|---|---|---|
| Age | 1978 | 1979 | 1980 |
| 0–15 | 80,000 | 82,000 | 86,000 |
| 16–44 | 60,000 | 65,000 | 68,000 |
| 45–64 | 50,000 | 56,000 | 62,000 |
| 65+ | 90,000 | 92,000 | 85,000 |

In a matrix, the position of an element determines its meaning. For example, the element 56,000, which appears in the third row and the second column, represents the number of days of care used by patients in the age category 45–64 during 1979. Thus, a given row represents the use of service by the corresponding age group during the three-year period, while a given column reflects the use of service by all age groups during the corresponding year.

Given this general description, consider now the notation for describing a matrix. As noted, a matrix is an array of numbers arranged in rows and columns. It is identified by enclosing the data in square brackets. The individual entries in a matrix are referred to as elements or terms of the matrix. In this text we follow the convention of denoting matrices by uppercase boldface letters and the elements of the matrix by lowercase italic letters. Thus, we might write

$$\mathbf{A} = \begin{bmatrix} a_{11} & a_{12} & a_{13} \\ a_{21} & a_{22} & a_{23} \end{bmatrix}$$

where $\mathbf{A}$ is a 2 × 3 matrix. The expression 2 × 3 is read "2 by 3" and means that there are 2 rows and 3 columns in the matrix. In general, a matrix with $r$ rows and $k$ columns is referred to as a *matrix of order* $r \times k$ ($r$ by $k$).

The elements of matrix $\mathbf{A}$ may be expressed generally by the term $a_{ij}$. The first subscript, $i$, refers to the row in which the element appears while the second subscript, $j$, indicates the column in which the term appears. For example, the element $a_{12}$ appears in the first row and second column of the matrix and $a_{23}$ in the second row and third column. In this way, the subscript attached to an element locates its position in the matrix.

By way of contrast, a matrix consisting of a single column is referred to as a *column vector* and is represented by a lowercase boldfaced letter. For example,

$$\mathbf{x} = \begin{bmatrix} 1 \\ 2 \\ 3 \end{bmatrix}$$

is a column vector of order 3. Similarly, a matrix consisting of a single row is called a *row vector* and we use a "prime" (′) to indicate a row vector. For example,

$$\mathbf{y}' = \begin{bmatrix} 1 & 2 & 3 & 4 \end{bmatrix}$$

is a row vector of order 4. We might have referred to $\mathbf{x}$ as a matrix of order 3 × 1 and $\mathbf{y}'$ as a matrix of order 1 × 4. The "prime" symbol often is called "transpose" and $\mathbf{y}'$ is read "y transpose."

A single number such as $3$, $\dfrac{1}{50}$ or $-12$ is called a *scalar*. Here, we might think of a scalar as a matrix of order $1 \times 1$.

## 4.3 MATRIX ADDITION

Having described matrices in general terms, we consider now the basic arithmetic operations of matrix algebra. Beginning with the operation of addition, we may write

$$\mathbf{A} = \begin{bmatrix} -1 & 6 & 7 \\ 9 & 14 & 12 \end{bmatrix} \quad \text{and} \quad \mathbf{B} = \begin{bmatrix} 5 & -3 & 6 \\ 10 & 14 & 8 \end{bmatrix} \tag{4.1}$$

The addition of these two matrices is given by

$$\mathbf{A} + \mathbf{B} = \begin{bmatrix} (-1 + 5) & (6 - 3) & (7 + 6) \\ (9 + 10) & (14 + 14) & (12 + 8) \end{bmatrix} = \begin{bmatrix} 4 & 3 & 13 \\ 19 & 28 & 20 \end{bmatrix} \tag{4.2}$$

Thus, the matrix representing the sum of $\mathbf{A}$ and $\mathbf{B}$ is formed by adding the two matrices, element by element.

As should be obvious, matrix addition is possible only when the two matrices involved are of the *same order*. That is, two matrices may be added if and only if they have the *same number of rows and columns*.

## 4.4 MATRIX SUBTRACTION

If we write the matrices $\mathbf{A}$ and $\mathbf{B}$ as

$$\mathbf{A} = \begin{bmatrix} 20 & 16 & 10 \\ 14 & 18 & 6 \end{bmatrix} \quad \text{and} \quad \mathbf{B} = \begin{bmatrix} 5 & 8 & 4 \\ 7 & 9 & 2 \end{bmatrix}$$

the matrix operation of subtraction may be illustrated by

$$\mathbf{A} - \mathbf{B} = \begin{bmatrix} (20 - 5) & (16 - 8) & (10 - 4) \\ (14 - 7) & (18 - 9) & (6 - 2) \end{bmatrix} = \begin{bmatrix} 15 & 8 & 6 \\ 7 & 9 & 4 \end{bmatrix} \tag{4.3}$$

Thus, the difference between two matrices is found by subtracting the two matrices, element by element. As in the case of matrix addition, matrix subtraction is possible if and only if the two matrices involved are of the same order.

## 4.5 MATRIX MULTIPLICATION

Referring to matrix addition, it can be shown that

$$\mathbf{A} + \mathbf{A} = 2\mathbf{A} \qquad (4.4)$$

Extending this finding to the case in which there are $\lambda \mathbf{A}'$s in the summation ($\lambda$ is the Greek letter lambda), we find that

$$\mathbf{A} + \mathbf{A} + \cdots + \mathbf{A} = \lambda \mathbf{A} \qquad (4.5)$$

This result applies to any value of $\lambda$ and constitutes the definition of *scalar multiplication*. When we multiply the matrix $\mathbf{A}$ by a scalar, every element in $\mathbf{A}$ is multiplied by $\lambda$. For example, letting $\lambda = 3$ and

$$\mathbf{A} = \begin{bmatrix} 1 & 2 & 3 \\ 4 & 5 & 6 \end{bmatrix}$$

we find

$$3\mathbf{A} = 3 \begin{bmatrix} 1 & 2 & 3 \\ 4 & 5 & 6 \end{bmatrix} = \begin{bmatrix} 3 & 6 & 9 \\ 12 & 15 & 18 \end{bmatrix}$$

Scalar multiplication is the simplest form of matrix multiplication.

We now turn to multiplication operations involving *vectors*, then consider the multiplication of matrices. Suppose we wrote

$$\mathbf{x}' = \begin{bmatrix} 12 & 10 & 6 \end{bmatrix}$$

and

$$\mathbf{a} = \begin{bmatrix} 7 \\ 4 \\ 3 \end{bmatrix}$$

The product $\mathbf{x}'\mathbf{a}$ that is given by

$$\mathbf{x'a} = \begin{bmatrix} 12 & 10 & 6 \end{bmatrix} \begin{bmatrix} 7 \\ 4 \\ 3 \end{bmatrix}$$

is calculated as follows

$$\mathbf{x'a} = 12(7) + 10(4) + 6(3) = 142$$

This example illustrates the procedure for obtaining $\mathbf{x'a}$. Observe that $\mathbf{x'a}$ is obtained by multiplying each element of $\mathbf{x'}$ by the corresponding element of $\mathbf{a}$ and summing the resultant products.

Consequently, if

$$\mathbf{x'} = \begin{bmatrix} x_1 x_2 \cdot \cdot \cdot x_n \end{bmatrix} \quad \text{and} \quad \mathbf{a} = \begin{bmatrix} a_1 \\ a_2 \\ \cdot \\ \cdot \\ \cdot \\ a_n \end{bmatrix}$$

$$\mathbf{x'a} = x_1 a_1 + x_2 a_2 + \cdot \cdot \cdot + x_n a_n \qquad (4.6.1)$$

$$= \sum_{i=1}^{n} x_i a_i \qquad (4.6.2)$$

In this case, the product of $\mathbf{x'a}$ is possible if and only if the vectors $\mathbf{x'}$ and $\mathbf{a}$ have the same number of elements.

Consider next *vector-matrix products*. If we defined the row vector $\mathbf{x'}$ as

$$\mathbf{x'} = \begin{bmatrix} 5 & 10 & 20 \end{bmatrix}$$

and the matrix $\mathbf{A}$ as

$$\mathbf{A} = \begin{bmatrix} 5 & 4 & 6 \\ 6 & 2 & 12 \\ 10 & 7 & 9 \end{bmatrix}$$

the product $\mathbf{x'A}$ is written in the form

$$\mathbf{x'A} = [5 \quad 10 \quad 20] \begin{bmatrix} 5 & 4 & 6 \\ 6 & 2 & 12 \\ 10 & 7 & 9 \end{bmatrix}$$

and we calculate $\mathbf{x'A}$ as follows

$$\mathbf{x'A} = [5(5) + 10(6) + 20(10) \quad 5(4) + 10(2) + 20(7) \quad 5(6) + 10(12) + 20(9)]$$

$$= [285 \quad 180 \quad 330]$$

The first element of the product vector is given by

$$[5 \quad 10 \quad 20] \begin{bmatrix} 5 \\ 6 \\ 10 \end{bmatrix} = 285$$

and the second element by

$$[5 \quad 10 \quad 20] \begin{bmatrix} 4 \\ 2 \\ 7 \end{bmatrix} = 180$$

Finally, the third element of the product vector is found by

$$[5 \quad 10 \quad 20] \begin{bmatrix} 6 \\ 12 \\ 9 \end{bmatrix} = 330$$

The elements of this vector are derived in the same way as the product $\mathbf{x'a}$. Here, however, we used each successive column of $\mathbf{A}$ as the vector $\mathbf{a}$. Thus, the product $\mathbf{x'A}$ is obtained by repetitions of the product $\mathbf{x'a}$ where the vector $\mathbf{a}$ is represented by successive columns of the matrix $\mathbf{A}$.

Multiplying two matrices can now be explained as a repetitive series of vector multiplications. To obtain the product of two matrices, say $\mathbf{A}$ and $\mathbf{B}$, we need only think of matrix **A** as consisting of a series of row vectors and matrix **B** of a series of column vectors. We assert that

$$\mathbf{AB} = \mathbf{C}$$

where

$$\mathbf{A} = \begin{bmatrix} 1 & 5 & 7 \\ 6 & 12 & 8 \end{bmatrix}; \quad \mathbf{B} = \begin{bmatrix} 3 & 5 & 8 \\ 2 & 4 & 11 \\ 6 & 9 & 2 \end{bmatrix} \quad \text{and}$$

$$\mathbf{C} = \begin{bmatrix} c_{11} & c_{12} & c_{13} \\ c_{21} & c_{22} & c_{23} \end{bmatrix}$$

The element $c_{11}$ of the product matrix **C** is obtained by multiplying the *first column* of **B** by the *first row* of **A**; thus the *first row* of **A** times the *first column* of **B** yields

$$c_{11} = \begin{bmatrix} 1 & 5 & 7 \end{bmatrix} \begin{bmatrix} 3 \\ 2 \\ 6 \end{bmatrix}$$

$$= 1(3) + 5(2) + 7(6)$$

$$= 55$$

Similarly, the element $c_{12}$ of the product matrix is obtained by multiplying the second column of **B** by the first row of **A**; thus,

$$c_{12} = \begin{bmatrix} 1 & 5 & 7 \end{bmatrix} \begin{bmatrix} 5 \\ 4 \\ 9 \end{bmatrix}$$

$$= 1(5) + 5(4) + 7(9)$$

$$= 88$$

The element $c_{13}$ is obtained by multiplying the third column of **B** by the first row of **A**; thus

$$c_{13} = \begin{bmatrix} 1 & 5 & 7 \end{bmatrix} \begin{bmatrix} 8 \\ 11 \\ 2 \end{bmatrix}$$

$$= 1(8) + 5(11) + 7(2)$$

$$= 77$$

Using the second row of **A**, we repeat the process to obtain the elements $c_{21}$, $c_{22}$, and $c_{23}$ of the product matrix **C** as follows:

$$c_{21} = \begin{bmatrix} 6 & 12 & 8 \end{bmatrix} \begin{bmatrix} 3 \\ 2 \\ 6 \end{bmatrix}$$

$$= 6(3) + 12(2) + 8(6)$$

$$= 90$$

$$c_{22} = \begin{bmatrix} 6 & 12 & 8 \end{bmatrix} \begin{bmatrix} 5 \\ 4 \\ 9 \end{bmatrix}$$

$$= 6(5) + 12(4) + 8(9)$$

$$= 150$$

$$c_{23} = \begin{bmatrix} 6 & 12 & 8 \end{bmatrix} \begin{bmatrix} 8 \\ 11 \\ 2 \end{bmatrix}$$

$$= [6(8) + 12(11) + 8(2)]$$

$$= 196$$

To summarize this example, we may express the multiplication of the matrices **A** and **B** by

$$\mathbf{AB} = \begin{bmatrix} 1 & 5 & 7 \\ 6 & 12 & 8 \end{bmatrix} \begin{bmatrix} 3 & 5 & 8 \\ 2 & 4 & 11 \\ 6 & 9 & 2 \end{bmatrix}$$

which yields

$$\mathbf{AB} = \begin{bmatrix} 1(3) + 5(2) + 7(6) & 1(5) + 5(4) + 7(9) & 1(8) + 5(11) + 7(2) \\ 6(3) + 12(2) + 8(6) & 6(5) + 12(4) + 8(9) & 6(8) + 12(11) + 8(2) \end{bmatrix}$$

$$= \begin{bmatrix} 55 & 88 & 77 \\ 90 & 150 & 196 \end{bmatrix}$$

Several additional comments concerning matrix multiplication are appropriate. First, the product **AB** is permitted if and only if the number of elements in each row of **A** is equal to the number of elements in each column of **B**. This implies that the number of columns in **A** must equal the number of rows in **B**. Although we were able to obtain the product **AB** in our example, the product **BA** does not exist. A second point concerning matrix multiplication is worthy of note. As seen above, when a matrix of order $2 \times 3$ was multiplied by a matrix of order $3 \times 3$, the product matrix was of the order $2 \times 3$. In general, we might express this relation in the form

$$\mathbf{A}_{r \times k} \mathbf{B}_{k \times m} = \mathbf{P}_{r \times m} \tag{4.7}$$

which allows us to ascertain the conformability of **A** and **B** for multiplication as well as the order of their product.

> At the heart of many of the calculations that we perform in this text is a special form of matrix multiplication. We frequently encounter a term similar to **A′B** which is the multiplication of the matrix **B** by the transpose of **A**.

In general, the transpose of matrix $\mathbf{A}$ is the matrix whose columns are the rows of $\mathbf{A}$. This implies that the order of the elements must be retained when deriving the transpose of a matrix. For example, if

$$\mathbf{A} = \begin{bmatrix} 1 & 7 & 10 \\ 6 & 4 & 14 \end{bmatrix}$$

the transpose of $\mathbf{A}$ is given by

$$\mathbf{A}' = \begin{bmatrix} 1 & 6 \\ 7 & 4 \\ 10 & 14 \end{bmatrix}$$

## 4.6 THE DETERMINANT AND INVERSE OF A MATRIX

We turn now to an operation that is appropriate for *square matrices* (i.e., matrices of order $r \times r$), which leads to a scalar value known as the *determinant*. This operation is of importance when finding the *inverse* of a matrix, which plays a role in the counterpart of division in matrix algebra, as well as in calculating measures of the variance exhibited by a set of data. In the following discussion we limit our analysis to $2 \times 2$ and $3 \times 3$ matrices since the calculation of the determinant and the inverse of higher order matrices is accomplished more easily by simple computer programs.

The determinant of matrix $\mathbf{A}$ usually is represented by $|\mathbf{A}|$, $\|\mathbf{A}\|$ or det $(\mathbf{A})$. However, $|\mathbf{A}|$ is more common and this notation is used throughout this text. The value of the determinant for a $2 \times 2$ matrix is the product of its diagonal terms less the product of the off-diagonal terms. Thus, if

$$\mathbf{A} = \begin{bmatrix} a_{11} & a_{12} \\ a_{21} & a_{22} \end{bmatrix}$$

the determinant of $\mathbf{A}$ is

$$|\mathbf{A}| = a_{11}a_{22} - a_{12}a_{21} \tag{4.8}$$

where $a_{11}$ and $a_{22}$ are the diagonal elements of the matrix while $a_{12}$ and $a_{21}$ are its off-diagonal elements. To illustrate, suppose that

$$\mathbf{A} = \begin{bmatrix} 7 & 10 \\ 4 & 20 \end{bmatrix}$$

The determinant of $\mathbf{A}$ is given by

$$|\mathbf{A}| = 7(20) - 4(10)$$

$$= 100$$

The determinant also plays a central role in deriving the *inverse* of a matrix. In previous sections we discussed the arithmetic operations of addition, subtraction, and multiplication. However, we have not discussed division because, in its usual sense, this operation does not exist in matrix algebra. To perform the operation of "division" in matrix algebra it is necessary to derive the inverse of a matrix. The inverse of the matrix $\mathbf{A}$ usually is denoted by the symbol $\mathbf{A}^{-1}$, which is read as "$\mathbf{A}$ inverse," "$\mathbf{A}$ to the minus one," or "the inverse of $\mathbf{A}$."

The use of the inverse in solving an algebraic expression is illustrated by the following example. If we were given the algebraic expression

$$ax = b \quad (a \neq 0) \tag{4.9}$$

we could solve for $x$ as follows

$$\frac{1}{a}(ax) = \frac{1}{a}b = a^{-1}b$$

Hence

$$x = a^{-1}b$$

where $a^{-1}$ is used to represent $1/a$.

Modifying this example, we might derive the simultaneous solution for two linear equations. For example, let

$$6x_1 + 4x_2 = 360$$

$$4x_1 + 16x_2 = 480$$

These equations could be solved simultaneously by substitution. In terms of our example, we find that

$$6(120 - 4x_2) + 4x_2 = 360$$

Hence, we find that $x_1 = 48$ and $x_2 = 18$.

However, we could have expressed this system in matrix notation:

$$\begin{bmatrix} 6 & 4 \\ 4 & 16 \end{bmatrix} \begin{bmatrix} x_1 \\ x_2 \end{bmatrix} = \begin{bmatrix} 360 \\ 480 \end{bmatrix}$$

Letting

$$\mathbf{A} = \begin{bmatrix} 6 & 4 \\ 4 & 16 \end{bmatrix}; \quad \mathbf{x} = \begin{bmatrix} x_1 \\ x_2 \end{bmatrix} \quad \text{and} \quad \mathbf{b} = \begin{bmatrix} 360 \\ 480 \end{bmatrix}$$

this system of equations may be expressed in the form

$$\mathbf{Ax} = \mathbf{b} \qquad (4.10)$$

which has the solution

$$\mathbf{x} = \mathbf{A}^{-1}\mathbf{b} \qquad (4.11)$$

Thus, to find the simultaneous solution to this system of linear equations, it is necessary to multiply the column vector $\mathbf{b}$ by the inverse of $\mathbf{A}$.

The inverse of $\mathbf{A}$ is defined as a matrix whose product with $\mathbf{A}$ is the identity matrix. The identity matrix is defined by

$$\mathbf{I} = \begin{bmatrix} 1 & 0 \\ 0 & 1 \end{bmatrix} \qquad (4.12)$$

Observe that

$$\mathbf{AI} = \mathbf{A} = \mathbf{IA} \qquad (4.13)$$

and that

$$\mathbf{AA}^{-1} = \mathbf{I} \qquad (4.14)$$

In terms of our example, we let

$$\mathbf{A}^{-1} = \begin{bmatrix} c_{11} & c_{12} \\ c_{21} & c_{22} \end{bmatrix}$$

$$\mathbf{A} = \begin{bmatrix} a_{11} & a_{12} \\ a_{21} & a_{22} \end{bmatrix} \quad \text{and} \quad \mathbf{I} = \begin{bmatrix} 1 & 0 \\ 0 & 1 \end{bmatrix}$$

Substituting, we find that

$$\begin{bmatrix} a_{11} & a_{12} \\ a_{21} & a_{22} \end{bmatrix} \begin{bmatrix} c_{11} & c_{12} \\ c_{21} & c_{22} \end{bmatrix} = \begin{bmatrix} 1 & 0 \\ 0 & 1 \end{bmatrix} \qquad \textbf{(4.15.1)}$$

Our problem is to find the values of $\mathbf{A}^{-1}$ such that Equation 4.15.1 is satisfied. Expanding Equation 4.15.1, we find that

$$a_{11}c_{11} + a_{12}c_{21} = 1 \qquad \textbf{(4.15.2)}$$

$$a_{21}c_{11} + a_{22}c_{21} = 0 \qquad \textbf{(4.15.3)}$$

$$a_{11}c_{12} + a_{12}c_{22} = 0 \qquad \textbf{(4.15.4)}$$

$$a_{21}c_{12} + a_{22}c_{22} = 1 \qquad \textbf{(4.15.5)}$$

If we multiply Equations 4.15.2 and 4.15.3 by $a_{21}$ and $a_{11}$, respectively, we obtain

$$a_{21}a_{11}c_{11} + a_{21}a_{12}c_{21} = a_{21}$$

$$a_{21}a_{11}c_{11} + a_{11}a_{22}c_{21} = 0$$

Solving for $c_{21}$ yields

$$c_{21} = \frac{-a_{21}}{a_{11}a_{22} - a_{21}a_{12}}$$

Recalling that $|\mathbf{A}| \ a_{11}a_{22} - a_{21}a_{12}$, we find that

$$c_{21} = \frac{-a_{21}}{|\mathbf{A}|}$$

Employing a similar procedure, we obtain

$$c_{12} = \frac{-a_{12}}{|\mathbf{A}|}$$

$$c_{11} = \frac{a_{22}}{|\mathbf{A}|}$$

$$c_{22} = \frac{a_{11}}{|\mathbf{A}|}$$

After substituting these values, we find that

$$\mathbf{A}^{-1} = \frac{1}{|\mathbf{A}|} \begin{bmatrix} a_{22} & -a_{12} \\ -a_{21} & a_{11} \end{bmatrix} \tag{4.16}$$

Even though the results expressed by Equation 4.16 pertain only to a $2 \times 2$ matrix, we make extensive use of this formula in subsequent chapters. Returning to our example, the determinant of $\mathbf{A}$ is found by

$$|\mathbf{A}| = 6(16) - 4(4)$$

$$= 80$$

The inverse of $\mathbf{A}$ is found to be

$$\mathbf{A}^{-1} = \frac{1}{80} \begin{bmatrix} 16 & -4 \\ -4 & 6 \end{bmatrix} = \begin{bmatrix} .20 & -.05 \\ -.05 & .075 \end{bmatrix}$$

The simultaneous solution to the system of linear equations is

$$\begin{bmatrix} x_1 \\ x_2 \end{bmatrix} = \begin{bmatrix} .20 & -.05 \\ -.05 & .075 \end{bmatrix} \begin{bmatrix} 360 \\ 480 \end{bmatrix}$$

$$\begin{bmatrix} x_1 \\ x_2 \end{bmatrix} = \begin{bmatrix} 48 \\ 18 \end{bmatrix}$$

These findings suggest that $x_1 = 48$ and $x_2 = 18$, which agrees with the results obtained earlier.

When finding the inverse of higher order matrices, it is simpler to employ a slightly different technique:

$$A = \begin{bmatrix} a_{11} & a_{12} & a_{13} \\ a_{21} & a_{22} & a_{23} \\ a_{31} & a_{32} & a_{33} \end{bmatrix}$$

Without providing a formal proof, we simply assert that

$$A^{-1} = \frac{1}{|A|} G'$$

where $G$ is a matrix of cofactors and

$$|A| = a_{11}a_{22}a_{33} - a_{12}a_{21}a_{33} + a_{12}a_{23}a_{31} - a_{13}a_{22}a_{31}$$

$$+ a_{13}a_{21}a_{32} - a_{11}a_{23}a_{32}$$

Concerning the matrix $G$, we define the cofactor $\mu_{ij}$ of element $a_{ij}$ by

$$\mu_{ij} = (-1)^{i+j} |M_{ij}|$$

where $M_{ij}$ is called the minor of $a_{ij}$ and is obtained by eliminating the row and the column in which $a_{ij}$ appears. For example, consider the element $a_{11}$. We eliminate the first row and first column of $A$ so that the elements $a_{22}$, $a_{23}$, $a_{32}$, and $a_{33}$ remain. As a result, we find that

$$\mu_{11} = (-1)^{1+1} \begin{vmatrix} a_{22} & a_{23} \\ a_{32} & a_{33} \end{vmatrix}$$

$$= (-1)^2 (a_{22}a_{33} - a_{23}a_{32})$$

Similarly, the cofactor of $a_{12}$ is given by

$$\mu_{12} = (-1)^{1+2} \begin{vmatrix} a_{21} & a_{23} \\ a_{31} & a_{33} \end{vmatrix}$$

$$= (-1)^3 (a_{21}a_{33} - a_{31}a_{23})$$

Once all cofactors have been obtained, we form the matrix

$$
\mathbf{G} = \begin{bmatrix} \mu_{11} & \mu_{12} & \mu_{13} \\ \mu_{21} & \mu_{22} & \mu_{23} \\ \mu_{31} & \mu_{32} & \mu_{33} \end{bmatrix}
$$

and, as indicated above, the inverse of **A** is obtained by the multiplication of the reciprocal of the determinant and the transposed matrix of cofactors. However, when finding the inverse of higher order matrices, it is quicker and simpler to use a high-speed computer to perform the required calculations.

---

**REFERENCES**

Broyles, R. W., and Lay, C. M. *Mathematics in Health Administration.* Germantown, Md.: Aspen Systems Corporation, 1980.

Searle, S. R., and Hausman, W. H. *Matrix Algebra for Business and Economics.* New York: John Wiley & Sons Inc., 1970.

**Part II**

# Working Capital Management

# Chapter 5

# Fundamentals of Working Capital Management

## Objectives

After completing this chapter, you should be able to:

1. Estimate working capital needs using the cash flow approach.
2. Estimate working capital needs using projected financial statements.
3. Differentiate between permanent and temporary working capital.
4. Describe the mechanisms by which working capital needs might be financed.
5. Determine the least costly mechanism of funding working capital needs.

This section of the text examines tools and techniques that may be used in the management of the various components of the hospital's working capital. More specifically, the primary purpose of this chapter is two-fold.

1. to examine the methods by which management may determine the amount of working capital required for a given period;
2. to investigate the various sources of financing working capital needs as well as the methods by which management may determine the least costly method of funding those requirements.

## 5.1 DEFINITIONS

Working capital is defined as the total current assets of the hospital enterprise. These assets consist of the cash balance, accounts receivable, investments in marketable securities, and inventory holdings. Thus, the working capital (*WC*) of the hospital is given by

$$WC = \text{Cash} + \frac{\text{Accounts}}{\text{Receivable}} + \frac{\text{Investments}}{\text{in Securities}} + \text{Inventory} \quad \textbf{(5.1)}$$

Net working capital, also a frequently used term, is defined as the working capital of the hospital less its current liabilities. Thus, the net working capital (NWC) of the hospital is given by

$$NWC = TCA - TCL \quad \textbf{(5.2)}$$

where

$$TCA = \text{Total Current Assets}$$

$$TCL = \text{Total Current Liabilities}$$

The major categories of the hospital's current liabilities are its accounts payable, accrued salaries and wages payable, and other short-term obligations.

The important issue is not the definition of the terms working capital and net working capital; rather, the critical issue is the role played by working capital management in achieving the goal of minimizing the cost of providing required services.

## 5.2 THE IMPORTANCE OF WORKING CAPITAL MANAGEMENT

To understand the importance of working capital management it is necessary first to examine the relationship between working capital and the goal of providing services required by the community. The word capital connotes the sum of the fixed or long-term assets and the liquid or current assets of the hospital. Long-term or fixed assets consist of such items as the land, land improvements, physical plant, equipment, and other tangible assets that management expects to hold for more than one year. Conversely, liquid or current assets consist of cash and such factors as inventories, accounts receivable, and short-term marketable securities that are expected to be converted into cash within a year.

To understand the relation between providing patient service and the total assets of the hospital, consider the functional relation

$$Y = f(K_i, L_j, S_g) \quad \textbf{(5.3)}$$

where

$Y$ = a composite measure of hospital output (i.e., patient care)

$K_i$ = units of fixed capital of type $i$

$L_j$ = hours of labor of type $j$

$S_g$ = units of supply item $g$

Such a relation is known as a production function and specifies the maximum amount of output obtainable when exactly $K_i^*$ units of input $K_i$, $L_j^*$ units of input $L_j$, and $S_g^*$ units of input $S_g$ are used in the production process. Obviously, patient services cannot be provided unless fixed assets, which are represented by $K_i$ in Equation 5.3, are available. However, the fixed capital of the hospital alone cannot provide patient care. Rather, the fixed capital represents only the capacity or the potential to produce care. To become productive, the fixed capital must be combined with labor and consumable supplies in a productive process that results in patient care.

To obtain the factor inputs required to provide patient care, the hospital must exchange cash for the use of these resources. If it is assumed that the working capital consists solely of cash, then that is the vehicle by which the hospital acquires the labor and consumable supplies needed to transform fixed assets into patient care. Thus, working capital is a vital and necessary element in providing patient care.

It then seems reasonable to argue that management must devote considerable time and energy in the administration of working capital. Further, because of the impact that efficient administration can exert on costs and on the financial solvency and continued existence of the hospital, working capital must be managed with the utmost care.

Working capital management consists of the administration not only of the current assets of the hospital but also of the liabilities incurred when these assets are acquired. To illustrate the relationship between assets and liabilities, consider the following example. Suppose the hospital purchases $20,000 worth of food supplies on credit. When the food is acquired, the hospital's assets obviously are increased by $20,000. However, its liabilities have increased by an equal amount. Thus, the hospital has acquired an asset (inventory) but also has incurred a liability (account payable) in the same amount. The account payable in effect has financed the purchase of the food supplies. Obviously, at some point the account payable will have to be paid, but for the moment it is the source of financing the inventory acquisition. For this reason, then, decisions concerning the acquisition of assets must take into account the effect of the source of funding on the financial position of the hospital as reflected in the balance sheet. Therefore, if management is to administer current assets properly, it must consider not only the hospital's assets but also the methods by which those assets may be financed.

If management is to minimize the total expense of providing patient care, the costs associated with the hospital's working capital also must be minimized. To minimize those costs, management must consider two interrelated factors:

1. It must determine the level or the quantity of working capital required to support hospital operations during a given period.
2. It must evaluate various sources of funding to determine which method of financing working capital needs minimizes the costs to the institution.

When considered jointly, the quantity of working capital coupled with the financing mechanism should be determined so that the costs are minimized. The problem of determining the quantity of working capital required during a given period is considered in the next section; sources of financing these needs are analyzed later.

## 5.3  WORKING CAPITAL NEEDS

When determining the working capital needs of the institution, it is convenient to obtain a solution for a situation that is simplified by a set of heuristic assumptions before considering a more realistic or complex situation. Accordingly, a cash flow approach to the determination of working capital needs is considered first, then the mechanics of projecting the income statement and balance sheet that provide the basis for determining those needs for a given period are examined.

### 5.3.1  A Cash Flow Approach

To illustrate the cash flow approach to the determination of working capital needs, let us return to the assumption that the current assets of the hospital consist solely of cash. Given this assumption, it is necessary to consider the sources, magnitude, and timing of both the cash receipts and cash disbursements.

The cash receipts of a hospital that is reimbursed under the retrospective method, as noted earlier, are generated primarily through payments by third party payers and patients. As a result, the cash inflow of such a hospital may be viewed as a random variable (i.e., a variable capable of assuming more than one value). On the other hand, the cash receipts of a hospital that receives reimbursement under the prospective method are generated primarily by a periodic payment from a third party payer (e.g., Blue Cross or a provincial plan) that is intended to finance a portion of operational activity on a current basis and, to a lesser extent, through payments made by third party payers and patients on outstanding accounts. Accordingly, the cash receipts of such an institution consist of both random and nonrandom components.

To simplify the analysis, assume that the cash disbursements of hospitals reimbursed under both of these systems are limited to payments associated with acquiring the services of labor and consumable supplies. Under the cash flow approach, determining the working capital needs of the institution can be viewed in terms of two streams—a cash inflow stream and a cash outflow stream. Under this simplifying assumption, the minimum amount of working capital required by the hospital is equal to the difference between the cash outflows and the cash inflows of the period.

### 5.3.1.1 Cash Outflows

As mentioned earlier, cash outflows may be represented by the cash payments required to obtain the services of labor and the consumable supplies used in providing care. As such, the cash disbursements may be viewed as consisting of wages and salaries plus payments required to acquire supplies. For illustration, assume that the timing and the magnitude of these two cash streams are as follows:

|  | Amount of Cash Outflow | |
| Day | Wage & Salaries | Supplies |
| --- | --- | --- |
| 15 | $7,500 | $   0 |
| 30 | 7,500 | 15,000 |
| | 15,000 | 15,000 |

Assume that the total wage and salary payments for the 30-day operating period are represented by a $7,500 cash outlay on day 15 and $7,500 on day 30. The supply expense for the period is assumed to be $15,000, and the associated cash disbursement occurs on day 30. Regarding the cash inflows and the resulting determination of minimum working capital needs, we assume that the amount of cash received by the institution is determined by the costs incurred in providing care.

### 5.3.1.2 Cash Inflows and Working Capital Needs: Retrospective Reimbursement

As seen above, the major share of the cash received by a hospital reimbursed under the retrospective method is generated through payments on outstanding receivables. Here, we assume that the cash inflow stream consists of two components. The first component may be viewed as a production cycle during which service is provided; the second component as an accounts receivable cycle that represents the time it takes to receive payment after service has been provided. Consequently, the timing of the institution's receipt of cash depends on: (1) the length of time required to provide service; and (2) the time required to convert outstanding receivables into cash. Returning to our example, suppose that the production cycle (the average length of stay) is 6 days and the accounts receivable cycle is 24 days. As a result, only one cash inflow occurs on day 30.

Concerning the magnitude of the cash inflows, it will be recalled that the reimbursement of the hospital is determined by costs incurred in providing care. Thus, given that the costs of the period have been found to be $30,000, the hospital will receive $1,000 per day ($30,000/30 days).

However, a difficulty arises when we compare the cash inflows and cash outflows of the 30-day operating cycle. As noted, two wage and salary payments plus one payment for supplies must be made during the period. On the other hand, due to the length of the production cycle and the accounts receivable cycle, only one cash inflow equal to the costs incurred in providing care during the first 6 days of the operating cycle is received. As a consequence, assuming that charges are equal to costs, the hospital must disburse $30,000 but will receive only $6,000 ($1,000/day × 6 days).

As mentioned, the quantity of working capital is equal to the difference between the cash receipts and cash disbursements during the inflow or outflow cycle, whichever is longer. In the following discussion, let $CI_t$ and $CO_t$ represent the cash inflows and cash outflows of period $t$, respectively, where $t$ is the time interval that is the longer of the cash inflow or cash outflow cycle. With this notation, the minimum working capital need, $MWCN$, may be expressed in the form

$$MWCN = CO_t - CI_t$$

Returning to the example, the cash inflows, cash outflows, and minimum working capital needs are as follows:

| Cash Outflows | | |
|---|---|---|
| Wages and Salaries (day 15) | $7,500 | |
| Wages and Salaries (day 30) | 7,500 | |
| Supplies | 15,000 | |
| Total | | $30,000 |
| Cash Inflows | | |
| Cash Receipts (day 30) | | 6,000 |
| Minimum Working Capital Needs | | 24,000 |

This result also is shown in Table 5-1, where we assume that the income statement and the balance sheet are prepared at the end of each 15-day period.

**Table 5-1** Quantity of Working Capital: Retrospective Reimbursement

| Day | Assets | | Liabilities & Equity | | Revenues | Expenses | Receipts | Disbursements |
|---|---|---|---|---|---|---|---|---|
| | | | Balance Sheet | | Income Statement | | Cash Flows | |
| 0 | Cash | $24,000 | Equity | $24,000 | | | | |
| 1 | Cash | 24,000 | Equity | 24,000 | | | | |
| | Inventory | 15,000 | A/P[1] | 15,000 | | | | |
| | | 39,000 | | 39,000 | | | | |
| 15 | Cash | 16,500 | Equity | 24,000 | | | | |
| | A/R[2] | 15,000 | | | | | | |
| | Inventory | 7,500 | A/P | 15,000 | $15,000 | $15,000 | | $7,500 |
| | | 39,000 | | 39,000 | | | | |
| 30 | Cash | 0 | Equity | 24,000 | | | | |
| | A/R | 24,000 | A/P | 0 | 15,000 | 15,000 | $6,000 | 22,500 |
| | | 24,000 | | 24,000 | 30,000 | 30,000 | 6,000 | 30,000 |

[1] A/P = Accounts payable.
[2] A/R = Accounts receivable.

The table shows the initial cash balance of the hospital is $24,000 and that inventories amounting to $15,000 were received on day 1. On the 15th day, the cash balance has declined from $24,000 to $16,500, which represents the wage and salary payment of $7,500. The inventory holdings of the institution have declined from $15,000 to $7,500, representing the use of supplies during the first 15 days of the operating cycle (i.e., $15,000 less $500/day for 15 days). In addition, the revenues earned during the first 15 days are equal to the expenses of the period and the accounts receivable reflect the revenue generated as of this day.

Consider next the financial statements prepared on the last day of the operating cycle. The cash balance now is zero because the cash balance of $16,500 plus the $6,000 payment on the outstanding receivables generated by providing care during the first 6 days of the operating cycle just offsets the $7,500 wage and salary payment plus the $15,000 payment for the supplies received on day 1. The hospital's accounts receivable now total $24,000, which represents the care provided during the second, third, fourth, and fifth production cycles of the 30-day period.

In this example, if the hospital has a beginning cash balance (working capital) of $24,000, it can satisfy its currently maturing obligations. Thus, the initial investment of $24,000 in cash represents a source of funding that, when coupled with the cash inflows of the period, is sufficient to finance the cash outflows.

Suppose that management is able to reduce the accounts receivable from 24 days to 18 days. Under this assumption, the cash outflows remain unchanged but the hospital now receives a cash inflow of $6,000 on day 24, representing payment for the care provided during the first 6-day production cycle *and* a $6,000 payment on day 30, which is payment for the care provided during the second production cycle. Thus, the cash inflows, cash outflows, and working capital needs associated with an accounts receivable cycle of 18 days are as follows:

| | |
|---|---|
| Cash Outflows | $30,000 |
| Cash Inflows | 12,000 |
| Working Capital Needs | 18,000 |

In this case, reducing the accounts receivable cycle by 6 days lowers the working capital needs of the institution by $6,000.

Similarly, if we now assume that the accounts receivable cycle is 12 days, the cash outflows still are $30,000 but the timing and magnitude of the cash receipts are as follows:

| Day | Amount | Explanation |
|---|---|---|
| 18 | $6,000 | payment for care provided during first production cycle |
| 24 | 6,000 | payment for care during second production cycle |
| 30 | 6,000 | payment for care during third production cycle |

Under this assumption, the working capital needs of the hospital are $12,000 ($30,000−$18,000).

This discussion illustrates a very important point: by reducing the length of the accounts receivable cycle (i.e., the period of time elapsing between the provision of service and the receipt of cash) the amount of working capital required before the hospital attains a self-sustaining position also is reduced. This should be kept in mind since we refer to this finding later. Before considering the operational implications of such a reduction on the financial status of the institution, consider the determination of working capital needs of a hospital that receives payment under the prospective method of reimbursement.

### 5.3.1.3 Cash Inflows and Working Capital Needs: Prospective Reimbursement

As mentioned, the cash receipts of a hospital that is reimbursed under the prospective system consist of both random and nonrandom components. The cash inflow stream may be viewed as consisting of two major components. With regard to the first, assume that the institution receives a cash payment on day 1 and that this cash inflow is intended to finance a portion of hospital activity on a current basis. The second component represents cash inflows generated through payments on outstanding accounts by other third party payers and self-responsible patients. As before, the stream of cash receipts generated by payments on receivables consists of a production cycle and an accounts receivable cycle.

The magnitude of the cash inflows is determined by the costs of providing care and the amount of the prepayment is found by multiplying the proportion of the total number of days of care financed prospectively by the total cost of operation. Thus, if 80 percent of the days of care is insured by the third party payer, a cash inflow of $24,000 (8 × $30,000) will be received on the first day of the 30-day operating cycle. As to cash receipts generated from the payment of accounts receivable, the hospital must finance $6,000 (.2 × $30,000), which is the difference between the total cost of providing care and the prospective payment. For each of the six-day periods in the 30-day cycle, then, the hospital must finance $1,200, which is determined by

1. calculating the total cost of operating the hospital per day (30,000/30 = $1,000);
2. multiplying the total cost of operating the hospital per day by the proportion of patients who are not insured under the prospective payer; this yields the proportion of the total cost of daily operation that is the responsibility of other payers ($1,000 × .2 = $200);
3. multiplying the cost of operating the hospital per day that is the responsibility of other payers by 6 days (the length of the production cycle); in this example, this value is given by $200 × 6 days = $1,200 for each 6-day production cycle.

Five of the six-day periods fall in the 30-day operating cycle. This implies that the hospital must finance $6,000 (5 × $1,200), which equals the difference between the total cost of operation and the amount of prepayments. These calculations permit us to determine the working capital required by the hospital during a typical 30-day operating cycle.

Returning to the situation in which the accounts receivable cycle is 24 days, we find the cash inflows for the 30-day operating cycle are given by

|  |  |  |
|---|---|---|
|  | Prospective Payment | $24,000 |
| Plus | Accounts Receivable Payments | 1,200 |
|  |  | 25,200 |

However, during the same period, the hospital must disburse $30,000 in cash. Thus, its working capital needs are $4,800 ($30,000 − $25,200), which is the difference between the cash outflows and cash inflows of the period (i.e., $CO_t − CI_t$). Under the assumption that the accounts receivable cycle is 24 days, the hospital does not receive cash payment for services to patients who are not covered by the prospective payer during the second, third, fourth, or fifth production cycles of the 30-day operating cycle. Therefore, the hospital must use funds derived from some other source to pay the costs of the care provided to such patients during the last four of the five production cycles. As before, the "other source" of funds is the working capital or cash the hospital must have available to meet its obligations and continue to operate until it achieves a self-sustaining position.

This result is shown in Table 5-2 where we assume that, as before, the hospital prepares a set of financial statements at the end of each 15-day period. With the possible exception of the liability account that appears in the liabilities and equity portion of the balance sheet, the interpretation of Table 5-2 is similar to the discussion of Table 5-1. When the hospital receives the prepayment, a liability is created that is extinguished by providing service to patients insured by the prospective payer during the 30-day operating cycle. As seen in the table, the liability account has declined from $24,000 to $12,000 by day 15. This

**Table 5-2** Quantity of Working Capital: Prospective Reimbursement

| Day | Assets | | Liabilities & Equity | | Revenues | Expenses | Receipts | Disbursements |
|-----|--------|------|----------|--------|----------|----------|----------|------|
| | | | Balance Sheet | | Income Statement | | Cash Flow | |
| 0 | Cash | $4,800 | Equity | $4,800 | | | | |
| 1 | Cash | 28,800 | Equity | 4,800 | | | $24,000 | |
| | Inventory | 15,000 | A/P[1] | 15,000 | | | | |
| | | 43,800 | Liability | 24,000 | | | | |
| | | | | 43,800 | | | | |
| 15 | Cash | 21,300 | Equity | 4,800 | | | | |
| | Inventory | 7,500 | A/P | 15,000 | | | | |
| | A/R[2] | 3,000 | Liability | 12,000 | $15,000 | $15,000 | — | $7,500 |
| | | 31,800 | | 31,800 | | | | |
| 30 | Cash | 0 | Equity | 4,800 | | | | |
| | Inventory | 0 | A/P | 0 | 15,000 | 15,000 | 1,200 | 22,500 |
| | A/R | 4,800 | Liability | 0 | | | | |
| | | 4,800 | | 4,800 | 30,000 | 30,000 | 25,200 | 30,000 |

[1] A/P = Accounts payable.
[2] A/R = Accounts receivable.

reduction represents the portion of the liability eliminated by operating the hospital for 15 days at a cost of $800/day, which is the portion of the daily costs that are insured by the prospective payer. It also is important to note that, as before, the cash balance of the institution on day 30 is zero. This is because the sum of the cash balance of $21,300 and the cash inflow of $1,200 on day 30 is just equal to the wage and salary payment of $7,500 plus the payment of $15,000 for the supplies received on day 1 of the operating cycle. The outstanding receivables total $4,800 on day 30, which represents the care provided to patients not covered by the prospective payer during the second, third, fourth, and fifth production cycles.

Consider now a slightly different case in which we assume that, with the exception of the length of the accounts receivable cycle, the timing and magnitude of cash disbursements are the same as before. In terms of the example, the accounts receivable cycle was assumed to be 24 days. For illustration, suppose the accounts receivable cycle is reduced to 18 days. In this situation, the hospital will receive payment of $1,200 for the first production cycle on day 24 as well as cash receipt of $1,200 for the second production cycle on day 30. Given a prospective payment of $24,000, the cash receipts of the institution are calculated as follows:

| | |
|---|---:|
| Prospective payment | $24,000 |
| Payment on day 24 | 1,200 |
| Payment on day 30 | 1,200 |
| | 26,400 |

Therefore, the minimum working capital needs of the hospital have been reduced from $4,800 to $3,600 ($30,000 − $26,400).

Similarly, if the accounts receivable cycle is reduced to 12 days, the cash receipts of the hospital are found to be

| | |
|---|---:|
| Prospective payment | $24,000 |
| Payment on day 18 | 1,200 |
| Payment on day 24 | 1,200 |
| Payment on day 30 | 1,200 |
| | 27,600 |

Therefore, the minimum working capital needs are reduced further from $3,600 (the needs associated with an 18-day accounts receivable cycle) to $30,000 − $27,600 or $2,400.

As in the discussion of the hospital that receives retrospective reimbursement, the reduction of the accounts receivable cycle also lowers the minimum working capital needs. By increasing the cash inflows of the period, management reduces not only its working capital needs but also the costs of care for which the community assumes financial responsibility. The relation between the quantity of working capital required by the institution and the costs of care to the community is discussed below.

### 5.3.1.4 Operational Results

When viewed from the perspective of the hospital that seeks to earn a net income, the cost of working capital may be defined in terms of foregone returns. Suppose that the efficiency of managing accounts receivable and inventories is held constant and that the rate of return earned on other current assets (cash and marketable securities) is less than the rate of return on the institution's investment in fixed assets such as land, buildings, and equipment. This is because the rate of return on the fixed assets, which could be expressed in terms of lives saved or improvements in the health status of patients, is higher than the return that could be earned from an investment in cash or marketable securities. Consequently, the investment in working capital involves an opportunity cost that is equal to the net return that is foregone when funds are invested in current assets as opposed to fixed assets. To minimize the opportunity costs associated with working capital, management should attempt to reduce the ratio of current assets to total assets.

Stated differently, the expenses for which the community bears financial responsibility can be defined in terms of net operating costs. Here, net operating costs are defined as the costs of operation less nonoperating revenue such as investment income. As nonoperating revenues increase and all other factors hold constant, the net operating costs, or those for which the community assumes financial responsibility, decline. To illustrate, let us return to the example of the hospital that is reimbursed prospectively. Suppose that the hospital originally required an investment of $4,800 in working capital, but the institution changed its credit and collection practices so that an investment of only $2,400 is required now. Other things being equal, the reduction in the accounts receivable cycle and the working capital needs release $2,400 that no longer is needed to finance day-to-day operations. Assuming this "cash" is invested in a long-term government bond that pays 10 percent per year, the cash surplus would earn an annual nonoperating revenue of $240.

Even though $240 is not a large sum, this analysis illustrates an important point: a reduction in the level of working capital enables management to take funds that previously were required in satisfying those needs and invest them in revenue-generating activities. The revenues from such investments may be used to meet operating costs that were financed previously by the community.

In summary, opportunity costs are incurred when funds are invested in working capital and these costs are equal to the rate of return that could have been obtained if the working capital of the hospital had been reduced and the excess funds invested in other assets. As before, the higher the investment in working capital, the higher the resulting opportunity costs. Therefore, to reduce the costs of care borne by the community, management should minimize the hospital's investment in working capital.

The quantity of working capital required by the hospital may be reduced by accelerating cash inflows and, as will be seen, by decelerating cash outflows. Therefore, to minimize cost, management must minimize the quantity of working capital by accelerating cash receipts and/or by decelerating cash disbursements.

One final observation on this topic is appropriate. A comparison of the results obtained for the institution that receives payment under the prospective method with the results obtained for the hospital that is paid retrospectively reveals that the working capital needs of the latter exceed those of the former. As a result, the opportunity costs associated with the investment in the receivables of the hospital receiving payment under the prospective method are lower than the corresponding opportunity costs of the hospital that receives a major share of its cash receipts retrospectively. This implies that the latter should emphasize monitoring and controlling its accounts receivable cycle. However, if working capital and operating costs are to be minimized, both groups of hospitals must devote considerable time and energy to managing outstanding receivables.

## 5.3.2 Working Capital Needs and Financial Statements

In the previous section, working capital needs were defined as the difference between the cash outflows and cash inflows of the period because it was assumed that cash was the hospital's only asset. In this section, this assumption is relaxed and the process of projecting working capital needs is discussed under more realistic conditions.

As mentioned earlier, one of the major functions of the manager is financial planning. The financial manager must determine the additional funding required not only for a single period but for several periods. The administrator then must be prepared to act on the basis of this information by reducing costs, obtaining additional funds, or postponing marginal investment projects.

Management may approach the problem of projecting working capital needs by estimating the financial statements that pertain to the period involved. Thus, management should develop a projected income statement from which the net income (loss) may be estimated by subtracting expected expenses from expected revenues. Once the expected net income or loss has been determined, management can construct a projected balance sheet from which the working capital needs of the period may be estimated. If the assumption that cash is the hospital's only current asset is relaxed, the additional funding required during the period is given by

$$
\begin{array}{c}
\textit{Anticipated} \\
\text{Residual Funding} \\
\text{(Working Capital} \\
\text{Needs)}
\end{array}
=
\begin{array}{c}
\textit{Estimated} \\
\text{Total} \\
\text{Assets}
\end{array}
-
\left(
\begin{array}{c}
\textit{Estimated} \\
\text{Liabilities}
\end{array}
+
\begin{array}{c}
\textit{Estimated} \\
\text{End-of-} \\
\text{Period Fund} \\
\text{Balance}
\end{array}
\right)
$$

To derive the end-of-period fund balance, it is necessary first to estimate the net income or loss of the period. This is because

$$
\begin{array}{c}
\textit{Estimated} \\
\text{End-of-} \\
\text{Period Fund} \\
\text{Balance}
\end{array}
=
\begin{array}{c}
\text{Beginning} \\
\text{Fund Balance}
\end{array}
+
\begin{array}{c}
\textit{Estimated} \\
\text{Net Income (Loss)}
\end{array}
$$

As a consequence, we first address the problem of estimating the income statement, then turn to projecting the balance sheet from which the working capital needs of the period may be estimated.

### 5.3.2.1 Break-Even Analysis and the Income Statement

As demonstrated in Tables 5-1 and 5-2, the revenues of the two hospitals were equal to expenses. Such a situation is defined as a break-even point, which implies that neither losses nor profits were realized. In this section, we examine break-even analysis as a tool for forecasting the hospital income statement.

For simplicity, assume that

1. total revenue is given by

$$TR = PV$$

   where $P$ corresponds to a fixed average charge per patient day and $V$ is the volume of patient care as measured by the number of days of care;
2. total revenue is zero when no patient care is provided;
3. total costs are linearly related to the volume of patient care; and
4. total economic costs are composed of a fixed and a variable component that may be identified or estimated statistically.

On the basis of these assumptions, we now consider in more detail the total revenue and total cost curves.

In accordance with the first two assumptions, the total revenue curve is a straight line that emanates from the origin and has as its slope the value assumed by $P$, which is the average daily charge. The relation between total revenue and the volume of care is seen in Figure 5-1. Given that $P$ is assumed to be constant, changes in total revenue ($\Delta TR$) are directly related to changes in volume ($\Delta V$). This relation is given by

$$\Delta TR = P(\Delta V) \tag{5.4}$$

Dividing both sides of Equation 5.4 by $\Delta V$, we find that $\Delta TR/\Delta V = P$, but, as can be seen in Figure 5-1, $\dfrac{\Delta TR}{\Delta V}$ is the slope of the total revenue curve. This implies that when specifying the total revenue curve under these simplifying assumptions, it is necessary only to calculate the value assumed by the constant $P$. Perhaps the simplest way of calculating the average charge per day is to divide total anticipated expenses by the corresponding number of patient-days of care provided. Such a calculation yields a prospective charge per patient day that then may be used to determine: (1) the revenues earned by the hospital and (2) in the case of the institution reimbursed prospectively, the amount of the hospital's liability that is liquidated by the provision of patient care.

The total cost function is assumed to be a linear function of the volume of patient care provided. The first step in estimating the relation between total cost and volume is an examination of the extent to which cost components vary in response to changes in volume. For example, it is convenient to divide costs into variable and fixed components. Fixed costs are those that are independent of the volume of patient care and do not vary with changes in the amount of service provided. Most fixed costs are associated with the existence of the hospital's plant and equipment and must be paid even if no care is provided.

**Figure 5-1** Revenue and Volume of Patient Care

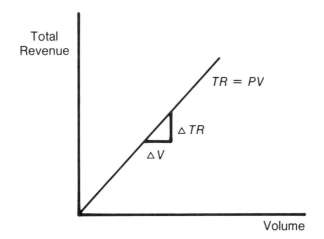

Other examples of fixed costs are long-term indebtedness, rental payments specified in long-term leases, a portion of the depreciation on the hospital's plant and equipment, insurance premiums, and the salaries of top management. In short, fixed costs remain constant at a given level and prevail at all volumes of patient care, including zero.

Variable costs are those that generally vary directly with the volume of care provided. Unfortunately, the largest component of costs—salaries and wages— may not vary directly with volume. Since different volumes of care may be provided with a given staffing pattern, it seems reasonable to assume that a *portion* of wage and salary costs is constant over a wide range of patient volume. It is equally true, however, that similar hospitals provide the same set of services with fairly divergent staffing levels. In this instance, assume that a portion of the total wage and salary costs varies with patient volume. Given the nature of wage and salary expenses, it is important to recognize that the ratio of the percent change in wage and salary costs to the percent change in patient volume probably is less than one.

Concerning the other expense components, it is reasonable to argue that supply costs change in proportion to differences in patient volume. This is tantamount to assuming that the number of services per day and the number of resources per service remain invariant from one period to the next.

This discussion suggests that the relation between total costs and the volume of patient care may be portrayed as in Figure 5-2. The general form of such a functional relation portrayed in the figure is given by

$$TC = b_0 + b_1V$$

where the coefficient $b_0$ represents fixed costs while the coefficient $b_1$, which is the slope of the function, represents the change in costs resulting from a unit change in output (i.e., the variable cost component).*

If the total revenue curve in Figure 5-1 is combined with the total cost curve in Figure 5-2, the break-even point (i.e., the point where total revenue equals total cost) can be ascertained easily. As seen in Figure 5-3, the total revenue curve intersects the total cost curve when the volume of patient care is $V^*$. Thus, total revenue is equal to total cost when the volume of patient care is $V^*$; this volume is called the break-even point. To determine the exact break-even point, we need only observe that

$$TR = PV$$

$$TC = b_0 + b_1V$$

---

* The appendix at the end of this chapter discusses the method by which the coefficients $b_0$ and $b_1$ might be estimated.

**Figure 5-2** Total Costs and Volume of Patient Care

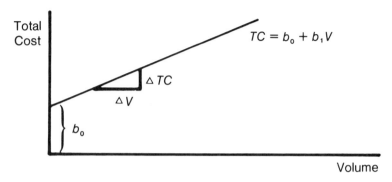

**Figure 5-3** Total Revenue and Total Cost Curves

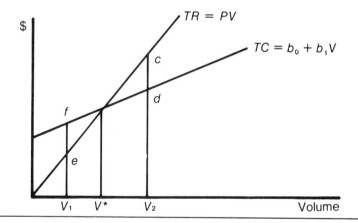

represent a system of linear equations that is solved simultaneously when

$$PV = b_0 + b_1V$$

As can be verified, the break-even point is found to be

$$V^* = \frac{b_0}{P - b_1}$$

where $P$ is assumed to be greater than $b_1$. Obviously, when $P$ is equal to $b_1$, the total revenue and total cost curves are parallel lines and the system of linear equations has no solution.

Under the assumptions described, total revenues are equal to total costs only when the volume of care is $V^*$. For example, the volume of care, $V_1$, is less than $V^*$. Figure 5-3 shows that when the volume of care is $V_1$, the total revenue of the hospital is given by the vertical distance $V_1e$, and the total costs corresponding to that rate of activity are represented by the vertical distance $V_1f$. Since $V_1f$ is greater than $V_1e$, we conclude that total costs exceed total revenues and the hospital sustains a loss. Thus, for all volumes of patient care that are less than $V^*$, total costs exceed total revenues. Conversely, consider a volume of care such as $V_2$ that is greater than $V^*$. For this volume, total revenue is represented by the vertical distance $V_2c$ and total cost by the vertical distance $V_2d$. Thus, for volumes of patient care in excess of $V^*$, the hospital earns a total revenue that exceeds total cost.

Such an analysis permits management to project a condensed income statement for various volumes of patient care. The total revenue and cost associated with a given volume of care is obtained by substituting the assumed number of patient days for the variable $V$ in the total revenue and total cost functions, respectively. The corresponding "profit" or loss is obtained by simply subtracting total costs from total revenues.

Consider the possibility that the volume of patient care will be less than $V^*$ and examine alternative courses of action to restore the equality of revenues and costs. Suppose there is a high probability that the volume will equal $V_1$. One alternative that may be available is simply to increase the charge per patient day while holding the expected cost structure constant. As can be seen in Figure 5-4, raising the charge per patient day from $P$ to $P'$, with no change in the cost structure, increases the slope of the total revenue curve. This is shown graphi-

---

**Figure 5-4** Raising Charges, Holding Costs Constant

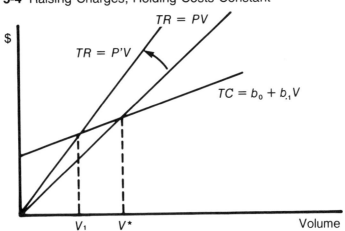

cally by rotating the total revenue function in a counterclockwise direction. With a cost per patient day of $P'$ and no change in the cost structure, total revenue generated by providing $V_1$ units of service is equal to the total costs associated with this rate of activity.

A second approach in redressing the excess of costs over revenues is to reduce fixed or variable costs while holding the charge per patient day constant. Although the distinction between fixed and variable costs may be somewhat academic because of the imprecise nature of hospital cost structures, it is worthwhile to explore the impact of a reduction in fixed costs as opposed to a drop in variable costs.

Consider first a reduction in fixed costs. As noted, the fixed costs of the hospital are represented graphically by the $y$ intercept of the total cost function. Thus, a reduction in the fixed costs results in a lessening of the vertical distance between the origin and the point at which the total cost curve intersects the $y$ axis (Figure 5-5). It is assumed that management is able to reduce fixed costs from $og$ to $ol$. Such a reduction simply lowers the total cost curve by the amount $og$-$ol$ for all volumes of patient care. This clearly eliminates the potential deficit and restores the balance between total revenues and total cost.

Finally, management might consider methods of lowering variable costs. A reduction in variable costs reduces the slope of the total cost function from $b_1$ to, say, $b_1'$. This decline is represented graphically (Figure 5-6) by rotating the total cost curve in a clockwise direction. At lower volumes of care where variable costs constitute a smaller proportion of total expenditures, the effect of the reduction is diminished. As can be seen in Figure 5-6, however, a reduction in variable costs and the corresponding decline in the slope of the total cost

**Figure 5-5** Effect of Reduction in Fixed Costs

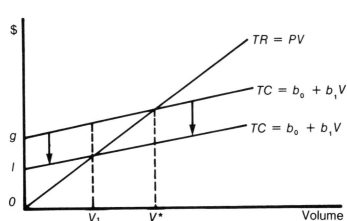

**Figure 5-6** Effect of Reduction in Variable Costs

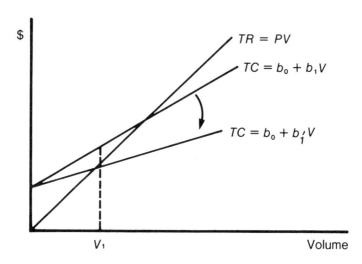

function from $b_1$ to $b_1'$ also will redress the imbalance between total revenues and total costs that results when the volume of patient care is $V_1$.

In summary, there are essentially three ways to lower the break-even point to the volume represented by $V_1$ and thereby eliminate an anticipated loss. Management may

1. raise the charge per patient day from $P$ to $P'$;
2. lower fixed costs from $og$ to $o\ell$;
3. lower variable costs so that the slope of the total cost function is reduced from $b_1$ to $b_1'$;

or some appropriate combination of these three approaches.

### 5.3.2.2 Ratio Analysis and the Balance Sheet

The previous section described how break-even analysis might be used in forecasting a hospital's income statement for various volumes of patient care. This section focuses on the use of ratio analysis in forecasting the balance sheet from which may be determined the institution's residual funding or working capital needs.

As before, suppose that a volume of care similar to $V_1$ is the most likely rate of activity and, on the basis of the analysis in the previous section, assume that the income statement in Table 5-3 has been projected for this level of activity. As seen earlier, the method of classifying the revenues of the hospital that receives reimbursement under the prospective system differs slightly from the method of grouping revenues of the hospital that receives retrospective reimbursement. These differences are reflected in Table 5-3, where the income of the hospital that receives retrospective reimbursement has been divided into inpatient and outpatient revenues. Conversely, the parentheses of the revenue section of the income statement list plan and nonplan revenue categories. The plan revenue category pertains to the income for service to patients who are insured by the prospective payer while the nonplan revenue category involves income earned from providing service to other patients. It is assumed that, apart from the system of reimbursement and classification of income, the two hospitals are similar.

This table reveals that a net operating loss of $640,000 will be incurred if the volume of care is $V_1$. That loss is given by the vertical difference between the total revenue and total cost curves of Figure 5-3. At first glance, it appears that this loss must be financed through some other source such as a bank loan, the sale of an asset, or a depletion of cash reserves. Although an accounting loss always is a serious matter, the anticipated loss shown in the table may not be as disastrous as it first appears. To be specific, net cash flow is not the same as operating net income or loss.

To see why this is so, consider each element of revenue or expense and determine whether or not it will result in a cash receipt or a cash disbursement. In the example in Table 5-3, depreciation charges, which are allowable costs under most third party contracts and are included in the revenues earned by providing service to insured patients, do not require a cash disbursement. This is true even though management regards the funding of depreciation as of considerable importance in providing capital for the future replacement of plant and equipment. During periods in which government and other third party payers demand economic restraint, even previously funded depreciation that has been invested in marketable securities must be regarded as a potential source to fi-

---

**Table 5-3** Projected Income Statement

| Revenues | | |
|---|---|---:|
| | Inpatient revenue (plan revenue) | $1,800,000 |
| | Outpatient revenue (nonplan revenue) | 200,000 |
| | Total revenue | 2,000,000 |
| Expenses | | |
| | Salaries (half variable) | 1,100,000 |
| | Supplies (variable) | 900,000 |
| | Other expenses (fixed) | 40,000 |
| | Depreciation (fixed) | 600,000 |
| | Total expense | 2,640,000 |
| | Net income (or loss) | (640,000) |

nance operating losses. If cash transactions alone are considered and depreciation charges are eliminated from the expense component of the income statement, the net cash flow is $-\$40,000$. Thus, a somewhat imperfect method of determining the operating cash flow is simply to add depreciation charges to the net income or loss that is projected on the basis of break-even analysis.

If the administrator knew the future level of investment in plant and equipment, accounts receivable, and inventories, as well as the amount that would have to be borrowed or repaid on existing indebtedness and the amount of credit that would be extended by suppliers, the net financial needs of the institution could be determined at this point. However, this seldom is the case and it is necessary to estimate each of these factors so as to project working capital needs.

When estimating the future value of balance sheet components, it is common practice to identify stable relationships between balance sheet items and factors that already have been estimated. Most of the stable relationships that are of primary interest in this regard involve the volume of care or a revenue variable to the balance sheet item that management wants to project. To the extent that the two factors are related in a fairly stable way, the forecast of the balance sheet item may be considered to be reasonably reliable. This approach is discussed next for estimating assets, liabilities, and working capital needs.

**Estimation of Current Assets.**   Consider first the estimation of the quantity and composition of current assets. Most of the current assets (i.e., accounts receivable, inventories, cash, and a few miscellaneous others) are related closely to volume or revenue variables. As mentioned earlier, such a relation may be used to estimate each component of the hospital's current assets.

This general approach can be applied to the problem of estimating the value of the accounts receivable that will appear on the projected balance sheet. In general, the revenues and accounts receivable of the hospital that is reimbursed on a retrospective basis will rise and fall together. Similarly, when the hospital reimbursed prospectively engages in revenue-generating activities that do not involve plan patients, its nonplan revenues and accounts receivable also will rise and fall together. As an example, suppose that the accounts receivable cycle of the two institutions is 30 days and that the analysis is limited to outstanding accounts receivable less bad debts, contractual allowances, etc. If revenues that originally are charged to an outstanding receivable are expected to increase by $240,000 during the coming period, 30 days of this revenue will remain uncollected at the end of the year. As a consequence, the end-of-period receivables associated with the current year are expected to increase by $20,000. This expected change results from the increase in revenue originally charged to an account receivable. In this case, the $20,000 represents 1/12 or one month's worth of the $240,000 that, on the average, will remain uncollected.

For purposes of illustration, bad debts, charity care, courtesy discounts, and contractual allowances are ignored temporarily. However, the impact of these factors on the determination of the value of the end-of-period receivables is considered later in this section. Returning to the problem of projecting the balance sheet from the estimated income statement in Table 5-3, suppose that, on the basis of historical data, the administrator of the hospital that is reimbursed retrospectively has determined that the ratio of accounts receivable to revenue is .02. This ratio implies that .02(365 days) = 7.3 days of revenue are invested in outstanding receivables. Given that the number of days' charges in receivables (NODCIR) has been estimated, the end of period receivables may be computed by

$$\text{NODCIR} = \frac{\text{End-of-Period Receivables}}{\text{Revenue}/365} \qquad \textbf{(5.5.1)}$$

Solving for the numerator of this fraction, we find that

$$\boxed{\text{End-of-Period Receivables} = \text{NODCIR (Revenue}/365) \qquad \textbf{(5.5.2)}}$$

Referring to Table 5-3, we find that the projected revenue for the period is $2,000,000. Given that NODCIR is assumed to equal 7.3 days, we may estimate the end-of-period receivables for the hospital reimbursed on a retrospective basis by

$$\text{End-of-Period Receivables} = 7.3 \ (\$2,000,000/365)$$

$$= \$40,000$$

A slightly different procedure is employed by a hospital reimbursed prospectively. In this case, it is necessary to differentiate plan revenues from those that are charged initially to an account receivable (i.e., nonplan revenues). For example, assume that on the basis of historical data the administrator of this hospital has determined that the ratio of accounts receivable to nonplan revenue is .20 rather than .02, as above. Such a ratio implies that .20(365 days) or 73 days of nonplan revenue are invested in outstanding receivables. By analogy it can be seen that

$$\text{NODCIR}^* = \frac{\text{End-of-Period Receivables}}{\text{Nonplan Revenue}/365} \qquad \textbf{(5.6.1)}$$

which, after solving for the term End-of-Period Receivables, yields

$$\frac{\text{End-of-Period}}{\text{Receivables}} = \text{NODCIR* (Nonplan Revenue/365)} \quad \textbf{(5.6.2)}$$

Referring to Table 5-3, we see that the revenues that are expected to be generated from nonplan sources is $200,000. Given that NODCIR is assumed to equal 73 days, we find

$$\text{Ending Accounts Receivable} = 73 \times \frac{\$200,000}{365}$$

$$= \$40,000$$

The expected level of accounts receivable will be greater or less than the end-of-period accounts receivable for the current period, depending on whether the expected value of the revenues initially charged to a receivable are greater or less than the corresponding income of the current period.

Throughout this discussion, bad debts, contractual allowances, charity care, and courtesy discounts have been ignored but it is possible to modify the analysis to accommodate these factors. As an example consider a hospital that: (1) is reimbursed prospectively, (2) uses full established rates to compute all revenues, and (3) expects to earn nonplan revenues of $280,000 in the coming year. Suppose further that the following data also are available:

| Deduction in Revenue | % of All Nonplan Revenue |
|---|---|
| Bad debt | 1.6 |
| Contractual allowances | .5 |
| Charity care | .2 |
| Courtesy discounts | .7 |

On the basis of these data, we may estimate the portion of the projected income statement pertaining to nonplan revenues as follows:

| | | |
|---|---|---|
| Nonplan Revenue | | $280,000 |
| less | | |
| Bad debts | $4,480 | |
| Contractual allowances | 1,400 | |
| Charity care | 560 | |
| Courtesy discounts | 1,960 | |
| | | 8,400 |
| Net nonplan revenue | | 271,600 |

If on the basis of historical data management finds that the ratio of outstanding receivables to revenue is .30, the end-of-period receivables will be $84,000. Accordingly, the accounts receivable section of the projected balance sheet might be presented as follows:

| Accounts Receivable | | $84,000 |
|---|---|---|
| less | | |
| Bad debts | $4,480 | |
| Contractual allowances | 1,400 | |
| Charity care | 560 | |
| Courtesy discounts | 1,960 | |
| | | 8,400 |
| Net accounts receivable | | 75,600 |

A hospital that is reimbursed retrospectively might follow this estimation procedure but in this case gross patient revenue might represent the unit of analysis. The remainder of this discussion ignores deductions in revenue so as to simplify the calculations.

Having estimated the end-of-period accounts receivable, we now consider the problem of estimating the other current assets of the hospital. When estimating the end-of-period inventories, we relate inventories to supply purchases by

$$\text{Inventory Ratio} = \frac{\text{Ending Inventory}}{\text{Total Purchases}/365}$$

The denominator of the inventory ratio involves the total purchases of a given period. Recognizing that the objective is to project the balance sheet from the income statement in Table 5-3, we may use supply expenses as a surrogate for the total purchases for the period. Following this procedure, we assume that the supply expenses incurred by the two hospitals amounted to $850,000 in the current period while the ending inventory was valued at $283,333. Thus, the inventory-purchase ratio is $\frac{\$283,333}{\$850,000}$ or .334, which implies that approximately 122 days of average supply usage are invested in the inventories of the institutions. If no changes are anticipated in the purchasing policy of the hospital or the internal distribution of supplies, we may use the inventory-purchase ratio of 1:3 to estimate the end-of-period inventory for the coming period. Returning to estimating balance sheet items from the income statement in Table 5-3, we observe that the supply expenses for the coming year are expected to be $900,000. If one-third of the year's supply expenses are invested in inventories, the end-of-period inventory would be $300,000 (1/3 × $900,000).

When estimating the end-of-period cash balance, it is possible to relate cash holdings to a revenue or volume variable. On the basis of this relationship and the estimated revenue or volume measure, the end-of-period cash balance could be forecast. However, several additional factors must be considered. One of the most important of these involves the potential earning power of idle cash. Cash on hand is required to meet currently maturing obligations and to satisfy other demands such as the payment of wages and salaries or the direct purchase of equipment or supplies. Unless the day-to-day cash demands fluctuate widely, there is no need to allow cash to remain idle in checking accounts where no interest is earned. As an example, if $100,000 is not needed for transactions and the annual interest rate is 10 percent, management could earn an additional $10,000 in interest income with little extra effort.

If past cash balances have been maintained at a minimum level that avoids frequent cash shortages, the historical ratio of cash to revenue or days of revenue invested in cash may be used in predicting the end-of-period cash holdings. Alternatively, management may employ the principles of mathematical expectation in determining the cash balance that minimizes the cost of holding cash (Chapter 7). This is referred to as the optimum cash balance. When the latter approach is used, the ending cash balance is given by the optimum cash balance. Since the issue of determining the optimum cash balance will be considered in detail later, assume here that a cash balance of $100,000 minimizes the total cost of holding cash and that this amount will be on hand at the end of the coming period.

To summarize this section, we have found that:

1. the end-of-period accounts receivable of a hospital reimbursed retrospectively may be estimated by

$$\text{NODCIR (Expected Revenue/365);}$$

2. the end-of-period accounts receivable of a hospital reimbursed prospectively may be estimated by

$$\text{NODCIR* (Expected Nonplan Revenue/365);}$$

3. the end-of-period inventory holdings may be estimated by

$$\text{Inventory Ratio} \times \frac{\text{Supply Expense}}{365}; \text{ and}$$

4. the end-of-period cash holdings were assumed to equal the optimum cash balance.

In terms of the forecasting problem, it is apparent from Table 5-4, which summarizes progress so far, that ratio analysis has been useful in estimating the current assets of the hospitals.

**Estimation of Long-Term Assets.** At this point in the analysis, projections concerning plant and equipment expenditures and liabilities have not been developed. With regard to the acquisition of plant and equipment, there is no mechanical method by which management may determine the amounts of related expenditures or liabilities. Rather, decisions to invest in fixed assets usually are a result of complex interactions among social, economic, and political factors. Many analysts assume that investment in plant and equipment will equal depreciation charges for the year. However, it must be remembered that depreciation is only an accounting device by which the cost of capitalized assets may be allocated over the useful lives of an institution's plant and equipment. New capital expenditures, on the other hand, should be determined on the basis of current and future needs. Clearly, there need not be any relation between de-

**Table 5-4** Current and Projected Balance Sheet

|  | Actual (current year) | Forecast (coming year) | Change |
|---|---|---|---|
| Current assets |  |  |  |
| Cash | $100,000 | $ 100,000 | $ 0 |
| Accounts receivable | 20,000 | 40,000 | 20,000 |
| Inventories | 283,333 | 300,000 | 16,667 |
| Total current assets | 403,333 | 440,000 | 36,667 |
| Long-term assets |  |  |  |
| Plant and equipment (at cost) | 3,900,000 | 3,900,000 | 0 |
| Accumulated depreciation | 600,000 | 1,200,000 |  |
| Net plant and equipment | 3,300,000 | 2,700,000 | (600,000) |
| Total assets | 3,703,333 | 3,140,000 | (563,333) |
| Liabilities |  |  |  |
| Accounts payable | 200,000 |  |  |
| Other liabilities (residual) | 200,000 |  |  |
| Total current liabilities | 400,000 |  |  |
| Long-term liabilities |  |  |  |
| Mortgage payable | 290,000 |  |  |
| Total liabilities | 690,000 |  |  |
| Fund balance | 3,013,333 | 2,373,333 | (640,000) |
| Total liabilities and fund balance | 3,703,333 | 3,140,000 | (563,333) |

preciation charges and the hospital's current or future capital needs. In terms of this example, it is assumed that the hospital's investment in fixed assets will remain constant during the coming year and that accumulated depreciation will have increased from $600,000 to $1,200,000 by the end of that year. Thus, the net plant and equipment of the hospital is expected to decrease by $600,000. These assumptions are reflected in Table 5-4.

At this point, the asset side of the projected balance sheet is complete. As seen in Table 5-4, the net projected change in total assets is −$563,333. This means that the sum of the institution's fund balance and liabilities must decrease by a like amount if the hospital's assets are to equal the sum of its liabilities and fund balance. However, a decline of $640,000 in the fund balance already has been projected—a sum equal to the projected net loss of the period (see Table 5-3).

As shown in Table 5-4, the only task remaining in the development of the balance sheet is the estimation of the current and long-term liabilities that are expected at the end of the coming period. The table indicates that the sum of the current and long-term liabilities must equal $766,667 ($3,140,000 − $2,373,333). Next, estimate the liability side of the balance sheet.

**Estimation of Liabilities.**   Consider first the problem of estimating the accounts payable that are expected to be outstanding at the end of the next period. Accounts payable represent, for the most part, unpaid bills that are accumulated as supplies are purchased; as a result, these liabilities should vary with patient volume. The ratio of accounts payable to supply expenses may be a useful way to predict the balance sheet value of accounts payable for the coming period. The general expression for the number of days of supply expenses financed by accounts payable (DOSEFAP) is

$$DOSEFAP = \frac{\text{Ending Accounts Payable}}{\text{Supply Expenses}/365} \qquad (5.7)$$

Table 5-4 demonstrates that the end-of-period accounts payable of the two institutions amounted to $200,000 and if, as before, the supply expenses were $850,000, DOSEFAP is

$$\frac{200,000}{850,000/365} \cong 86 \text{ days}$$

Thus, the ratio of accounts payable to supply expense is

$$\frac{86}{365} \text{ or } \frac{\$200,000}{\$850,000}$$

and the accounts payable at the end of the coming year would be approximately $211,500 (.235 × $900,000).

**Working Capital Needs.** If it also is known with certainty that the mortgage payment for the coming year will be $40,000, the administrator can determine the working capital needs for the coming period. As in any balance sheet, the assets of the institution must equal its liabilities plus the fund balance. The total assets of the hospital have been estimated to be $3,140,000 while the estimated fund balance of $2,373,333 was found by subtracting the expected operating loss of $640,000 from the current fund balance of $3,703,333. Given that the accounts payable are expected to total $210,000 and that the mortgage payment of $40,000 will reduce the mortgage payable from $290,000 to $250,000, the residual amount of required funding, which represents the working capital needs of the institution, can be found by

| | |
|---|---|
| Total Assets | $3,140,000 |
| less | |
| Accounts payable | (211,500) |
| Mortgage payable | (250,000) |
| Fund balance | (2,373,333) |
| Residual funding required = | 305,167 |

As seen here and in Table 5-5, the difference between total assets and the sum of all other liabilities and the fund balance is $305,167. This value represents the increase in other liabilities or other sources of funding required if assets are to equal total liabilities plus the fund balance. As a consequence, it can be concluded from this analysis that the hospital should expect to seek additional financing of $305,167 by increasing the level of its indebtedness.

## 5.4 FINANCING WORKING CAPITAL

As noted, the management of working capital involves two separate but interrelated problems. If the costs of working capital are to be minimized, management not only must determine the quantity of such capital that will be required for a given period but also must decide on the appropriate mechanism by which these assets are to be financed. Thus far, the discussion has been limited to an analysis of the methods by which management may estimate the quantity of working capital needs for a given period. This section shifts focus to concentrate on the mechanisms that may be used to finance the working capital needs of the institution. First, however, the nature of working capital is examined.

## 5.4.1 Nature of Working Capital

The assets held by the hospital may be divided into essentially three major components: fixed assets, permanent current assets, and variable current assets. Figure 5-7 is an example of the composition of the assets of a typical hospital during a reasonably short period of time. As can be seen, fixed assets and current permanent assets are assumed to be constant during the period even though the volume of care provided by the hospital may have varied considerably. Thus, in the short run, fixed assets and permanent current assets do not vary in response to changes in the volume of care. On the other hand, variable current assets exhibit considerable volatility. Since other factors are held constant, the volatility in this component is attributable to changes in the volume of patient care during the period. In the discussion that follows, we refer to the fixed assets and permanent current assets as the hospital's permanent working capital and, conversely, to the variable current assets as the temporary working capital.

**Table 5-5** Current and Projected Balance Sheet—Funding Need

|  | Actual (current year) | Forecast (current year) | Change |
|---|---|---|---|
| Current assets |  |  |  |
| Cash | $100,000 | $100,000 | $      0 |
| Accounts receivable | 20,000 | 40,000 | 20,000 |
| Inventories | 283,333 | 300,000 | 16,667 |
| Total current assets | 403,333 | 440,000 | 36,667 |
| Long-term assets |  |  |  |
| Plant and equipment (at cost) | 3,900,000 | 3,900,000 | 0 |
| Accumulated depreciation | 600,000 | 1,200,000 | (600,000) |
| Net plant and equipment | 3,300,000 | 2,700,000 | (600,000) |
| Total assets | 3,703,333 | 3,140,000 | (563,333) |
| Liabilities |  |  |  |
| Accounts payable | 200,000 | 211,500 | 11,500 |
| Other liabilities (residual) | 200,000 | 305,167 | 105,167 |
| Total current liabilities | 400,000 | 516,667 | 116,667 |
| Long-term liabilities |  |  |  |
| Mortgage payable | 290,000 | 250,000 | (40,000) |
| Total liabilities | 690,000 | 766,667 | 76,667 |
| Fund balance | 3,013,333 | 2,373,333 | (640,000) |
| Total liabilities and fund balance | 3,703,333 | 3,140,000 | (563,333) |

**Figure 5-7** Components of a Hospital's Assets

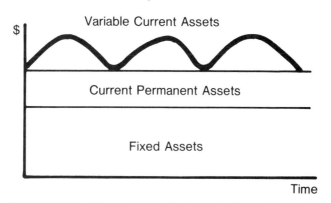

One of the most important characteristics of temporary working capital is its volatile nature. When examining working capital needs, it is important to recognize that, in the absence of changes in the policies of third party payers or management of the hospital, these needs are self-liquidating in the short run. Similar to other industries, a hospital experiences periods in which the demand for service increases. To satisfy these demands, the hospital may be forced to hire additional personnel and purchase additional supplies. As seen earlier, however, additional working capital is required to obtain these resources, and the financial needs can be satisfied eventually through the internal operations of the institution. However, recognizing that cash inflows and cash outflows may not be perfectly synchronized, the need for funding may arise before it becomes available. Thus, in addition to determining the best method of financing permanent working capital, management also must assess various methods of satisfying temporary needs until internally generated financing becomes available.

### 5.4.2 Sources of Funding

The hospital's working capital needs may be financed by various mechanisms. In general, these sources of funding are as follows:

1. equity
2. long-term liabilities
3. short-term liabilities
   a. accounts payable
   b. cash borrowing

This classification suggests that the working capital needs may be financed from two basic sources of funds—debt and/or equity.

### 5.4.2.1 Equity

The equity of the institution may be viewed as the funding that is given to the hospital to acquire land, buildings, and equipment as well as maintaining operations until the enterprise becomes self-sustaining. Given that the equity represents an investment of the community in the hospital, this source of funding need not be repaid unless the assets are liquidated. Thus, an important characteristic of equity is that it represents a relatively permanent source of funding for the hospital.

Since permanent working capital represents a permanent asset that is required if the hospital is to sustain operations for an indefinite period, it should be financed through a permanent source of funds. If the hospital is to operate indefinitely, permanent working capital should not be financed by either long-term or short-term debt, which represent obligations that must be paid. When these liabilities are paid, the hospital is denied the funding it requires to finance its permanent working capital needs. Thus, when considering alternate methods, equity represents the only certain source of permanent funding and should be used in financing permanent working capital needs.

### 5.4.2.2 Long-Term and Short-Term Borrowing

Hospital management may rely on debt as a mechanism of funding working capital needs. When examining debt as a financing mechanism, management should differentiate between trade credit and cash borrowing. With regard to cash borrowing, the debt instruments available to the hospital may be regarded as being either long-term or short-term loans that are extended by banks and other financial institutions. If a loan matures and must be repaid within a short time, usually one year, it is regarded as a short-term or current liability. On the other hand, if the loan matures and must be repaid over a longer period, usually in excess of one year, it usually is regarded as a long-term or noncurrent liability. The basic difference between equity and cash borrowing is that the former need not be repaid while the latter requires the hospital to make payments on predetermined dates.

### 5.4.2.3 Trade Credit

The second important method of financing working capital needs is trade credit, which may be viewed as a short-term loan extended to the hospital by firms that supply goods and services required in day-to-day operations. Trade credit is carried in the hospital's records as an account payable. Technically, an account payable is a current liability that is generated by operational activity as opposed to cash borrowing that may be thought of as a purely financial transaction. For example, inventory items are received and used before the hospital pays the supplier; in such a situation, the seller extends trade credit to the institution for a short period.

Recall, for a moment, the discussion in section 5.3.1 describing a cash flow approach to the determination of working capital needs. In both examples described in this section, it was assumed that the hospital's cash disbursements consisted of a single payment for supplies on day 30 and a wage and salary payment on days 15 and 30. The working capital needs during this period are reduced by the amount of the supply expenses if the payment for supplies is delayed until, say, day 60. The extension of the payment period is, in effect, a 60-day loan to the hospital. As a result, the use of trade credit enables the hospital to support operational activity since it has used a short-term liability (an account payable) to finance a portion of its working capital needs. Given that the hospital is able to finance working capital needs with less of its own funds, the use of trade credit releases cash assets that may be invested in interest-earning securities. Such an approach appears to be ideal when viewed from the perspective of the hospital and it might be argued that trade credit should be used wherever and whenever possible.

From the perspective of the vendor, however, essentially two problems emerge. On the one hand, suppliers recognize that it is not possible to require cash payments when goods are delivered and, as a result, they must extend trade credit. On the other hand, suppliers also realize that, when they do so, they incur certain costs. These costs consist of out-of-pocket expenditures equal to the interest charges required to support the loan as well as opportunity costs equal to the earnings vendors could have obtained by investing the funds committed to outstanding receivables in interest-bearing securities.

Since the extension of credit is an operating necessity, many suppliers offer trade credit that provides a purchase discount if payment is made within a specified period. As the name implies, a purchase discount is a reduction in the price the hospital must pay. These discounts induce the purchaser to make payment before the expiration of the discount period.

The terms of trade credit depend on the nature of the industry, the credit standing of the purchaser, and the financial position of the seller. In general, however, the terms usually are expressed by 2/10/30 which means that if the hospital pays for a purchase within 10 days of the invoice date, which is referred to as the discount period, the price of the purchased goods can be reduced by 2 percent. Thus, if on a $1,000 purchase, payment occurs within the discount period, the hospital only pays $980 for the supply items. If payment does not occur within the discount period, the hospital must pay $1,000 by the 30th day, which is the end of the net period.

Assuming that a $1,000 purchase is made and terms of 2/10/30 are extended, the cost of trade credit is $20 for the use of $980 for a 20-day period (day 11–day 30). In this situation, the cost of $20 can be viewed as an interest charge;

when evaluating these terms, it is convenient to express the cost of credit as an annual rate of interest. The general expression for interest (cost of credit) is given by

$$\text{Cost of Credit} = \text{Principal} \times \frac{\text{Annual Rate}}{\text{of Interest}} \times \frac{a}{365} \qquad (5.8)$$

where the term $a/365$ corresponds to the fraction of a year for which interest is charged. Given that the cost of credit, principal, and the term $a/365$ are known, Equation 5.8 may be rearranged to determine the annual rate of interest as follows:

$$\frac{\text{Annual Rate}}{\text{of Interest}} = \frac{\text{Cost of Credit}}{\text{Principal}} \times \frac{365}{a} \qquad (5.9)$$

Returning to our example, suppose the hospital ignores the discount and pays for the $1,000 purchase on day 30. Such a decision means that the hospital pays $20 for the use of $980 for 20 days and the annual rate of interest is

$$\frac{\text{Annual Rate}}{\text{of Interest}} = \frac{\$20}{\$980} \times \frac{365}{20} = 37.2\%$$

As can be seen from this example, when the hospital takes the discount, there is no cost for the use of credit during the discount period. However, if the terms of 2/10/30 are offered and the hospital ignores the discount, an opportunity cost is incurred. Table 5-6 lists the implicit interest rates incurred when payment is made 30, 60, 90, and 120 days after the invoice date. This table shows that,

**Table 5-6** Implicit Annual Rate of Interest for the Terms of Credit

| Payment Made on Day | Calculation | Annual Interest |
|---|---|---|
| 30 | $\frac{20}{980} \times \frac{365}{20}$ | 37.2 |
| 60 | $\frac{20}{980} \times \frac{365}{50}$ | 14.9 |
| 90 | $\frac{20}{980} \times \frac{365}{80}$ | 9.3 |
| 120 | $\frac{20}{980} \times \frac{365}{110}$ | 6.8 |

after the discount period, the annual rate of interest decreases as the net period increases.

The relationship between the annual rate of interest, as expressed in percentage terms, and the number of days between the end of the discount period and the net period is presented in Figure 5-8. Essentially two characteristics of this figure should be noted. First, there are no explicit costs associated with the extension of trade credit during the discount period. As a result, between day 1 and day 10 trade credit may be regarded as an interest-free loan because the price remains constant even though payment is made on day 1, day 10, or any of the intervening days of the discount period. After the discount period, the hospital incurs an explicit cost for the use of trade credit but the annual interest rate decreases as the net period increases. Thus, the second point is that, if the hospital ignores the discount, the annual rate of interest declines so long as the institution postpones payment.

On the basis of these observations it can be concluded that payment should be made either at the *end* of the discount period or at the *end* of the net period. In both cases, emphasis is placed on paying at the end of the period because, if the hospital elects to take advantage of the discount, the cost of the goods is the same irrespective of whether payment is made on the first or last day of the discount period. As a result, there is no financial incentive for management to pay before the end of either the discount period or the net period; instead, the financial incentive is to delay payment. By doing so until the end of the discount or net period, management avoids the commitment of funds to an investment in inventories, which implies that assets are released and may be invested in interest-bearing securities or other revenue-generating activities.

**Figure 5-8** Trade Credit and Discount Interest Rate

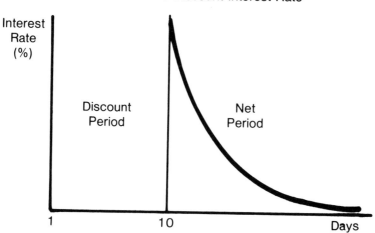

Given the configuration of the curve in Figure 5-8, it might be argued that it is in the hospital's financial interests to postpone payment indefinitely. However, suppliers will attempt to prevent the annual rate of interest from declining by engaging in normal collection efforts as well as turning over unpaid accounts to a lawyer or a collection agency. Thus, unless outstanding accounts are paid on a timely basis, the hospital's credit rating will suffer, which may make suppliers and other lenders less willing to extend credit. Such an unwillingness probably will increase the cost of future purchases since the hospital may have to pay cash when goods are delivered or deal with vendors who charge a higher price to compensate for those who delay in making payment.

### 5.4.3 Financing Temporary Working Capital Needs

Since a hospital should devote its equity to financing its permanent capital assets, management should use long-term or short-term debt, including trade credit, to fund temporary working capital needs. The following discussion focuses on this mechanism.

When considering temporary working capital needs, short-term debt is an acceptable financing alternative because the needs usually are self-liquidating in a short time. When only short-term debt is used, management runs the risk of encountering periods of economic inflation or recession or tight monetary policies. Under these circumstances, short-term funding might not be renewed, which could force the hospital to close. Even if it is not necessary to liquidate its assets, the withdrawal of short-term financing may mean that the hospital is forced to reduce its services as bankers, suppliers, and other financial institutions reduce the availability of funding. Another risk is that the current rate of interest normally applies only to the current debt instrument. Since interest rates fluctuate over time, uncertainty regarding the rate of interest complicates the process of financial planning.

On the other hand, when long-term debt is used to finance temporary working capital needs, management avoids much of the uncertainty concerning the availability of funding. However, when viewed in terms of interest charges and the creation of excess cash, financing the temporary needs through long-term debt usually is the most costly. This is seen in Figure 5-9, where the temporary capital needs of the institution are represented by the arcs AB and CD. This figure assumes that these needs are financed through the issuance of a long-term debt instrument that matures at time $t$. It also demonstrates that the use of long-term debt will force the hospital to pay for the use of funds during periods in which the financing is not required. As a result, the hospital needlessly incurs additional operating costs.

Of course, the institution can invest the surplus funds in marketable securities during the periods in which the borrowed funds are not needed. While such a

**Figure 5-9** Financing Working Capital Needs

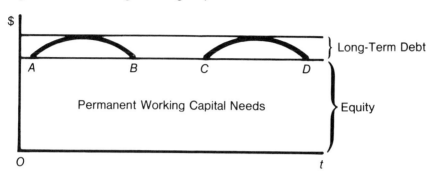

procedure might earn a return, it usually will not be as much as the interest charges associated with the debt. Since the timing of long-term debt and temporary working capital needs do not necessarily coincide, the use of long-term debt increases the cost of financing the hospital's short-term needs. As a result, if management is to minimize the cost of working capital, short-term needs should be financed through short-term debt.

The primary advantage of short-term debt in financing temporary working capital needs is that management can synchronize the maturity of debt instrument with the hospital's demand for temporary funds. This advantage suggests that temporary needs should be financed by short-term debt having a maturity schedule that exactly matches the fluctuations in working capital. Unfortunately, such a rule is not completely valid because it does not consider the uncertainties associated with cash inflows from payments on outstanding receivables.

Debt, whether long-term or short-term, constitutes a fixed obligation and both the amount and timing of related payments are known with certainty. However, apart from nonrandom prospective payments, the cash inflows from payment of accounts receivable are not known with certainty. As a consequence, the amount and timing of the funds required to liquidate a debt are known approximately but, due to several factors, the exact amount and timing cannot be projected with complete accuracy. A fixed obligation therefore must be satisfied with an uncertain cash flow.

This situation represents a real and potentially costly hazard to the hospital. As an example, suppose that the maturity of the debt coincides with the anticipated time when funds are required and that cash inflows are not received when expected. In such a situation, the hospital may be unable to pay the debt. At best, a failure to extinguish the liability will cast doubt on the hospital's credit standing and, at worst, may result in financial failure. As a result, the hospital must minimize the risk of default.

This consideration suggests that management should adjust the maturity of the short-term debt so as to provide a short time between the end of the period during which a funding need is anticipated and the date on which the debt instrument matures.

### 5.4.4  Choice of Short-Term Finance

Having identified short-term debt as the appropriate technique of financing temporary working capital needs, we now consider the form of the short-term financing mechanism. This section analyzes short-term cash borrowing, trade credit, and, in certain circumstances, the liquidation of temporary investments in marketable securities as potential methods of financing these needs. When evaluating these alternate methods, it is necessary to consider the costs of financing in both dollar and percentage terms.

First, assume that the temporary working capital needs of the institution may be financed through trade credit or through short-term cash borrowing. In this situation, it might be argued that if the interest rate for the latter is below the minimum point of the cost-of-credit curve, the prudent decision is to take the discount and engage in cash borrowing to pay the invoice before the end of the discount period. Alternatively, if the interest rate exceeds the minimum point of the cost-of-credit curve, the hospital should use trade credit to finance temporary working capital needs.

To illustrate, suppose the hospital requires additional funding to finance a $1,000 purchase. Assume also that the terms of credit extended by the supplier are 2/10/30 and that the hospital is able to negotiate an 8 percent, 30-day loan for $1,000. Under these assumptions, the cost of trade credit is $20 and the interest rate is approximately 37 percent. Conversely, the dollar cost of the bank loan is $6.57 $\left(\dfrac{30}{365} \times 1,000 \times .08\right)$. In this situation, the interest rate on cash borrowing (.08) is below the minimum point of the cost-of-credit curve ($\sim.37$). Similarly, the dollar cost of cash borrowing ($6.57) is less than the dollar costs of trade credit ($20). Consequently, short-term cash borrowing is the least costly alternative, which implies that the discount should be taken and the working capital needs financed through the short-term bank loan.

Now, assume that the hospital is able to finance this inventory acquisition through trade credit or through the use of available funds. In this situation, the mechanism by which these needs should be financed depends on

1. the terms of trade credit
2. the cost of short-term borrowing
3. the rate of return that can be earned by investing available funds in assets other than inventories

Here, let $r$ represent the rate of return that can be earned from investments in assets other than inventories and $C^*$ represent the charges associated with the least costly form of debt, which in this case is limited to trade credit and short-term cash borrowing. If $r$ is greater than $C^*$, the prudent decision is to maintain the investment and finance inventories through the least costly credit alternative. Conversely, if $r$ is less than $C^*$, the prudent action is to take the discount and finance the purchase through available funds or assets.

To illustrate, suppose that, as before, the hospital makes a $1,000 purchase that may be financed by

1. trade credit in which the terms are 2/10/30
2. selling marketable securities yielding 14 percent, which is payable in 10 days if the investment is retained by the hospital or
3. cash borrowing by negotiating a 30-day, 6 percent loan for $1,000

As before, the cost of trade credit is $20 and the interest rate is approximately 37 percent. The annual interest rate on investment in a marketable security is 14 percent and the opportunity cost of selling this security prematurely is $140. Similarly, the annual interest rate on short-term cash borrowing is 6 percent and the cost of the bank loan is approximately $5.00. On the basis of these calculations, the prudent financial decision is to

1. retain the investment in marketable securities
2. take the discount and
3. finance the purchase through cash borrowing, which in this case is the least costly alternative

In a slightly different example, suppose management is faced with the same situation except that the investment in marketable securities earns an annual yield of only .1 percent. The costs of the three sources of finance are as follows:

| | |
|---|---|
| Trade credit | $20.00 |
| Investment | 1.00 |
| Bank loan | 4.93 |

In this case, the least costly alternative is to take the discount and finance the purchase through the sale of the short-term investment.

This discussion suggests that, if costs are to be minimized, the least expensive funding mechanism must be identified and used when financing a hospital's temporary working capital needs. The method of obtaining funding is a separate issue that may be addressed only after management has examined the costs of each alternative to determine the least costly financing mechanism.

# Appendix 5-1

As seen in the discussion of break-even analysis, it is necessary to estimate the parameters of a linear equation that assumes the form

$$y = b_0 + b_1 x$$

where $b_0$ represents fixed costs and $b_1$ corresponds to the variable cost component. As in any standard statistical text, the "normal" equations pertaining to $b_0$ and $b_1$ are given by

$$b_0 n + b_1 \sum_{i=1}^{i=n} x_i = \sum_{i=1}^{i=n} y_i$$

$$b_0 \sum_{i=1}^{i=n} x_i + b_1 \sum_{i=1}^{i=n} x_i^2 = \sum_{i=1}^{i=n} x_i y_i$$

As should be verified, these equations may be expressed in the form

$$(\mathbf{X'X})\mathbf{b} = \mathbf{X'y}$$

where

$$\mathbf{X'} = \begin{bmatrix} 1 & \cdots & 1 \\ x_1 & \cdots & x_n \end{bmatrix}; \qquad \mathbf{y} = \begin{bmatrix} y_1 \\ \vdots \\ y_n \end{bmatrix}$$

and

$$\mathbf{b} = \begin{bmatrix} b_0 \\ b_1 \end{bmatrix}$$

Hence, the coefficients $b_0$ and $b_1$ are given by

$$\mathbf{b} = (\mathbf{X'X})^{-1}\mathbf{X'y}$$

Alternatively, the calculation of $b_1$ and $b_0$ might be expressed in the form

$$b_1 = \frac{\sum_{i=1}^{i=n} x_i y_i - \left[ \left( \sum_{i=1}^{i=n} x_i \right) \left( \sum_{i=1}^{i=n} y_i \right) \right] / n}{\sum_{i=1}^{i=n} x_i^2 - (\Sigma x_i)^2 / n}$$

and

$$b_0 = \bar{y} - b_1\overline{X}$$

In these formulations, the $x$'s correspond to observed rates of operation (e.g., number of days of care per period) and the $y$'s represent the corresponding total costs. For a further analysis of the resulting equation, a standard statistics text should be consulted.

---

**REFERENCES**

Archer, S. H. "A Model for the Determination of Firm Cash Balances." *The Journal of Financial and Quantitative Analysis,* vol. 1, no. 1, March 1966, pp. 1–11.

Berman, H., and Weeks, L. *The Financial Management of Hospitals*, 3rd ed. Ann Arbor, Mich.: Health Administration Press, 1976, ch. 9, 10.

Barbatelli, E. "Using Depreciation to Provide for Future Hospital Needs." *Hospitals,* JAHA, vol. 41, no. 14, July 16, 1967.

Knight, W. D. "Working Capital Management—Satisficing Versus Optimization." *Financial Management,* vol. 1, no. 2, Spring 1972, pp. 33–40.

Miller, R. F. "Price and Volume Changes Will Influence Your Working Capital Needs." *Hospital Financial Management,* vol. 26, no. 6, June 1972, pp. 3–6.

Smith, K. V. "State of the Art of Working Capital Management." *Financial Management,* vol. 2, no. 4, Autumn 1973, pp. 50–55.

# Chapter 6

# Management of Accounts Receivable

**Objectives**

After completing this chapter, you should be able to:

1. Understand the nature and necessity of extending credit in the hospital industry.
2. Describe the costs of extending credit.
3. Understand and describe the objectives of managing accounts receivable.
4. Understand, describe, and implement the basic approaches to the administration of outstanding receivables.
5. Estimate the timing and magnitude of cash receipts from payments made on receivables from institutional and noninstitutional sources.

## 6.1 INTRODUCTION

The method of reimbursing the hospital exerts an impact on its investment in accounts receivable. This investment by an institution that is reimbursed on a prospective basis will be less than the corresponding investment by a hospital that is reimbursed retrospectively. On the other hand, the examination of the cash flow approach to determining minimum working capital needs revealed that, in both cases, a reduction in the accounts receivable cycle released assets that could be invested in interest-earning securities that, in turn, could increase the hospital's cash receipts. Thus, if the costs of working capital are to be minimized, management must exercise control over the size of the hospital's investment in accounts receivable.

## 6.2 CHARACTERISTICS OF ACCOUNTS RECEIVABLE

Accounts receivable may be defined as the amounts of money owed to a hospital by patients, agents of patients, or other institutions for goods or services. Hospital accounts receivable represent accounts payable by entities that reimburse the institution for goods and services provided. If accounts payable represent business loans received, outstanding receivables must be regarded as an extension of business credit.

As will be seen, it is convenient to categorize hospital accounts receivable in terms of institutional and noninstitutional sources of payment. Following this procedure, institutional and noninstitutional sources of outstanding receivables are presented in Tables 6-1 and 6-2, respectively. As shown in Table 6-1, hospitals in the United States and Canada are likely to generate outstanding receivables whose payment is guaranteed by an institutional payer. The common denominator of these sources of receivables involves the certainty with which management might expect to receive payment in full. Conversely, management is far less certain of receiving payment in full from the sources in Table 6-2. It is well recognized that the portion of the bill for which the patient is responsible may prove to be uncollectable; hence, the probability of receiving payment in full is less than one. Although the lists in these tables are not exhaustive, such a grouping is useful when estimating the timing and magnitude of the cash flows arising from the various components of the hospital's receivables.

As noted in Chapter 5, working capital needs could be funded through accounts payable but such a practice was found to be costly. Conversely, if accounts payable are costly to the borrower, accounts receivable should be an

**Table 6-1** Institutional Sources of Hospital Receivables, by Country and Revenue Category

| Country and Major Source of Receivable | Revenue Category |
| --- | --- |
| United States | |
| Blue Cross | Insured inpatient and outpatient services |
| Medicare and Medicaid | Insured inpatient and outpatient services |
| Commercial insurance company | Insured inpatient and outpatient services |
| Workmen's Compensation | Insured inpatient and outpatient services |
| Canada | |
| Workmen's Compensation Board | Services provided to insured patients |
| Department of Veteran's Affairs | Services provided to insured patients |
| Other provincial plans | Insured service to nonresidents |
| Other municipal, provincial, and federal programs | Patient services |
| Other nongovernmental agencies and institutions | Recoveries |

**Table 6-2** Major Noninstitutional Sources of Accounts Receivable, by Country

| Major Source of Receivable | Revenue Category |
|---|---|
| United States | |
| Insured patient | Use of uninsured inpatient and outpatient services; deductibles, coinsurance |
| Uninsured patient | Inpatient and outpatient services |
| Canada | |
| Uninsured patient | Inpatient and outpatient services as well as authorized and differential charges |
| Insured patient | Use of uninsured outpatient services as well as authorized and differential charges |

attractive investment alternative to the lender. Therefore, lenders should be anxious to extend credit. However, this is not the case, and to understand why accounts receivable are not as good an investment as might appear at first glance, it is necessary to examine the costs of extending credit.

## 6.3 THE COST OF ACCOUNTS RECEIVABLE: THE GENERAL CASE

Assuming payment is made on day 30, the interest on trade credit with terms 2/10/30 was approximately 37 percent. This is a substantial return that would delight most lenders. However, 37 percent is not the interest rate the lender actually receives since it does not consider costs of extending credit. Thus, to obtain the effective or the net rate of interest, the gross interest rate of 37 percent must be adjusted to reflect the cost of extending trade credit. Lenders' costs of credit may be divided into three major categories: (1) opportunity costs, (2) routine credit and collection costs, and (3) delinquency costs.

### 6.3.1 Opportunity Costs

Opportunity costs arise from the fact that, when credit is extended, assets are committed to accounts receivable as opposed to some other investment alternative. As a result, the lender incurs an opportunity cost equal to the rate of return that could have been earned if the funds invested in accounts receivable had been diverted to some other alternative. It also should be noted that lenders forced to borrow funds to finance their investment in accounts receivable incur out-of-pocket costs. These also vary directly with the investment in accounts receivable and are equal to the interest charges assessed by banks and other financial institutions.

Since the lender's assets are invested in accounts receivable throughout the credit period, opportunity costs accrue during the entire time that credit is extended. However, if borrowers elect to ignore the discount and to pay for the use of credit, the opportunity costs are offset by the associated returns to the lender. Thus, if opportunity costs were the only ones incurred when extending credit, accounts receivable might represent a potential profit to the lender. As mentioned earlier, however, lenders incur other costs when they extend credit.

## 6.3.2 Routine Credit and Collection Costs

The second category of costs associated with accounts receivable involves routine credit and collection expenses. These are operating expenditures incurred in making knowledgeable credit decisions and in protecting the lender's income and operating position. In achieving these objectives, the lender should operate a credit department, responsible for identifying poor credit risks, and a collection department responsible for keeping track of billings, due dates, sending payment notices, and taking other action to obtain payment.

The necessity of maintaining a credit and collection department results in operational expenditures that require cash disbursements. One of the primary objectives of these units is to avoid delinquency costs and the need to write off accounts as uncollectable.

## 6.3.3 Delinquency Costs

It is just as naive to believe that all bills will be paid on time as it is to believe that the credit department will be completely successful in identifying poor credit risks. Despite the efforts of the credit and collection department, some individuals invariably will fail to pay their bills. When this occurs, the lender must attempt to collect past due accounts. It is at this point that delinquency costs are encountered, since the actions that must be taken add to the expense of extending credit.

When an account becomes overdue, the first step generally involves a follow-up by the collection department, which reminds the individual that the account is past due and requests prompt payment. If this is successful, delinquency costs are not large. However, if the collection department is not successful, additional and more costly steps are necessary. For example, the account might be turned over to a collection agency that may charge 10 to 15 percent of the receivable for its efforts. Another alternative is to retain a lawyer who probably will charge at least 10 percent of the balance. Finally, if all efforts fail, the lender may have to write off the account as a bad debt. In that case, the delinquency cost is equal to the value of the goods or services sold. Regardless of the steps taken, it should be clear that delinquency costs can be significant; because of these costs, the extension of trade credit is not a particularly attractive investment alternative to lenders.

## 6.4  ADVANTAGES OF TRADE CREDIT

As might be expected, the operation of the credit and collection department, plus delinquency costs, represent items that detract from earnings—which of course reduces net income. Furthermore, since these costs are incurred only if the lender extends credit, the reasons underlying hospitals' extension of credit merit inquiry.

As mentioned, the magnitude of a hospital's investment in outstanding receivables is influenced to a significant extent by the method of reimbursement. Under retrospective reimbursement, a large investment in accounts receivable is an operational necessity. On the other hand, under prospective reimbursement, the receivables are attributable, at least in part, to transactions involving the provision of services not covered by the prospective payer. In both cases, it must be noted that the hospital is a community resource that cannot deny care to patients who are unable to pay on a cash basis. In most cases, the need for care is unexpected and the patient frequently is ill-prepared to finance the cost of uninsured care on a current basis. This suggests that the hospital's extension of credit is an unavoidable operating necessity.

Since hospitals are forced to extend credit, they incur the same costs as commercial companies. Unlike commercial firms, however, the hospital cannot use credit to expand sales volume or profits to justify the costs of trade credit. Because of the stochastic nature of the demand for service, the hospital cannot use trade credit or liberalize credit terms to increase patient care. Even if hospitals could increase volume by liberalizing credit policies, this would not necessarily result in additional profits because the magnitude of hospital revenues usually is determined by the costs of providing service and does not include a profit factor. As a result, the profit-generating potential of trade credit does not exist for hospitals.

Hospitals also traditionally have felt that it is unwise to charge interest, either in the form of offering credit on terms or of assessing carrying charges on accounts receivable. Many administrators feel that, because of the indiscriminate nature of illness and demand for care, charging an implicit or explicit rate of interest is morally wrong and, since the hospital is a community resource, charging interest would jeopardize seriously the relation between the institution and the population served. This suggests that in order to become competitive for the debtor's dollar, hospitals may be forced to charge interest on long overdue accounts.

Since credit cannot be used as a mechanism to increase patient volume and profits, the advantages of offering trade credit are not available to hospitals as they are to commercial companies. As a result, only the costs and none of the benefits of extending credit accrue to the hospital. Given this situation, then, the objective of accounts receivable management is clear. If the costs of operation are to be minimized, accounts receivable and the granting of credit should be reduced to the lowest possible level. The next section reviews managerial policies and practices that may help accomplish this task.

## 6.5 MANAGEMENT AND CONTROL OF ACCOUNTS RECEIVABLE

The management of accounts receivable should be viewed as a process that begins before the patient is admitted to the hospital and continues until the bill is paid or a decision is reached to write it off as uncollectable. During this period, a number of problems emerge that require managerial action to minimize the costs of extending credit.

The problem of minimizing the accounts receivable cycle is central to the objective of reducing the costs of extending credit. All other factors holding constant, a reduction in this cycle reduces the hospital's investment in outstanding receivables; in turn, this decreases opportunity costs and credit and collection expenses associated with outstanding accounts. In addition, the probability of incurring a bad debt usually increases as the account ages. As a result, a reduction in the accounts receivable cycle also is likely to reduce delinquency costs to the hospital. If the total costs of extending credit are to be minimized, the length of the accounts receivable cycle should be kept as short as possible.

When considering minimizing the length of the accounts receivable cycle, management should recognize that a single hospital can do little to increase the speed with which third parties pay their debts, but the collection department can influence the rapidity with which self-responsible patients pay. Germane to both considerations, however, is the possibility of the hospital's accelerating internal processing and submission of bills to the institutional and noninstitutional entities responsible for payment.

The following discussion examines policies and procedures that should be implemented during each phase of the process by which accounts receivable are managed as well as the methods of evaluating the effectiveness of accounts receivable management.

### 6.5.1 The Preadmission Phase

Figure 6-1 is an example of the decisions that may be reached on the financial status of a patient before admission to the hospital. As this figure indicates, management should distinguish first between patients insured under a third party contract and those who have no insurance.

**Figure 6-1** Preadmission Phase

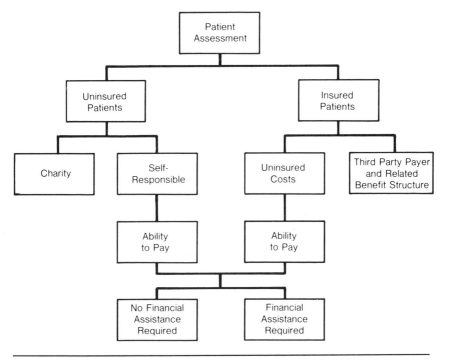

Consider first patients covered by a third party payer. For these individuals, it is necessary not only to identify the responsible third party payer (Blue Cross, Medicare, the provincial plan, etc.) but also to assess the extent to which anticipated costs represent an insured benefit under the contract. Obviously, the difference between the anticipated costs of hospital care and costs insured by the third party payer represents the patient's financial liability. Uninsured costs are related to the use of care that exceeds the maximum benefits provided by the third party payer as well as coinsurance charges, deductibles and, in Canada, authorized and differential charges. After estimating the costs for which the patient is responsible, management should evaluate the individual's ability to pay. This involves an assessment of the person's income and liquid assets in relation to the level of the uninsured costs as well as the individual's other debts. On the basis of this assessment, management may identify patients who are likely to require assistance in paying their portion of the hospital bill. For this group of patients, management may consult with the individuals, and perhaps a financial intermediary, to arrange bank financing or a personal payment plan. Such a procedure not only reduces the probability of writing off the account as a bad debt but also reduces the accounts receivable cycle.

The second group involves patients who are not insured by a third party payer. For this group, one of the major purposes of preadmission processing is to identify indigent patients who will receive free or charity care. Even though such persons normally constitute a small proportion of the patient population, the hospital should be aware of their existence. If it is ascertained that the probability of receiving payment is zero, the account should not be classified as a normal or regular receivable. When accounts are classified inappropriately as regular or normal receivables, collection efforts are wasted and the hospital's bad debts are inflated artificially. Thus, if management is to avoid wasting the efforts of the credit and collection department and if an accurate picture of the hospital's receivables is to be presented in the balance sheet, free or charity patients should be identified and classified appropriately.

As for the third group—individuals not classified as charity patients—management should evaluate their ability to pay. As before, this evaluation can identify patients who require special assistance in obtaining funding or in arranging a personal payment plan.

## 6.5.2 The Admission Phase

The information developed in the preadmission phase provides the basis for the admission phase of managing accounts receivable. The information required to assess the insurance status and ability to pay also constitutes the basis for preparing admission forms as well as the records required by third party payers. For elective admissions, then, the second phase of managing accounts receivable should consist of the patient's signing admission forms as well as any other documents required by the hospital.

## 6.5.3 The Production Phase

After the patient has been admitted to the hospital, management must address a slightly different set of problems. During the production phase (i.e., the length of stay, the provision of ambulatory care, and so on), management may accelerate internal processing by ensuring that the accounting system records all requests for service and that all services provided are entered promptly and accurately in the patient's account. The importance of prompt recording of service should be clear: (1) if it is necessary to identify services provided, the time required for internal processing must increase; (2) if correct charges are not billed, the time required for internal processing also must increase. To avoid such delays, a system of checks and balances must exist to provide internal control over the process by which entries are recorded. Such a control system should be characterized by at least the following features:

1. The internal control system should ensure that all charges are made in accordance with the hospital's established rate schedule.
2. A subsidiary record should be established for each patient and should be checked against the admission register.
3. Service departments should follow routine procedures to ensure prompt and accurate reporting of all services involving charges.
4. The accuracy of the type of service provided during the period covered, the rates used, and extensions calculated should be validated routinely.
5. Control totals should be developed from charge media and balanced against the posting of accounts receivable.
6. Statistical data should be maintained and compared with recorded revenue.
7. The total of the accounts receivable appearing in subsidiary records should be reconciled with the general ledger control accounts. Such a reconciliation should be prepared periodically by a responsible person.
8. Such functions as recording transactions involving accounts receivable should be performed independently of handling the corresponding cash receipts.
9. Persons independent of accounts receivable and the credit department should confirm accounts by mail and by
   a. comparing statements with the patient's account,
   b. keeping statements under control until mailing, and
   c. investigating any discrepancies.

It should be noted that this list is not exhaustive but is intended to indicate control procedures that may accelerate internal processing. The task of designing the hospital's accounts receivable system is primarily the responsibility of the industrial engineer, the auditor, and the chief financial officer. The primary responsibility of hospital administration, however, is to review the design of the system and its results to ensure that management objectives are being attained.

### 6.5.4 The Discharge Phase

Assuming that the accounting system has promptly and accurately recorded the quantity, composition, and costs of services provided during the production phase, a statement of hospital charges as well as the portion of the bill that is the responsibility of the patient should be available at the time of discharge. The hospital should be prepared to accept cash payments from patients at the time of their departure. In the case of a hospital reimbursed retrospectively, these procedures should enable management to bill the third party payer for the insured portion of hospital charges upon or immediately following the patient's discharge.

### 6.5.5 The Post-Discharge Phase

During the post-discharge phase of managing outstanding receivables, administration's primary focus is on prompt payment. By improving the performance of the collection department, management may reduce both the opportunity costs and the delinquency costs incurred when credit is extended. When monitoring the performance of this department, management must ensure that the information, procedures, and policies that determine the organization and timing of collection efforts as well as the policies that specify the criteria for writing off an account as uncollectable are stated clearly and used appropriately by line personnel. A number of books and articles have been written on the mechanics of developing and implementing sound collection techniques for hospitals. Given the volume and quality of material available, the literature is not summarized here; readers are directed to the references at the end of this chapter.

An observation on the role of administration in managing the credit and collection department is appropriate. The hospital administrator should not assume the day-to-day responsibility of operating the credit and collection system. Rather, this should be the joint responsibility of the patient accounts manager and the chief financial officer. After consulting with financial personnel, the administrator should assume the responsibility for establishing policies on writing off bad debts, identifying free service patients, granting discounts and rebates, and monitoring the functioning of the accounts receivable system.

One final point concerning the administration and control of accounts receivable should be considered. A major management objective is to minimize the cost of accounts receivable. At first glance, it would seem that one approach to achieving such a goal is to minimize the costs of credit and collection. However, this fails to recognize that the opportunity costs and delinquency costs of outstanding accounts might be reduced by increasing the hospital's credit and collection efforts, thus reducing those costs. How much a hospital should expend on credit and collection is an empirical question that may be answered by examining the costs and savings of various levels of activity. Optimally, however, these efforts should be increased until the marginal savings are equal to the marginal costs.

### 6.5.6 Evaluation of Accounts Receivable Management

One of the principal objectives of management is to minimize the hospital's investment in accounts receivable. Essential to this is an adequate management information system that portrays both the composition and quantity of credit granted by the hospital. In the absence of such a system, overdue accounts probably will be neglected, which may result in an increase in bad debt expenses as well as in the costs associated with collection activities. Apart from the proper recording of transactions involving accounts receivable, a number of summary analyses should be provided to indicate the state of the institution's receivables. The most frequently encountered statements are ratios reflecting the rate at which accounts receivable are collected and ratios that indicate the number of days' charges in receivables. A number of these ratios were discussed earlier and are reintroduced here to indicate their value in controlling receivables.

One of the ratios used in evaluating the management of receivables related to providing patient care is the accounts receivable turnover ratio (*ART*), which is given by

$$ART = \frac{\text{Net Patient Service Revenue}}{\text{Net Patient Receivables}} \qquad \textbf{(6.1)}$$

The term "net patient service revenue" appears in the numerator of *ART*. This term refers only to revenues generated by providing patient revenue that involve a charge to an account receivable. In addition, when calculating *ART*, the manager should exclude bad debts, charity care, courtesy discounts, and contractual agreements from the numerator and denominator.

As noted, many hospitals engage in revenue-generating activities that do not involve patient care. For example, a hospital may sell laundry services, dietary services, steam, heat, and so on to entities other than patients. These revenue-generating activities usually occur prior to the receipt of cash, which implies that the income earned is accompanied by a charge to an account receivable. Designating the accounts receivable turnover ratio associated with this dimension of hospital operations by *ART** we find

$$ART^* = \frac{\text{Net Recovery Income}}{\text{Recovery Receivables}} \qquad \textbf{(6.2)}$$

where the term "recovery" refers to income-generating activities that do not involve patient care. As in Equation 6.1, the numerator of *ART** consists only of revenues that involve a charge to an account receivable. Again, the values in the numerator and denominator of *ART** should be adjusted to eliminate the effects of bad debts, contractual agreements, and so on.

The ratios *ART* and *ART** indicate the number of times that outstanding receivables were collected or "turned over" during the period. In terms of the simplified cash flow model presented earlier, an increase in these ratios indicates that cash inflows have increased during the period, which of course is one of the primary objectives of managing accounts receivable.

Another indicator for evaluating accounts receivable management is the number of days' charges in receivables (*NODCIR*). With respect to receivables generated by providing patient care, *NODCIR* is given by

$$NODCIR = \frac{\text{Number of Days in the Year}}{ART} \qquad \textbf{(6.3)}$$

Similarly, we define NODCIR* as

$$NODCIR* = \frac{\text{Number of Days in Year}}{ART*} \qquad \textbf{(6.4)}$$

which pertains to receivables related to revenues generated through the sale of laundry service, dietary service, steam, heat, or the rental of buildings to agents other than patients. NODCIR and NODCIR* indicate the average age of receivables associated with the provision of patient and nonpatient services. Thus, they provide a crude measure of the hospital's accounts receivable cycle. As a result, a reduction in these ratios implies that cash inflows have been increased and, other factors remaining constant, the opportunity costs incurred during the credit period have been reduced.

Once these ratios have been computed, they may be compared against similar ratios that have prevailed during previous periods as well as against ratios that are calculated using data from the hospital's budget. On the basis of these comparisons, management may identify problem areas that require investigation and take immediate action to avoid additional credit costs. As an example, if the standard or expected credit period is 30 days, a potential problem may be identified if the actual credit period is found to be 90 or 120 days.

It should be recognized that NODCIR and NODCIR* indicate only the average age of outstanding accounts. To obtain a more detailed picture of the age composition of those accounts, management should develop an accounts receivable profile similar to the one in Table 6-3. As the table shows, the hospital's receivables have been grouped in terms of the number of days the account has been outstanding. The first column lists the number of accounts in each of the age groupings, the second column the percentage of the total number of receivables in each age category.

As an example, the table shows that 30 of the receivables are more than 70 days old and that these 30 accounts represent 3.5 percent of 860 outstanding receivables. The third column contains the dollar value of the accounts receivable in each category and the fourth column the percentage of the total dollar value of receivables in each. Thus, the 30 accounts that are more than 70 days old have a total value of $30,000, which represents 30 percent of the total dollar value of the hospital's receivables. If the values in the second column are compared with the corresponding values in the fourth column, it is clear that the accounts that are more than 70 days old comprise only 3.5 percent of the hospital's receivable accounts but 30 percent of the total dollar amount owed.

However, the other ratios in the fourth column are less than the corresponding percentages in the second column. This suggests that the manager might focus collection efforts on the 30 accounts that have been outstanding for more than 70 days.

Before proceeding with such a policy, the manager might consider the expected payoffs from an increased collection effort. This assessment may be facilitated by using the principles of mathematical expectation. The fifth column of Table 6-3 lists the average value of the accounts in each category while the last column gives the probability that the average account in each age group will be collected. The expected payoff associated with age category $i$ is given by

$$E(R_i) = P_i \bar{V}_i \qquad (6.5)$$

where

$E(R_i)$ = expected dollar return associated with age category $i$,
$P_i$ = probability of collecting on an account in category $i$,
$\bar{V}_i$ = the average value of outstanding accounts in category $i$.

Performing the indicated calculations for each of the age groups, we find the expected payoffs are as follows:

| Age Group | Expected Payoff | Ordinal Ranking |
|---|---|---|
| Less than 30 | $73.34 | 2 |
| 30–40 | 75.83 | 1 |
| 41–50 | 40.00 | 4 |
| 51–60 | 13.75 | 5 |
| 61–70 | 33.33 | 6 |
| More than 70 | 50.00 | 3 |

**Table 6-3** Age Composition of Accounts Receivable

| Number of Days Account Has Been Outstanding | Number of Accounts (1) | % (2) | Total Amount of Accounts (3) | % (4) | Average Amount (5) | P[1] (6) |
|---|---|---|---|---|---|---|
| Less than 30 | 480 | 55.8 | $44,000 | 44.0 | $91.67 | .80 |
| 30–40 | 120 | 14.0 | 13,000 | 13.0 | 108.33 | .70 |
| 41–50 | 90 | 10.5 | 6,000 | 6.0 | 66.67 | .60 |
| 51–60 | 80 | 9.2 | 2,000 | 2.0 | 25.00 | .55 |
| 61–70 | 60 | 7.0 | 5,000 | 5.0 | 83.33 | .40 |
| More than 70 | 30 | 3.5 | 30,000 | 30.0 | 1,000.00 | .05 |
| Total Average | 860 | 100.0 | 100,000 | 100.0 | 229.17 | .52 |

[1] P = probability of collecting.

Thus, if the objective of management is to maximize the hospital's cash receipts, the efforts of the credit and collection department should be focused on age categories that have the highest expected payoff, and, if we rank the expected payoffs, ordinally, it can be seen that the collection should concentrate on accounts that are 30 to 40 days old first, accounts less than 30 days old second, accounts more than 70 days old third, etc.

On the other hand, if management's objective is to reduce the *number* of accounts receivable, as opposed to their *value*, it should develop a different set of expectations. In this case, the number of accounts associated with each age group that management expects to collect is given by

$$E(N_i) = P_i N_i \qquad (6.6)$$

where

$E(N_i)$ = expected number of accounts collected,
$P_i$    = probability of collection in category $i$,
$N_i$    = number of accounts in category $i$.

Performing the indicated calculation for each category and ranking the results ordinally, we find the expected payoffs are as follows:

| Age Category | $E(N_i)$ | Ordinal Ranking |
|---|---|---|
| Less than 30 | 384 | 1 |
| 30–40 | 84 | 2 |
| 41–50 | 54 | 3 |
| 51–60 | 44 | 4 |
| 61–70 | 24 | 5 |
| More than 70 | 1 | 6 |

These findings suggest that management should focus efforts on the youngest accounts first, accounts 30 to 40 days old second, accounts 41 to 50 days old third, etc.

This discussion should not be interpreted to mean that the credit and collection department should ignore age categories with a low ordinal ranking. Rather, standard collection procedures should be applied to all age categories, with special or additional attention to those with a high ordinal ranking.

As seen throughout this section, the primary purpose of managing outstanding receivables is to reduce the time required to convert the account into cash. A closely related problem is estimating the magnitude and timing of payments on the institution's receivables by patients or their third party representatives. The next section is devoted to this issue.

## 6.6 ESTIMATION OF CASH RECEIPTS

A primary function of management is financial planning and forecasting. Of particular importance to ensuring the financial viability and solvency of the institution is the availability of cash to meet currently maturing obligations. Given that the realization of outstanding receivables represents a major source of cash, an estimation of these receipts is important in ensuring the solvency of the hospital. This section considers techniques of estimating the cash from payments on receivables by institutional and noninstitutional sources.

### 6.6.1 Institutional Sources

As noted earlier, two major problems in the management of accounts receivable involve the timing and the magnitude of the corresponding cash flows during a given period. Closely related to the magnitude of such flows is the probability that an account will result in a bad debt or in full or partial payment. The institutional components of the accounts receivable generated by hospitals in the United States and Canada were summarized in Table 6-1. With regard to these third party payers, it seems reasonable to assume that the probability of receiving payment in full is equal to one, so the probability that one of these accounts will result in a bad debt is zero. Thus, the problem confronting management when estimating these cash flows is not confounded by the possibility that one of these accounts will be uncollectable.

Assuming that management is certain of receiving payment in full from the third parties summarized in Table 6-1, a simple model based on the principles of mathematical expectation may be used when estimating cash receipts from these sources. For illustration, assume that

1. the accounts receivable cycle for this category of receivables has been found to be 30 days;
2. the potential pay period extends from day 31 to day 35 (i.e., the hospital never receives payment before the 31st day nor later than the 35th day);
3. the hospital submits bills amounting to $K$ each day and the third party payer begins to process the bill immediately after receipt (note: $K$ may assume the value zero);
4. for each day during the potential pay period the probability of receiving payment has been computed to be $P_1, P_2, P_3, P_4, P_5$, and the sum of these probabilities is equal to one. Here the probabilities $P_1, \cdots, P_5$ are the relative frequencies with which payment is received during each day of the potential pay period;

5. management wants to estimate the cash flows for a planning period that corresponds to the potential pay period associated with the submission represented by $\$K_t$.

These assumptions are summarized in Figure 6-2. As this shows, $\$K_t$ are submitted for payment at time $t$ and pass through the potential pay period of day 31 to day 35 that corresponds to the planning period. Since the sum of the probabilities $P_1$, $P_2$, $P_3$, $P_4$, and $P_5$ equals one by assumption, the cash inflow during the planning period associated with the submission of $\$K_t$ at time $t$ is given by:

$$(P_1 + P_2 + P_3 + P_4 + P_5)\$K_t = \$K_t \qquad (6.7)$$

Recall, however, that $\$K$ are submitted for payment daily, which implies that $\$K_t$ represents only a portion of the expected cash receipts.

Thus, to obtain an accurate estimate of the cash receipts expected during the planning period, management must consider bills submitted before and after time $t$. Using time $t$ as the base period, we may depict the submission of bills before and after time $t$ as follows:

| Day | Value of Bills Submitted |
|-----|--------------------------|
| $t - 4$ | $\$K_{t-4}$ |
| $t - 3$ | $\$K_{t-3}$ |
| $t - 2$ | $\$K_{t-2}$ |
| $t - 1$ | $\$K_{t-1}$ |
| $t$ | $\$K_t$ |
| $t + 1$ | $\$K_{t+1}$ |
| $t + 2$ | $\$K_{t+2}$ |
| $t + 3$ | $\$K_{t+3}$ |
| $t + 4$ | $\$K_{t+4}$ |

Here, the subscripts $t + j$ and $t - j$ for $j = 1, \cdots, 4$ refer to the date on which the submission occurs. Also note that $\$K_{t-j}$ and $\$K_{t+j}$ need not equal $\$K_{t-i}$ and $\$K_{t+i}$ respectively, for $i \neq j$. Rather, the value of the bills submitted for payment will reflect the volume of care rendered prior to the submission date.

**Figure 6-2** Mathematical Expectation of Accounts Receivable

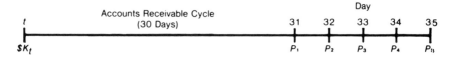

Now, consider the relation between the various potential pay periods associated with billings before and after time $t$ and the planning period. The potential pay period of $\$K_{t-1}$ in relation to the planning period is presented in Figure 6-3. As can be seen, the second day of the potential pay period of $\$K_{t-1}$ corresponds to the first day of the planning period and the third day of the potential pay period to the second day of the planning period. Similarly, the fifth day of the potential pay period of $\$K_{t-1}$ corresponds to the fourth day of the planning period. During the planning period, then, we would expect to receive

$$(P_2 + P_3 + P_4 + P_5)\$K_{t-1}$$

from third parties in payment of the bills amounting to $\$K_{t-1}$ that were submitted on day $t - 1$. Using a similar analysis we would expect to receive

$$(P_3 + P_4 + P_5)\$K_{t-2}$$

during the planning period. Here, however, the expected cash receipt of $(P_3 + P_4 + P_5)\$K_{t-2}$ is related to the bills amounting to $\$K_{t-2}$ that were submitted on day $t - 2$. A similar analysis can be used in deriving a set of expectations for the other bills submitted before and after time $t$. For example, payments expected during the planning period on bills amounting to $\$K_{t+3}$ submitted on day $t + 3$ are given by

$$(P_1 + P_2)\$K_{t+3}$$

As should be verified, this expectation is based on the finding that the first day of the potential pay period corresponds to the fourth day of the planning period, while the second day of the potential pay period of $\$K_{t+3}$ corresponds to the last day of the planning period.

After making all such calculations and rearranging the resulting data slightly, management may estimate the cash flows during each day of the planning period. As can be seen in Table 6-4, payments expected on day 1 of the planning period are given by

---

**Figure 6-3** Relationship of Pay and Planning Periods

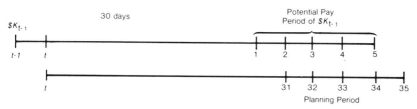

$$P_1 \$K_t + P_2 \$K_{t-1} + P_3 \$K_{t-2} + P_4 \$K_{t-3} + P_5 \$K_{t-4}$$

which is nothing more than column summation. Similarly, the totals of the other columns provide an estimate of the cash receipts for the remaining days of the planning period. Summing over all days in the planning period gives an estimate of the total cash receipts expected during that time. Such an estimate is given by

$$E(CI) = \$K_{t-4}(P_5) + \$K_{t-3}(P_4 + P_5) + \$K_{t-2}(P_3 + P_4 + P_5)$$

$$+ \$K_{t-1}(P_2 + P_3 + P_4 + P_5) + \$K_t(P_1 + P_2 + P_3 + P_4 + P_5)$$

$$+ \$K_{t+1}(P_1 + P_2 + P_3 + P_4) + \$K_{t+2}(P_1 + P_2 + P_3)$$

$$+ \$K_{t+3}(P_1 + P_2) + \$K_{t+4}(P_1) \qquad (6.8)$$

Several other comments concerning Table 6-4 are in order. The diagonal of the table lists the expected payments associated with the submission of bills amounting to $\$K_t$ on day $t$. Thus, summing elements along the diagonal gives cash receipts of $\$K_t$ that management knows with certainty will be received during the planning period. Elements above and to the right of the diagonal correspond to expected payments generated by the submission of bills after time $t$. Similarly, the elements below and to the left of the diagonal correspond to expected payments generated by the submission of bills before time $t$.

The calculations in Table 6-4 may be simplified considerably when the notation and operations of matrix algebra are employed. To illustrate, we let

$$\mathbf{p}' = \begin{bmatrix} P_1 & P_2 & P_3 & P_4 & P_5 \end{bmatrix} \quad \text{and}$$

$$\mathbf{K} = \begin{bmatrix} K_t & K_{t+1} & K_{t+2} & K_{t+3} & K_{t+4} \\ K_{t-1} & K_t & K_{t+1} & K_{t+2} & K_{t+3} \\ K_{t-2} & K_{t-1} & K_t & K_{t+1} & K_{t+2} \\ K_{t-3} & K_{t-2} & K_{t-1} & K_t & K_{t+1} \\ K_{t-4} & K_{t-3} & K_{t-2} & K_{t-1} & K_t \end{bmatrix}$$

As should be verified, the equation

$$\mathbf{c} = \mathbf{p}'\mathbf{K} \qquad (6.9)$$

**Table 6-4** Expected Cash Flows During Each Day of the Planning Period

| Day of Potential Pay Period | Day of Planning Period | | | | |
|---|---|---|---|---|---|
| | 1 | 2 | 3 | 4 | 5 |
| 1 | $P_1 \, \$K_t$ | $P_1 \, \$K_{t+1}$ | $P_1 \, \$K_{t+2}$ | $P_1 \, \$K_{t+3}$ | $P_1 \, \$K_{t+4}$ |
| 2 | $P_2 \, \$K_{t-1}$ | $P_2 \, \$K_t$ | $P_2 \, \$K_{t+1}$ | $P_2 \, \$K_{t+2}$ | $P_2 \, \$K_{t+3}$ |
| 3 | $P_3 \, \$K_{t-2}$ | $P_3 \, \$K_{t-1}$ | $P_3 \, \$K_t$ | $P_3 \, \$K_{t+1}$ | $P_3 \, \$K_{t+2}$ |
| 4 | $P_4 \, \$K_{t-3}$ | $P_4 \, \$K_{t-2}$ | $P_4 \, \$K_{t-1}$ | $P_4 \, \$K_t$ | $P_4 \, \$K_{t+1}$ |
| 5 | $P_5 \, \$K_{t-4}$ | $P_5 \, \$K_{t-3}$ | $P_5 \, \$K_{t-2}$ | $P_5 \, \$K_{t-1}$ | $P_5 \, \$K_t$ |

yields a row vector that has the following interpretation. The first element corresponds to the cash flow expected on the first day of the planning period, the second element the second day, and so on. Summing the elements of the row vector **c** therefore provides an estimate of the cash inflows expected from third party payers during the planning period.

The importance of these detailed calculations might be questioned. However, it should be recognized that when the principles of mathematical expectation are used in estimating expected cash receipts during the planning period, management explicitly takes into account the distribution and amount of previous billings as well as the probability distribution indicating the likelihood of receiving payment on a given day. Implicit in this analysis is the notion that expected cash receipts are influenced by the corresponding distribution of payments as well as by the distribution depicting the probability of receiving the corresponding cash inflow. To show how the distribution depicting the probability of receiving payment and the distribution of previous billings might influence expected cash flows, consider the following situation. Using the same assumptions as described earlier, suppose that the distribution of billings is as follows:

| Day | Value of Bills Submitted |
|---|---|
| $t - 4$ | $24,000 |
| $t - 3$ | 20,000 |
| $t - 2$ | 16,000 |
| $t - 1$ | 14,000 |
| $t$ | 12,000 |
| $t + 1$ | 10,000 |
| $t + 2$ | 8,000 |
| $t + 3$ | 6,000 |
| $t + 4$ | 4,000 |
| | 114,000 |

Further, suppose that the distribution depicting the probability of receiving payment during the potential pay period is given by

$$P_1 = .6$$
$$P_2 = .2$$
$$P_3 = .1$$
$$P_4 = .05$$
$$P_5 = .05$$

Given these distributions, the expected cash inflow during each day of the planning period is found by

$$\mathbf{c}_1' = [.6 \quad .2 \quad .1 \quad .05 \quad .05] \begin{bmatrix} \$12,000 & \$10,000 & \$8,000 & \$6,000 & \$4,000 \\ 14,000 & 12,000 & 10,000 & 8,000 & 6,000 \\ 16,000 & 14,000 & 12,000 & 10,000 & 8,000 \\ 20,000 & 16,000 & 14,000 & 12,000 & 10,000 \\ 24,000 & 20,000 & 16,000 & 14,000 & 12,000 \end{bmatrix}$$

$$= [\$13,800 \quad \$11,600 \quad \$9,500 \quad \$7,500 \quad \$5,500]$$

On the basis of these calculations, the hospital would expect to receive $13,800 on the first day of the planning period, $11,600 on the second day, $9,500 on the third day, and so on. Summing all elements in the row vector **c**, we find that management expects to receive a total of $47,900 from third party payers during the planning period.

Now, consider a slightly different situation. Suppose that the distribution of billings is the same as before, but the distribution depicting the probability of receiving payment is given by

$$P_1 = .05$$
$$P_2 = .05$$
$$P_3 = .05$$
$$P_4 = .05$$
$$P_5 = .8$$

Under this assumption, the cash receipts expected during the planning period are given by

$$\mathbf{c}_2' = [.05 \quad .05 \quad .05 \quad .05 \quad .8] \begin{bmatrix} \$12,000 & \$10,000 & \$8,000 & \$6,000 & \$4,000 \\ 14,000 & 12,000 & 10,000 & 8,000 & 6,000 \\ 16,000 & 14,000 & 12,000 & 10,000 & 8,000 \\ 20,000 & 16,000 & 14,000 & 12,000 & 10,000 \\ 24,000 & 20,000 & 16,000 & 14,000 & 12,000 \end{bmatrix}$$

$$= [\$22,300 \quad \$18,600 \quad \$15,000 \quad \$13,000 \quad \$11,000]$$

Summing the elements of the row vector $c_2'$, the total cash receipts expected during the planning period are \$79,900, as opposed to the \$47,900 estimated earlier.

Suppose further that a projection of cash needs indicates that \$150,000 will be required during the planning period. Also assume that, apart from the cash from institutional payers, \$100,000 is available to the institution. Thus, depending on which distribution depicting the probability of receiving payment is appropriate, the hospital can expect to have either a cash surplus of \$29,900 or a cash shortage of \$2,100. In the first case, management can evaluate alternate investment opportunities in which to invest the expected surplus to earn additional income, while in the second, management should investigate alternate sources of credit that may be required to finance the shortage. As can be seen from this example, then, when both the distribution of billings and the distribution depicting the probability of receiving payment are considered, management may improve both its financial forecasts and the institution's financial plans.

The relationship of financial forecasting and planning to operational results should be mentioned. If, on the basis of the financial forecast, a cash shortage is expected, management should explore sources of funding to satisfy the cash needs. Obviously, such an investigation facilitates the selection of the least cost alternative, which in turn reduces the hospital's operating cost. Alternatively, if a cash surplus is expected, management can investigate investment possibilities and select the security that provides a maximum rate of return subject to the risk that the administration is willing to assume. Obviously, such a procedure also will have a favorable effect on the operating position of the hospital.

## 6.6.2 Noninstitutional Sources

When cash flows from noninstitutional sources are estimated, an additional factor must be considered. In the case of institutional accounts receivable, the probability that a debt will prove uncollectable was seen to be zero. When estimating cash flow from noninstitutional accounts receivable, management must recognize the possibility that some patients will not pay and that it may be necessary to write off those receivables as bad debts.

Hence the problem of estimating the cash receipts for the categories of accounts receivable summarized in Table 6-2 is complicated by the possibility that an account may prove uncollectable. Thus, in addition to the problems of estimating the timing and magnitude of cash receipts, management also must estimate the value of outstanding uncollectable accounts.

These concerns are complicated further by the nature of the accounts in Table 6-2. In many situations, only a portion of the hospital bill represents the patient's financial responsibility. In the United States, many of the receivables in this group are generated through deductibles or coinsurance charges as well as hospital services that are in excess of the maximum benefits offered by a third party payer. In Canadian hospitals, the majority of the outstanding receivables that are the responsibility of the patient are generated through differential and authorized charges as well as through charges for the use of services that are not insured under the provincial plan. These observations suggest that the receivables in Table 6-2 will be large in number but small in value. As a result, the technique for estimating cash receipts from this source must accommodate accounts that are large in number but small in dollar volume. The method also must be capable of estimating: (1) the timing of cash receipts, (2) the magnitude of cash receipts, and (3) the value of receivables that will prove to be uncollectable. As will be seen, an absorbing Markov chain is such a technique.

### 6.6.2.1 Introduction to Markov Chains

Markov chains are a specific class of probability models that are appropriate to a broad spectrum of decision-making problems. When a Markov chain is used, the set of variables under examination is divided into several clearly defined and *mutually exclusive* states. At any point in time, the system is said to be in one of these states. Assume that at a moment in time the system is in state A. The major assumption of Markov chain analysis is that the probability of observing the system in the same state or one of the other states at the next point in time depends only on the state in which the system is found currently. That is, the probability depicting the transition of the system from one state to another or remaining in the same state is independent of how the system reached its present state.

To illustrate this technique, consider the problem of estimating the probability that a person will require health care. The human body might be viewed as a system composed of several subsystems such as respiratory, digestive, and cardiovascular systems, central nervous system, etc. In turn, the individual may be healthy, in which case the system and all of the subsystems are operating properly; or the person may be in need of medical care, in which case one or more of the subsystems are not operating properly and are in need of "repair."

Regarding the human body as a system, suppose that, if the individual is healthy today there is a probability of .8 that the person will be healthy tomorrow and a probability of .2 that medical care will be required tomorrow. Also assume that the human body has a self-adjusting mechanism that operates imperfectly so that, if the person requires medical care today, there is a probability of .6 that the individual will be healthy tomorrow and a probability of .4 that the person will require medical care tomorrow. If we let state 1 correspond to the situation in which the person is healthy and state 2 represent the situation in which the individual is in need of medical care, we may summarize these assumptions as seen in Table 6-5.

**Table 6-5** Probabilities Involving the Body's Health

| From ➔ To | Healthy (State 1) | In Need of Medical Care (State 2) |
|---|---|---|
| Healthy (State 1) | .8 | .2 |
| In Need of Medical Care (State 2) | .6 | .4 |

The probabilities in Table 6-5 are conditional and may be written as $P(j|i)$ or $P_{ij}$ where $i$ and $j$ correspond to one of the designated states. The interpretation of $P_{ij}$ is as follows: If the system is in state $i$ at the beginning of the period, $P_{ij}$ is the probability that the system will be in state $j$ at the end of the period.

The information in Table 6-5 may be summarized in matrix form as follows

$$\mathbf{P} = \begin{bmatrix} P_{11} & P_{12} \\ P_{21} & P_{22} \end{bmatrix} \qquad (6.10)$$

This is referred to as a transitional probability matrix. As before, $P_{11}$ corresponds to the probability that the system will be in state 1 at the end of the period, given that it was in state 1 at the beginning. Similarly, $P_{12}$ is the probability that the system will be in state 2 at the end of the period if it was in state 1 at the start. In terms of our example, we find that

$$\mathbf{P} = \begin{bmatrix} .8 & .2 \\ .6 & .4 \end{bmatrix} \qquad (6.11)$$

Suppose we know with certainty that the person is healthy at the beginning of the initial period (period 0). Thus, at that time there is a probability of one that the individual is healthy and a probability of zero that medical care is required. This assumption may be summarized by introducing a vector that consists of the initial state probabilities. Thus, we define the initial state probability vector $\mathbf{x}'_0$ by

$$\mathbf{x}'_0 = \begin{bmatrix} 1 & 0 \end{bmatrix} \qquad (6.12)$$

where the elements 1 and 0 represent the probabilities of the individual's being healthy or requiring medical care respectively. The subscript 0 in $\mathbf{x}'_0$ refers to the period of reference that, in this case, is the beginning of the initial period. Hereafter, we refer to state probability vectors as state vectors.

Given the assumption of independence introduced earlier, the state vector for period 1 (i.e., $x'_1$) is given by

$$x'_1 = x'_0 P$$

$$= [1 \quad 0] \begin{bmatrix} .8 & .2 \\ .6 & .4 \end{bmatrix}$$

$$= [.8 \quad .2]$$

Thus, the state vector $x'_1$ indicates that in period 1 there is a probability of .8 and a probability of .2 that the individual will be healthy or will require medical care, respectively. Similarly, we find the state vector for period 2 is

$$x'_2 = x'_1 P = x'_0 P^2$$

$$= [.76 \quad .24]$$

while the state vector for period 3 is

$$x'_3 = x'_2 P = x'_0 P^3$$

$$= [.752 \quad .248]$$

In general, then, we find

$$x'_n = x'_0 P^n$$

which implies that the state vector for the person in period $n$ is equal to the product of the state vector in period 0 and the $n$th power of the transitional probability matrix.

The behavior of the system over time as described by the transitional probability matrix and the sequence of state vectors $x'_0, x'_1, \cdots, x'_n$ is called a Markov chain. An important aspect of Markov chain is the long-run behavior of the system after the effects of the initial conditions have been dissipated. Suppose that after a very large number of periods (transitions), the state vector $x'_n$ is equal to the state vector $x'_{n-1}$ and is independent of $x'_0$. Eliminating the subscript, we call the vector $x'$ the steady state vector for the Markov chain described by $P$ and the elements of $x'$ are the *steady state probabilities*. Thus, the steady state vector $x'$ is the state vector that satisfies the equation

$$x' = x' P \qquad (6.13)$$

Returning to our example, we assumed that the system started in state 1 ($x'_0$ = [1   0]) and obtained

$$x'_1 = [.8 \quad .2]$$

$$x'_2 = [.76 \quad .24]$$

$$x'_3 = [.752 \quad .248]$$

Hence, it appears that the state vector eventually will converge to [.75   .25].

To confirm these results, assume the system started in state 2 ($x'_0$ = [0   1]). Here, we find

$$x'_1 = x'_0 P = [.6 \quad .4]$$

$$x'_2 = x'_0 P^2 = [.72 \quad .28]$$

$$x'_3 = x'_0 P^3 = [.744 \quad .256]$$

which also implies that the state vector will converge to [.75   .25] regardless of the initial state.

Consider now the steady state vector that may be written in the form $x' = x'P$. Employing the transitional matrix $P$, the equation $x' = x'P$ may be expressed in the form

$$x' = x' \begin{bmatrix} .8 & .2 \\ .6 & .4 \end{bmatrix}$$

Letting $x' = [P^*_1 \quad P^*_2]$, where $P^*_1$ and $P^*_2$ correspond to the steady state probabilities, we may write

$$[P^*_1 \quad P^*_2] \begin{bmatrix} .8 & .2 \\ .6 & .4 \end{bmatrix} = \begin{bmatrix} .8P^*_1 + .6P^*_2 \\ .2P^*_1 + .4P^*_2 \end{bmatrix}$$

As a result, we find that

$$P^*_1 = .8P^*_1 + .6P^*_2$$

$$P^*_2 = .2P^*_1 + .4P^*_2 \qquad \qquad (6.14.1)$$

One of these equations is redundant because they both reduce to

$$P_1^* = \frac{.6}{.2} P_2^* = 3P_2^* \qquad (6.14.2)$$

$$P_1^* - 3P_2^* = 0 \qquad (6.14.3)$$

However, since the system must be found in one of the designated states, the sum of the steady state probabilities must equal one, which implies that

$$P_1^* + P_2^* = 1$$

Using this fact in combination with Equation 6.14.3, we may now express the equations

$$P_1^* - 3P_2^* = 0$$

$$P_1^* + P_2^* = 1$$

in matrix notation as follows

$$\begin{bmatrix} 1 & -3 \\ 1 & 1 \end{bmatrix} \begin{bmatrix} P_1^* \\ P_2^* \end{bmatrix} = \begin{bmatrix} 0 \\ 1 \end{bmatrix}$$

This system of equations has the solution

$$\begin{bmatrix} P_1^* \\ P_2^* \end{bmatrix} = \begin{bmatrix} 1 & -3 \\ 1 & 1 \end{bmatrix}^{-1} \begin{bmatrix} 0 \\ 1 \end{bmatrix}$$

$$= \begin{bmatrix} \frac{1}{4} & \frac{3}{4} \\ -\frac{1}{4} & \frac{1}{4} \end{bmatrix} \begin{bmatrix} 0 \\ 1 \end{bmatrix} = \begin{bmatrix} \frac{3}{4} \\ \frac{1}{4} \end{bmatrix}$$

These findings suggest that the long-term probability of the person's being in state 1 (i.e., healthy) is .75 and of being in state 2 (i.e., in need of medical care) is .25. These results are independent of the state assumed during the initial period.

### 6.6.2.2 Estimation Procedures

On the basis of this understanding, Markov chain analysis may be applied to the problem of estimating the timing and magnitude of the cash inflows from payments by patients on their outstanding accounts. The primary purpose of such an analysis is to estimate: (1) the timing of the cash receipts, (2) the magnitude of the cash receipts, and (3) the value of the uncollectables associated with the accounts summarized in Table 6-2.

The outstanding account of a patient may be quite active. For example, the individual may visit the outpatient clinic of the hospital several times during the month and, on each occasion, may use services that are not insured by a third party payer. In addition, the individual may make several payments to the hospital during the same period. In most cases, a payment by the patient is applied to the oldest account first, with any extra amount being applied to the next oldest charge, and so on.

For example, an account that consists only of current charges will be regarded as zero months old. If the oldest charge is one month delinquent, the account is one month old, and so on for the remaining possibilities. If a patient makes no payment during a month, the age of the account is said to have increased by one month. On the other hand, if the patient makes payments during the month, but they are insufficient to cover the oldest account, then at the end of the month the age of account has increased by one month. Similarly, if the patient makes a payment equal to or greater than the oldest charge, the age of the account remains stationary or is reduced to some age less than what it was at the beginning of the month.

Similar to the discussion in section 6.6.2.1, the accounts receivable of the hospital are described in terms of well-defined and mutually exclusive states. In this section, however, transitional or nonabsorbing states and absorbing or trapping states are used to describe the institution's accounts receivable. Accounts that are current or one month old are said to be in a transitional or nonabsorbing state while accounts that are paid in full or are written off as bad debts are in a trapping or absorbing state. The reason for this distinction is made clear later in this section.

Similar to the earlier discussion, we use the notation $P_{ij}$ to represent the transition of an account from state $i$ to state $j$ in one month. Here, as before, we assume that the transitional probability $P_{ij}$ depends only on the state of the account at the beginning of the period. For example, letting 0 and 1 correspond to current accounts and accounts that are one month delinquent, respectively, $P_{01}$ represents the probability that an account consisting only of current charges at the beginning of the period will be one month delinquent at the end. Similarly, the notation $P_{00}$ represents the probability that an account consisting only of current charges at the beginning of the period will involve only current charges at the end. In this situation, the patient might pay all charges that were due at the beginning of the period and incur additional charges during the period.

To complete the notation regarding the states in the Markov chain, we use the symbol $F$ to represent accounts that are paid in full and the letter $B$ to represent accounts that are written off as uncollectable. Employing this notation, we observe that $P_{0F}$ corresponds to the probability that an account that consists of only current charges will be paid in full and $P_{1B}$ to the probability that an account that is one month delinquent will result in a bad debt.

For illustration, assume that the hospital follows the practice of writing off as bad debts those accounts that are more than one month delinquent. As a result, there are four states that are relevant to this analysis (0, 1, $F$, or $B$) and we may summarize the transitional or conditional probabilities pertaining to these states in matrix form as follows

$$
P = \begin{bmatrix} P_{FF} & P_{FB} & P_{F0} & P_{F1} \\ P_{BF} & P_{BB} & P_{B0} & P_{B1} \\ P_{0F} & P_{0B} & P_{00} & P_{01} \\ P_{1F} & P_{1B} & P_{10} & P_{11} \end{bmatrix}
$$

Consider first the probabilities that correspond to accounts consisting only of current charges at the beginning of the month. On the basis of historical data, suppose that management has estimated $P_{0B}$, $P_{0F}$, $P_{00}$, and $P_{01}$ as follows

$$P_{0F} = .8$$

$$P_{0B} = 0$$

$$P_{00} = .1$$

$$P_{01} = .1$$

Here, $P_{0B}$ is equal to zero, a result that deserves clarification. As will be recalled, we assumed that only accounts more than one month delinquent are written off as bad debts. As a result, it is not possible for an account to pass from state 0 to state $B$ in one month. Given that it is not possible to write off a current account as a bad debt, the probability $P_{0B}$ must equal zero. In a similar fashion, suppose that the probabilities corresponding to an account that is one month old have been estimated as follows:

$$P_{1A} = .7$$

$$P_{1B} = .1$$

$$P_{10} = .1$$

$$P_{11} = .1$$

Consider next the probabilities that correspond to accounts in one of the absorbing states at the beginning of the period. Here, we assume that, if a patient pays the account in full and new charges are incurred in a given period, we create a new account. As a consequence, if an account is paid in full at the beginning of the period, it must be paid in full at the end of the period. Thus, when an account begins the period in state $F$, we have

$$P_{FF} = 1$$

$$P_{FB} = 0$$

$$P_{F0} = 0$$

$$P_{F1} = 0$$

Similarly, we assume that if an account becomes a bad debt it remains in state $B$. Thus, we have

$$P_{BF} = 0$$

$$P_{BB} = 1$$

$$P_{B0} = 0$$

$$P_{B1} = 0$$

We may summarize these assumptions by forming the transitional probability matrix

$$\mathbf{P} = \begin{bmatrix} 1 & 0 & 0 & 0 \\ 0 & 1 & 0 & 0 \\ .8 & 0 & .1 & .1 \\ .7 & .1 & .1 & .1 \end{bmatrix} \tag{6.15}$$

Several properties concerning the transitional probability matrix are worthy of note. First, the probabilities in the matrix satisfy the condition

$$0 \leqslant \mathbf{P}_{ij} \leqslant 1$$

which implies that the probabilities lie between zero and one. Further, since the account must remain in one of the states or move to one of the other possible states by the end of the month, it follows that the sum of the probabilities in a row must equal one. Thus, each row constitutes a conditional probability distribution for which the conditions

$$0 \leq P_{ij} \leq 1$$

and

$$\Sigma P_{ij} = 1$$

are satisfied.

States $F$ and $B$ are referred to as absorbing states because, once an account is paid in full or becomes a bad debt, it is said to have been absorbed (i.e., the account cannot move from these two states). If a Markov chain is characterized by at least one absorbing state and it is possible to move from the transient states to the absorbing state, it is called an absorbing Markov chain. The probability matrix introduced above, therefore, is an absorbing Markov chain.

Returning to the earlier example, let us examine the transitional probability matrix after the passage of one month. If an account starts in state 0, the possible states in which it might be found after two months are shown in the tree diagram in Figure 6-4. The corresponding probabilities also are shown in this figure. In the following, we denote the probability that an account that starts in state $i$ will be in state $j$ after $n$ months by $P_{ij}^n$. As a result, $P_{00}^2$ is the probability that an account that starts in state 0 will be found in state 0 after two months. Referring to the tree diagram, we find that there are essentially four paths that lead to this result: 0 to $F$ to 0; 0 to $B$ to 0; 0 to 0 to 0, and 0 to 1 to 0. The probabilities of these four paths' occurring are as follows:

$$
\begin{array}{llll}
0 \rightarrow F \rightarrow 0 = (.8)\,(0) & = & 0 \\
0 \rightarrow B \rightarrow 0 = (0)\,(0) & = & 0 \\
0 \rightarrow 0 \rightarrow 0 = (.1)\,(.1) & = & .01 \\
0 \rightarrow 1 \rightarrow 0 = (1.)\,(.1) & = & \underline{.01} \\
& & .02
\end{array}
$$

This result is equivalent to

$$P_{00}^2 = \begin{bmatrix} .8 & 0 & .1 & .1 \end{bmatrix} \begin{bmatrix} 0 \\ 0 \\ .1 \\ .1 \end{bmatrix} = .02$$

**Figure 6-4** Tree Diagram Showing Possible Paths a Current Account May Follow during Two Months

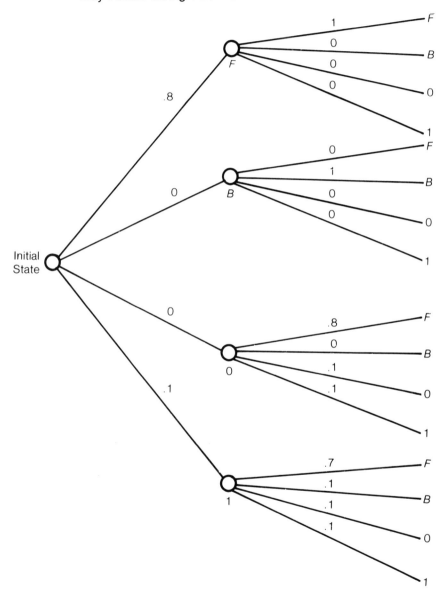

Proceeding in a similar fashion, we find

$$P_{01}^2 = \begin{bmatrix} .8 & 0 & .1 & .1 \end{bmatrix} \begin{bmatrix} 0 \\ 0 \\ .1 \\ .1 \end{bmatrix} = .02$$

while

$$P_{0F}^2 = \begin{bmatrix} .8 & 0 & .1 & .1 \end{bmatrix} \begin{bmatrix} 1 \\ 0 \\ .8 \\ .7 \end{bmatrix} = .95$$

and

$$P_{0B}^2 = \begin{bmatrix} .8 & 0 & .1 & .1 \end{bmatrix} \begin{bmatrix} 0 \\ 1 \\ 0 \\ .1 \end{bmatrix} = .01$$

As can be verified, the sum $P_{00}^2 + P_{01}^2 + P_{0F}^2 + P_{0B}^2$ is equal to one. The element $P_{0B}^2$ is obtained by multiplying elements appearing in the corresponding row by successive columns in the matrix $\mathbf{P}$. In general, then, to find $\mathbf{P}^2$, which is the transitional probability matrix after two periods, we need only compute

$$\mathbf{P} \cdot \mathbf{P}$$

which yields

$$\mathbf{P}^2 = \begin{bmatrix} 1 & 0 & 0 & 0 \\ 0 & 1 & 0 & 0 \\ .95 & .01 & .02 & .02 \\ .85 & .11 & .02 & .02 \end{bmatrix}$$

Several aspects of the matrix $\mathbf{P}^2$ should be observed. First, compare the probabilities $P_{ij}^2$ and $P_{ij}$ where $i$ and $j$ are nonabsorbing states. These comparisons suggest that

$$P_{00}^2 < P_{00}$$

$$P_{01}^2 < P_{01}$$

$$P_{10}^2 < P_{10}$$

$$P_{11}^2 < P_{11}$$

On the other hand, if we compared $P_{ik}^2$ with $P_{ik}$, where $i$ corresponds to a nonabsorbing state and $k$ is an absorbing state, we find that

$$P_{0F}^2 > P_{0F}$$

$$P_{0B}^2 > P_{0B}$$

$$P_{1F}^2 > P_{1F}$$

$$P_{1B}^2 > P_{1B}$$

These comparisons imply that the probability of an account's moving from one transient state to another decreases as the number of periods increases, while the probability it will move from a transitional state to an absorbing state increases as the number of transitions increases. Consequently, as $n$ approaches $\infty$, $P_{00} + P_{01}$ approaches zero while $P_{0F} + P_{0B}$ approaches one. Similarly, as $n$ approaches $\infty$, $P_{10} + P_{11}$ approaches zero while $P_{1F} + P_{1B}$ approaches one.

With these properties in mind, we turn to the estimation of the number of months that will pass before an account enters an absorbing state. Consider as an example the average number of months an account is expected to begin the period in one transient state, say current, and will be one month delinquent at the end of the period. Recognizing that $0 < P_{01} < 1$ and that $P_{01}^n$ approaches zero, this expectation is given by

$$P_{01}(1) + P_{01}^2(1) + \cdots + P_{01}^n(1) \tag{6.16}$$

where the values in parentheses represent a period of one month.

Such a solution might be expressed more generally by letting $X$ represent a number that satisfies the condition $0 < X < 1$. We assert that the sum

$$S = 1 + X + \cdots + X^n \qquad (6.17)$$

may be expressed by $1/1 - X$. This result is obtained by multiplying this sum by $X$ and subtracting the results from both sides of Equation 6.17. Thus, we find that

$$S - XS = 1 - X^{n-1}$$

and

$$S = \frac{1 - X^{n-1}}{1 - X}$$

Recalling that $0 < X < 1$, it will be observed that $X^{n-1}$ approaches zero as $n$ increases indefinitely. Hence, $S = 1/1 - X$ as mentioned earlier.

We might obtain a similar result by partitioning the matrix $\mathbf{P}$ as follows:

$$\mathbf{P} = \left[\begin{array}{cc|cc} 1 & 0 & 0 & 0 \\ 0 & 1 & 0 & 0 \\ \hline .8 & 0 & .1 & .1 \\ .7 & .1 & .1 & .1 \end{array}\right] = \left[\begin{array}{c|c} \mathbf{I} & \mathbf{O} \\ \hline \mathbf{X} & \mathbf{W} \end{array}\right]$$

The submatrix in the northwest corner of $P$ (**I**) consists solely of the absorbing states and will be recognized as an identity matrix. The matrix in the northeast corner (**O**) consist of zeros and is referred to as a null matrix. In the southeast quadrant is

the $2 \times 2$ matrix $\begin{bmatrix} .1 & .1 \\ .1 & .1 \end{bmatrix}$ that contains the transitional probabilities that pertain

to the nonabsorbing states; this is labeled matrix **W**. The final submatrix, in the southwest quadrant, consists solely of the transitional probabilities that relate the nonabsorbing states to the trapping states. This is labeled matrix **X**.

Similar to our earlier work in which we found that $S = (1 - X)^{-1}$, we may express the sum

$$\mathbf{I} + \mathbf{W} + \mathbf{W}^2 + \cdots + \mathbf{W}^n$$

in the form $(\mathbf{I} - \mathbf{W})^{-1}$ where $n$ is allowed to increase indefinitely.[1] Implicit in this expression is the multiplication of the identity matrix by $\mathbf{W}$, $\mathbf{W}^2$, $\cdots$, $\mathbf{W}^n$.

---

[1] See appendix at the end of this chapter for a discussion of this finding.

In this case, the identity matrix corresponds to a period of time (i.e., one month) just as the values in the parentheses of Equation 6.17 represented one month. Hence, $(\mathbf{I} - \mathbf{W})^{-1}$ provides the basis for estimating the length of time an account will remain in a given transient state before it is paid in full or written off as a bad debt.

The next task, then, is to find the matrix $\mathbf{I} - \mathbf{W}$, and derive its inverse. Referring to the first set of calculations, we find that $\mathbf{I} - \mathbf{W}$ is given by

$$\begin{bmatrix} 1 & 0 \\ 0 & 1 \end{bmatrix} - \begin{bmatrix} .1 & .1 \\ .1 & .1 \end{bmatrix} = \begin{bmatrix} .9 & -.1 \\ -.1 & .9 \end{bmatrix}$$

As can be verified by referring to Chapter 4, the inverse of $(\mathbf{I} - \mathbf{W})$ is given by

$$(\mathbf{I} - \mathbf{W})^{-1} = \frac{1}{.8} \begin{bmatrix} .9 & .1 \\ .1 & .9 \end{bmatrix}$$

$$= \begin{bmatrix} 9/8 & 1/8 \\ 1/8 & 9/8 \end{bmatrix}$$

As implied earlier, each element of $(\mathbf{I} - \mathbf{W})^{-1}$ represents the average number of months an account will remain in one of the transient states, given that it initially was found in a nonabsorbing state. For example, an account found initially in state 0 is expected to remain in a current state for 1.125 months (i.e., 9/8 months). Similarly, an account found initially in state 0 is expected to remain in state 1 for .125 months (1/8 month). The values that pertain to an account that is found initially in state 1 are given a similar interpretation.

We consider next the process of estimating the value of accounts that ultimately will result in a cash inflow and the value of those that will be written off as bad debts. Similar to the discussion in the previous section, these estimates require the steady state values assumed by the elements of the matrix $\mathbf{P}$. In deriving the required steady state probabilities, recall that the matrix $\mathbf{P}$ may be partitioned as follows

$$\mathbf{P} = \left[ \begin{array}{cc|cc} 1 & 0 & 0 & 0 \\ 0 & 1 & 0 & 0 \\ \hline .8 & 0 & .1 & .1 \\ .7 & .1 & .1 & .1 \end{array} \right] = \left[ \begin{array}{c|c} \mathbf{I} & \mathbf{O} \\ \hline \mathbf{X} & \mathbf{W} \end{array} \right]$$

Employing the partitioned matrix, we obtain $\mathbf{P}^2$ (i.e., the value of $\mathbf{P}$ after two transitions) by

$$\mathbf{P}^2 = \mathbf{P} \cdot \mathbf{P} = \left[\begin{array}{c|c} \mathbf{I} & \mathbf{O} \\ \hline \mathbf{X} & \mathbf{W} \end{array}\right]\left[\begin{array}{c|c} \mathbf{I} & \mathbf{O} \\ \hline \mathbf{X} & \mathbf{W} \end{array}\right] = \left[\begin{array}{c|c} \mathbf{I} & \mathbf{O} \\ \hline (\mathbf{I} + \mathbf{W})\mathbf{X} & \mathbf{W}^2 \end{array}\right]$$

Similarly, the matrix $\mathbf{P}^3$ is given by

$$\mathbf{P}^3 = \mathbf{P}^2 \cdot \mathbf{P} = \left[\begin{array}{c|c} \mathbf{I} & \mathbf{O} \\ \hline (\mathbf{I} + \mathbf{W})\mathbf{X} & \mathbf{W}^2 \end{array}\right]\left[\begin{array}{c|c} \mathbf{I} & \mathbf{O} \\ \hline \mathbf{X} & \mathbf{W} \end{array}\right]$$

$$= \left[\begin{array}{c|c} \mathbf{I} & \mathbf{O} \\ \hline (\mathbf{I} + \mathbf{W} + \mathbf{W}^2)\mathbf{X} & \mathbf{W}^3 \end{array}\right]$$

Observing the general pattern formed by these results, we may let the number of transitions equal $n$ and obtain $\mathbf{P}^n$ as follows

$$\mathbf{P}^n = \left[\begin{array}{c|c} \mathbf{I} & \mathbf{O} \\ \hline (\mathbf{I} + \mathbf{W} + \mathbf{W}^2 + \cdots + \mathbf{W}^{n-1})\mathbf{X} & \mathbf{W}^n \end{array}\right]$$

Recall that, as the number of transitions, $n$, increases indefinitely, $\mathbf{W}^n$ approaches zero and, when $\mathbf{W}^n = \mathbf{0}$, the appendix at the end of this chapter reveals that

$$(\mathbf{I} + \mathbf{W} + \mathbf{W}^2 + \cdots + \mathbf{W}^{n-1}) = (\mathbf{I} - \mathbf{W})^{-1}$$

Substituting $(\mathbf{I} - \mathbf{W})^{-1}$ for the sum $(\mathbf{I} + \mathbf{W} + \cdots + \mathbf{W}^{n-1})$ in $\mathbf{P}^n$ we obtain

$$\mathbf{P}^n = \left[\begin{array}{c|c} \mathbf{I} & \mathbf{O} \\ \hline (\mathbf{I} - \mathbf{W})^{-1}\mathbf{X} & \mathbf{O} \end{array}\right]$$

As seen earlier, the southwest quadrant of the matrix relates the transitional states to the absorbing states. As a consequence, the submatrix given by

$$(\mathbf{I} - \mathbf{W})^{-1}\mathbf{X}$$

represents the steady state probabilities that relate the transitional states to the absorbing states. Returning to our example, we find that

$$\mathbf{K} = (\mathbf{I} - \mathbf{W})^{-1}\mathbf{X} = \begin{bmatrix} 9/8 & 1/8 \\ 1/8 & 9/8 \end{bmatrix}\begin{bmatrix} 8/10 & 0 \\ 7/10 & 1/10 \end{bmatrix} = \begin{bmatrix} 79/80 & 1/80 \\ 71/80 & 9/80 \end{bmatrix}$$

These calculations indicate that if an account begins in state 0, the probability is 79/80 that it will be paid in full and 1/80 that it will be written off as a bad debt. On the other hand, if an account is first observed in state 1 (i.e., one month delinquent) the probability is 71/80 that it will be paid in full and 9/80 that it will be written off as a bad debt.

Each row in $\mathbf{K}$ sums to one which reflects the fact that, in the long run, the account will be absorbed. In general, this finding is characteristic of any absorbing Markov chain.

Having estimated the elements of $(\mathbf{I} - \mathbf{W})^{-1}\mathbf{X}$, let us now estimate the value of accounts that, during the month, will be paid in full and the value of those that will be written off as bad debts. Suppose that at an instant in time management knows that accounts totaling $96,000 are outstanding and that these accounts are distributed as follows

$$\text{Current accounts:} \quad \$80,000$$

$$\text{One month delinquent: } \$16,000$$

Letting

$$\mathbf{v}' = [80,000 \quad 16,000]$$

the expected collections and bad debts are given by

$$\mathbf{v}^* = \mathbf{v}'\mathbf{K}$$

$$= [80,000 \quad 16,000] \begin{bmatrix} 79/80 & 1/80 \\ 71/80 & 9/80 \end{bmatrix}$$

$$= [93,200 \quad 2,800]$$

Hence the amount we expect to collect is $93,200 and the amount expected to be uncollectable is $2,800.

In summary, this section has discussed techniques that may be used in estimating cash flows from the institutional and noninstitutional debtors of the hospital. The principles of mathematical expectation were used when estimating the cash receipts associated with the third party payers for whom the probability of a bad debt is zero. On the other hand, an absorbing Markov chain was used in estimating (1) the timing of cash receipts, (2) the value of cash receipts, and (3) the value of the bad debt expense associated with the accounts receivable of noninstitutional payers. Summing the cash expected from (1) third party payers,

(2) self-pay patients, and, in the case of the hospital that is reimbursed prospectively, (3) the amount of the prepayment, yields an estimate of the hospital's total expected cash receipts. On the basis of this understanding, the next chapter discusses cash management.

---

**REFERENCES**

Barnes, E. H. *Barnes on Credit and Collection*. Englewood Cliffs, N.J.: Prentice-Hall, Inc., 1961.

Berman, H. J., and Weeks, L. *The Financial Management of Hospitals,* 3rd ed. Ann Arbor, Mich.: Health Administration Press, 1976, Ch. 12.

Craig, C. R. "Patient Accounts Management: How a Small Hospital Does It Successfully." *Hospital Financial Management,* vol. 30, no. 11, November 1976, pp. 42–47.

Deva, R. "Collect That Account Beforehand." *Hospital Financial Management,* vol. 30, no. 1, January 1976, pp. 22–26.

Fairall, J. W. "Outpatient Collections Need Not Be A Problem." *Hospital Financial Management,* vol. 28, no. 6, June 1974, pp. 26–28.

Hall, J. "Analysis the Key to Better Management of Accounts Receivable." *Hospital Financial Management,* vol. 24, no. 3, March 1970, p. 7.

Happach, B. "Problems in Receivables." *Topics In Health Care Financing,* vol. 3, no. 1, Fall 1976, pp. 11–25.

Hospital Financial Management Association. *Patient Account Management Techniques.* Chicago: Hospital Financial Management Association, 1977.

Kenneth, R. J. "Set Goals for Proper Receivables Management." *Hospital Financial Management,* vol. 27, no. 3, March 1973, pp. 18–25.

# Appendix 6-1

This appendix demonstrates that the sum $I + W + W^2 + \cdots$ may be expressed in the form $(I - W)^{-1}$. To prove this, we write

$$(I - W)(I + W + W^2 + \cdots + W^{n-1})$$

Since $IW^n = W^n$, expanding this expression yields

$$I + W + W^2 + \cdots + W^{n-1} - W - W^2 - \cdots - W^n = I - W^n$$

Thus, we find

$$(I - W)(I + W + W^2 - \cdots + W^{n-1}) = I - W^n$$

Now if $n$ increases, we say that the elements of $W$ decrease. Letting $n$ be the smallest value such that the elements of $W = 0$, and hence $W = 0$, we find

$$(I - W)(I + W + W^2 + \cdots + W^{n-1}) = I$$

and

$$(I + W + W^2 + W^3 + \cdots + W^{n-1}) = (I - W)^{-1}$$

Chapter 7

# Management of Cash

**Objectives**

After completing this chapter, you should be able to:

1. Describe the functions of money.
2. Describe the importance and composition of cash.
3. Describe the system by which cash receipts and disbursements might be controlled by the hospital.
4. Describe the motives for holding cash.
5. Understand and describe the basic elements of the cash balance decision.
6. Determine the cash balance under conditions of certainty.
7. Determine the cash balance under conditions of uncertainty.

The previous chapter discussed briefly the relation between the management of accounts receivable and the management of cash, as well as techniques for estimating the timing and magnitude of cash flows that arise when payments are made by debtors of the hospital. This chapter examines the basic principles and procedures that management should use in minimizing the cost of holding cash and thereby increase the likelihood of providing service at a minimum cost. Before turning to a formal discussion of cash management, it is desirable first to discuss the functions performed by money and the importance of cash in the operations of the hospital enterprise.

## 7.1 THE FUNCTIONS OF MONEY

Money serves essentially four basic functions: as a unit of value, as a medium of exchange, as the standard of deferred payment, and as a store of value. The first two usually are referred to as the primary functions of money while the last two are called the derivative functions because they emanate from the primary functions.

### 7.1.1 Unit of Value

The first function of money has been given many names, of which the most common are "unit of value" and "standard of value." Each of these implies that the value of each good or service is measured and expressed in terms of monetary units. That is, the value of each good or service can be expressed as a price that indicates the number of monetary units for which it can be exchanged in a market transaction. As an example, suppose the hospital routinely purchases supply items $x$ and $y$. If item $x$ has a price of \$16 and item $y$ of \$2, it follows that one unit of $x$ is worth 8 units of $y$. Thus, the problem of expressing the relative value of items purchased is simplified by measuring the value of those goods or services in monetary units.

### 7.1.2 Medium of Exchange

Cash also is a medium of exchange. This function is served by anything that is generally accepted in exchange for goods and services. In this sense, money is referred to as generalized purchasing power since the possession of cash permits an individual or an enterprise to purchase needed items from suppliers who offer the most favorable terms.

### 7.1.3 Standard of Deferred Payments

A hospital may encounter periods in which short-term debt is required to finance working capital needs. On the other hand, it frequently is required to extend credit to patients or third party payers when care is used. As a result, the hospital both extends and receives credit in the course of normal day-to-day operations.

Consider, as an example, a situation in which the hospital is forced to engage in cash borrowing to finance working capital needs. The hospital must issue a short-term debt instrument that requires it to make payments that are expressed in monetary units and represent the principal as well as explicit or implicit interest charges. Some of these debt instruments mature in a few days or a few months while long-term debt may mature in ten years or more. In addition, many contracts require the payment of fixed or semifixed amounts at some future date. Examples of these kinds of agreements include long-term leases and salary contracts. In each of these examples, money is the unit in which deferred or future payments are expressed.

Money is a standard of deferred payments only to the extent that its purchasing power is maintained at a constant level through time. When the purchasing power of money increases (i.e., prices of goods and services fall), groups that have promised to pay fixed amounts return more purchasing power than was borrowed, while those that receive the fixed amounts experience a windfall gain. Conversely, if the purchasing power of money declines (as in inflation), groups that promise to pay fixed amounts return less purchasing power than was borrowed and those that receive the fixed amounts suffer the economic consequences of an increasing price level.

### 7.1.4 Store of Value

The cash holdings of the hospital represent purchasing power that may be spent over time for the goods and services that management wishes to buy. Thus, the decision to hold cash is predicated on the belief that money will be accepted at any time in exchange for goods and services required in operational activity. This suggests that cash represents a store of value that may be used to meet unpredicted emergencies and to pay debts that are expressed in monetary units.

Money is not, of course, the only store of value since this function can be served by any valuable asset. In this sense, the hospital can store value for future use by holding promissory notes, bonds, mortgages, or any other asset whose value may be expressed in monetary terms. The major advantage of these other assets is that, unlike cash, they usually earn income in the form of interest, rent, or usefulness and the hospital may experience a windfall gain through appreciation. On the other hand, they are characterized by certain disadvantages:

1. they may involve storage costs,
2. they may depreciate in terms of money,
3. they may not be accepted in exchange transactions,
4. they may not be convertible into cash without an economic loss.

Given the advantages and disadvantages of nonmonetary assets, the hospital is free to determine the composition of stored value (money vs. nonmoney assets) and to alter the composition of stored wealth so as to achieve the most advantageous ratio of money to nonmonetary assets while taking into account such factors as income-earning potential, security, and liquidity. To a significant extent such decisions also are influenced by expectations concerning the future behavior of prices. As an example, if it is expected that prices are more likely to rise than fall, less wealth will be held in the form of money and more in the form of other assets. On the other hand, if prices are expected to fall, a higher proportion of stored value will be held as cash and a lesser proportion in other forms. These issues and other related considerations are examined in detail later.

## 7.2 THE COMPOSITION AND IMPORTANCE OF CASH

The objective of this section is to provide a basic understanding of the composition and importance of cash. Such an understanding provides the foundation for an examination of the methods by which cash may be controlled as well as the techniques that may be used to determine the cash balance.

### 7.2.1 The Composition of Cash

Cash may be defined as consisting of actual money as well as other resources and credit instruments that are used as monetary equivalents. This definition includes coin and paper currency, demand deposits in banks, checks, and other nonmonetary forms of cash or cash equivalents that are accepted readily in exchange transactions and in the settlement of obligations. Perhaps the most important characteristic of cash, then, is its common acceptance as a medium of exchange and as the unit in which general purchasing power is expressed.

In terms of this definition, items such as postage stamps, postdated checks, and IOUs must be excluded from the cash classification. Similarly, term deposits, temporary investments in bank savings accounts, or other securities should be regarded as investments rather than cash. These items normally are not used as monetary equivalents and therefore should not be regarded as cash.

### 7.2.2 The Importance of Cash

The importance of cash arises from its highly active characteristic, its rather obvious value in financing activity, and its susceptibility to misappropriation. From the perspective of the hospital, almost every transaction is related directly or indirectly to a cash receipt or disbursement. Since the providing of service is related, directly or indirectly, to a cash receipt and most expenses sooner or later require a cash disbursement, the daily activities of the hospital result in a more or less continuous flow of cash. Thus, cash inflows and cash outflows either initiate or complete substantially all of the hospital's transactions. Given that cash is perhaps the most active of all assets and represents the hospital's lifeblood, the administrator must devote considerable time and energy to its effective management.

Cash is, of course, a necessity in the operation of any enterprise. In the case of a hospital, an adequate cash balance is a necessary ingredient in providing adequate patient care in that a sufficient amount must be available to pay employees and creditors. The hospital's credit standing depends to a significant extent on the promptness with which it pays its debts. A supplier may react to a history of unpaid bills and late payments by charging higher prices, limiting the amount of credit extended, and eliminating trade discounts. Any or all of these reactions can result in significantly higher costs that must be paid for supplies and purchased services. Needless to say, if such consequences are to be avoided, the hospital must have sufficient cash to discharge its financial obligations on a timely basis.

On the other hand, it must be recognized that, when held idle in excessive amounts, cash is unproductive and earns nothing of benefit for the hospital. As mentioned earlier, the earning power of idle cash is negative during periods of inflation. As the prices of goods and services purchased by the hospital increase, the purchasing power of cash declines. Thus, given that cash serves as a medium of exchange and a store of value, a rise in prices implies that more dollars must be expended to obtain a fixed set of real resources. These consequences suggest that the cash balance must be regulated so as to avoid holding too little or too much cash. Effective cash management requires that all available cash must be used either in discharging obligations or in earning a positive return for the hospital.

Cash is also susceptible to misappropriation by employees and others because it is: (1) small in bulk, (2) easily concealed and transported, and (3) readily exchanged for other goods and services. Moreover, ownership normally is established by possession, which implies that cash is subject to misappropriation. These factors, coupled with the highly active characteristics of cash, suggest that considerable effort must be devoted to the design and maintenance of an internal control system that safeguards the movement of cash from the time it is received until it is disbursed.

## 7.3 THE MANAGEMENT AND CONTROL OF CASH

Internal cash controls are essential in the hospital's business office and at all locations where cash is received or disbursed. An effective cash control system is a necessity if cash resources are to be protected from error and fraud. The following discussion outlines the basic components of an internal cash control system and considers the advantages of implementing such a system.

### 7.3.1 General Guidelines

Management should consider several basic guidelines when developing or revising the system by which cash is controlled. Among the more important are:

1. All employees who have access to cash or routinely handle cash should be bonded.

2. The number of imprest funds (i.e., petty cash funds, change funds, etc.) as well as the number of persons who have access to cash should be limited.

3. The bank accounts maintained by the hospital should be reconciled by responsible employees who do not have access to cash.

4. There should be a distinct separation of responsibility for cash handling and cash accounting. For example, persons who handle incoming cash should not have access to or control over accounts receivable records.

5. Definite responsibility should be assigned for handling cash and the custody of cash funds.

6. All forms pertaining to cash receipts and cash disbursements should be prenumbered and accounted for in numerical sequence.

7. Internal audits and surprise checks should be made by responsible employees at irregular intervals.

8. Business office responsibilities should be arranged so that an error or misappropriation by one employee will be discovered by another.

9. Physical protection in the form of vaults, cash registers, and locked cashier's facilities should be provided.

10. Specific methods of handling receipts and disbursements of cash should be established in writing, while decisions regarding nonroutine cash transactions should be made by the chief financial officer.

11. The system by which cash is controlled should be the subject of continuous evaluation and review.

The observance of sound internal controls is conducive to promoting the efficiency and the effectiveness of the business office. By implementing sound internal cash controls, daily and monthly reports are more timely and accurate since errors and imbalances are minimized. More importantly, any system of internal control will deter attempts to misappropriate hospital funds. It should be noted that no system is perfect but even the simplest internal control system can discourage the potential wrongdoer.

## 7.3.2 An Internal Control System

This section outlines the basic parameters of the system by which cash may be controlled by management, including the separation of functions that must be performed when cash is received and disbursed.

### 7.3.2.1 Cash Receipts

Hospital cash receipts are divisible into two main categories: (1) mail receipts and (2) over-the-counter cash receipts. To be effective, the internal cash control system must address the peculiarities of each.

Figure 7-1 displays a basic system by which mail receipts can be controlled. The control begins with the receipt of cash and the preparation of a mail remittance form by a bonded employee who is independent of the accounting department and the general cashier.

At this point in the system, two functions must be performed. First, all checks received through the mail should be endorsed immediately and the instruction "for deposit only" should be recorded on each. Second, the mail clerk should prepare a prenumbered cash receipt slip that is sent to the maker of the check, and should record the amount and the name of the payer in a daily mail remittance report.

The system in Figure 7-1 assumes that the mail remittance report is completed in triplicate. The distribution of this report is as follows:

1. The original and any relevant correspondence are forwarded to the accounting department, where these documents are used to record the cash receipts in the hospital books.
2. The second copy and the cash receipts are sent to the chief cashier, who compares the cash receipts with the mail remittance form. The purpose of

**Figure 7-1** Control over Mail Receipts

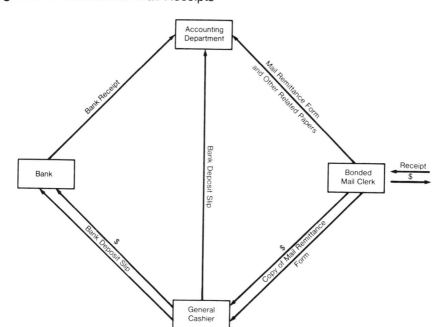

this comparison is to ensure that the cash items in the report are listed properly.

3. The third copy, which should be verified and signed by the chief cashier, is retained by the mail clerk.

Once the general cashier has validated the mail remittance report, a daily bank deposit is prepared in duplicate. The original along with the cash or endorsed checks are forwarded to the bank. The duplicate of the bank deposit slip goes to the accounting department, where the mail remittance report and the bank deposit slip are compared. At a later point, the bank will send a deposit receipt to the accounting department, which will compare the mail remittance report and bank deposit slip with the bank deposit receipt.

If this system is used, misappropriation is difficult unless several hospital employees act in collusion. For example, the mail clerk cannot appropriate mail receipts without omitting them from the mail remittance report. If the receipt of cash is omitted from that report, the appropriate account will not be credited by the accounting department and subsequent billings will lead the patient or other entities to file a complaint with the hospital. Similarly, mail receipts cannot be misappropriated by the cashier since the accounting department must verify all mail receipts by an independent comparison of the mail remittance report with bank deposit slips. Finally, employees in the accounting department cannot misappropriate funds since they have no access to the cash.

Controlling cash received over the counter is a more difficult task than controlling mail receipts because over-the-counter receipts are collected by cashiers in several locations in the hospital such as the cafeteria, gift shops, barber shops, etc. It almost goes without saying that the number of such locations should be minimized and, to the extent possible, the receipt of cash should be centralized.

Figure 7-2 presents a system for controlling over-the-counter receipts. As mentioned, cash control requires a separation of custody and recordkeeping functions. The control process begins with ensuring that each transaction is recorded properly on a cash register tape to which the cashier does not have access. For obvious reasons, a cashier who has access to the cash should not have access to the register tape. The system in Figure 7-2 assumes that the cashier is required to count the cash in the register at the end of each day and prepare a cashier's report recording the results of the count. The cash and the daily cashier's report are sent to the head cashier, who also has access to the cash but not to the register tape. The head cashier compares the cash items with the daily cashier's report and, in the absence of discrepancies, prepares a bank deposit slip in duplicate. The original along with the cash items go to the bank for deposit and the duplicate is sent to the accounting department. Concurrently, an employee from the accounting department who does not have access to cash should obtain the cash register tape, which then may be compared with the bank

**Figure 7-2** Control of Over-the-Counter Receipts

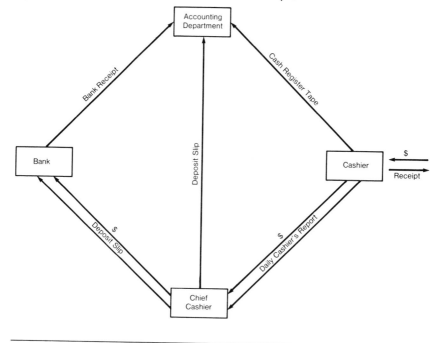

deposit slip and the bank receipt to ensure that cash has been deposited accurately and promptly in the bank.

The employee in the accounting department has access to the cash register tape but not to the cash. As a result, this individual is unable to misappropriate cash without the participation of the sales clerk and the head cashier. Conversely, the sales clerk and the head cashier have access to cash but not to the register tape. Since the cash register tape, the bank deposit slip, and the bank receipt are compared by employees in the accounting department, the sales clerk and the head cashier cannot misappropriate cash unless they win the assistance of others. As in the case of mail receipts, the implementation of a control system similar to this one makes the misappropriation of funds difficult in the absence of collusion.

### 7.3.2.2 Cash Disbursements

The key to controlling cash disbursements is determining the authenticity of hospital liabilities and the amounts to be paid at the time they are recorded in the hospital books. The proper recording of liabilities generally leads to the proper disbursement of funds, while the improper recording of liabilities is just as likely to result in an improper disbursement of cash. Thus, much care must be exercised to ensure that liabilities are recorded properly.

With the exception of imprest funds, which are handled on a cash basis, all cash disbursements should be made by prenumbered checks written on protective paper. Definite authority and responsibility for signing checks should be given to only a few individuals and, in certain circumstances, it may be desirable to require two signatures.

---

**Figure 7-3** Controlling Cash Disbursements

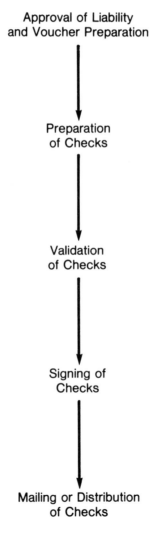

As in controlling cash receipts, there should be a division of duties in disbursing hospital cash. Figure 7-3 outlines a possible segregation of disbursing duties.

The first step involves the validation of the liability and the preparation of the voucher. The voucher is the central control document that authorizes the disbursement of funds. No disbursement should be made without the proper execution of a voucher, which of course requires the examination of all supporting documents such as the purchase orders, invoices, and receiving reports. The voucher bears witness to the fact that all authorizations, prices, quantities, and extensions have been examined and, to the extent possible, have been found to be correct and accurate. As such, the voucher indicates the amount of cash to be disbursed and thereby constitutes the basis for preparing the check. Once prepared, the check, along with the voucher and all related papers, are presented to the disbursing authority, who reviews all documents to ensure that the check has been prepared properly. Once satisfied that all is in order, the disbursing officer signs the check, which is mailed to the recipient directly from the disbursing office. The voucher and related documents should then be marked "paid" so that they cannot be presented again for payment and forwarded to the accounting department so they may be recorded in the hospital's books.

Regarding cash disbursements related to the hospital's payroll, the person responsible for signing payroll checks should have nothing to do with the compilation, validation, preparation, or recording of employee earnings. Before signing payroll checks, the disbursing officer should examine a sample of all payroll checks to ensure that they have been prepared properly.

## 7.3.3 Evaluation of the Control System

Table 7-1 lists components that should be in most cash control systems. The *internal auditor*, like the external auditor, should use such a list in evaluating the hospital's internal control system. Answers to the questions in this table usually are obtained by investigation and by interviews with hospital employees. The objectives of the internal auditor are to: (1) be acquainted with employees and the functions each performs, (2) acquire an understanding of hospital operations, (3) determine existing internal control methods, (4) identify apparent weaknesses and areas requiring closer investigation, and (5) obtain information required for the development of internal audit procedures. In accomplishing these objectives, valuable impressions concerning the efficiency of individual employees and the role played by each in the internal control system may be obtained by completing the checklist in the table.

An evaluation of the internal control system is the primary responsibility of the *external auditor*. The time spent by this auditor is related directly to the effectiveness and completeness of the hospital's internal control system. It is in

**Table 7-1** Internal Cash Control Checklist

| Component | Item |
|---|---|
| General | 1. Has the governing board authorized all bank checking accounts? |
| | 2. Do inactive checking accounts exist and, if so, why are they maintained? |
| | 3. How many different checking accounts are maintained and what is the purpose of each? |
| | 4. Has the responsibility for the receipt and deposit of cash been centralized? |
| | 5. Are all persons handling cash<br>a. bonded?<br>b. required to take an annual vacation? |
| | 6. Are employees in departments such as billing, credit and collection, purchasing, and others who might participate in irregularities or fraudulent behavior bonded? |
| | 7. Is access to cash properly limited? |
| | 8. Do employees of the cashier's department:<br>a. prepare charge tickets or other revenue documents?<br>b. keep or have access to patient records?<br>c. assist in balancing patient ledgers with general ledger accounts?<br>d. participate in making statements?<br>e. approve rebates or discounts?<br>f. approve or participate in determining which accounts to write off as bad debts?<br>g. prepare or approve vouchers or sign checks?<br>h. prepare or sign payroll checks?<br>i. keep or have access to petty cash? |
| | 9. Are bank statements and cancelled checks received from the bank by the person who prepares the bank reconciliation? |
| | 10. Are bank reconciliations made by persons who do not participate in the receipt and disbursement of cash? |
| | 11. Are bank reconciliations received periodically by persons who are not responsible for receiving and disbursing cash? |
| Cash Receipts | 1. At how many locations and by whom is cash received? |
| | 2. What kind of cash receipt records are maintained and who keeps them? |
| | 3. Is the mail opened by a person<br>a. who does not prepare bank deposits?<br>b. who does not have access to accounts receivable records? |

**Table 7-1** continued

| Component | Item |
|---|---|
| | 4. Are cash receipts listed in detail by the person who opens the mail? |
| | 5. Is the mail receipt list compared with the accounting records by an independent person? |
| | 6. Are cash receipts deposited daily and intact? |
| | 7. Does the cashier retain control over cash until deposited? |
| | 8. Does someone, independent of the cashier and having no access to cash, make surprise checks of cash items and the bank deposit slips after the deposit has been prepared but before the deposit actually has been made? |
| | 9. Are authenticated bank deposit slips compared with cash receipt records? |
| | 10. Have bankers been instructed to cash no checks made payable to the hospital? |
| | 11. If cash register tapes, cash receipt slips, and daily cash logs are used to validate cash receipts, is the validation performed by an employee independent of the cashier? |
| | 12. Is an independent control established outside the cashier's office over miscellaneous cash receipts such as interest, dividends, etc.? |
| Cash Disbursements | 1. What kinds of cash disbursement records are maintained and who keeps them? |
| | 2. Are all cash disbursements, except for petty cash items, made by checks? |
| | 3. Is a voucher system in operation and are all cash disbursements validated by a voucher and supporting documents? |
| | 4. Are vouchers and supporting documents reviewed before checks are signed? |
| | 5. Is notation of payment made on voucher and supporting documents so that duplicate payments are not possible? |
| | 6. Who is responsible for signing checks? |
| | 7. How many signatures are required on checks? |
| | 8. Are checks prenumbered and written on protective paper? |
| | 9. Are voided checks mutilated to avoid reuse? |
| | 10. Are voided checks retained and properly filed? |
| | 11. Are unused checks controlled properly? |
| | 12. Are all checks made payable to a person or a company? |
| | 13. Are checks signed only after preparation has been completed? |

**Table 7-1** continued

| Component | Item |
|---|---|
| | 14. Does any person who is responsible for signing checks have any of the following duties?<br>a. open mail or list mail receipts?<br>b. act as cashier or have access to cash?<br>c. prepare bank reconciliations?<br>d. prepare or audit disbursement vouchers?<br>e. have custody of petty cash?<br>15. Who is responsible for preparing checks?<br>16. Does the person responsible for reconciling the bank statement<br>a. account for all check numbers?<br>b. examine signatures?<br>c. examine endorsements?<br>d. compare cancelled checks with entries in accounting records?<br>17. Regarding checks that have been outstanding for long periods of time<br>a. are such checks investigated?<br>b. is payment on such checks stopped? |

this regard that the hospital may realize substantial savings in audit fees by developing and implementing a complete and effective internal control system. In addition, some of the procedures performed by the external auditor can be carried out less expensively by hospital employees. For example, it is not necessary to pay the external auditor to reconcile the hospital's bank statement or petty cash funds when the same procedure can be performed just as well and far less expensively by a hospital employee. Even though the auditor will want to examine these reconciliations, such a review may be facilitated by providing appropriate schedules and adding machine tapes or subsidiary records when the audit is begun. In fact, the external auditors should provide a list of schedules and tapes they will require that can be prepared so as to reduce audit time.

In addition to reducing the cost of external audits, the development and implementation of a sound internal control system will promote efficiency in the business office. It is in this regard that an internal control system reduces errors and out-of-balance situations so that daily and monthly reports are both more accurate and timely.

A sophisticated internal control system sometimes is difficult to implement in a small institution since it may not be possible to provide for an entirely satisfactory division of duties. In such a situation, increased attention must be given to the application of the other principles and procedures such as bonding, job rotation, surprise cash counts, and similar practices. The administrator should ensure that as many additional internal controls are implemented as are feasible, given the existing situation.

## 7.4 THE CASH BALANCE DECISION

Since holding cash earns nothing for the hospital and, in times of inflation, may even earn a negative return, it seems legitimate to inquire into the reasons or motives that may induce management to retain cash. The answer is related to the functions served by money described earlier. Three reasons or motives for holding cash can be identified.

## 7.4.1 Motives for Holding Cash

The first motive is related closely to the fact that money is a medium of exchange and is the unit in which deferred payments are stated. These functions suggest that cash may be held by an institution to meet demands that arise out of normal operations. The need to meet currently maturing obligations is referred to as the *transaction motive* or the *transaction demand for cash*. As an example of the transaction motive, the employment of labor, the purchase of supplies, and the acquisition of equipment represent sources of demand for cash that must be satisfied if the hospital is to preserve its credit rating and assure its continued operation.

The second motive is related to the fact that cash also serves as a store of value that may be used to meet unforeseen or unpredicted contingencies. This function of money suggests that a cash buffer may be held as a precautionary balance that can be used to satisfy an unpredicted demand. The need to hold such a balance is referred to as the *precautionary motive* or the *precautionary demand for cash*. Thus, the precautionary motive for holding cash is defined as the need to hold a portion of the institution's assets in that form to meet unforeseen contingencies.

The final motive is that money serves as a store of value and is the unit in which goods and services are measured. As mentioned earlier, when it is expected that the prices of goods and services will rise (fall), less (more) wealth will be held in the form of cash and a higher (lower) proportion in the form of nonmonetary assets. At the risk of oversimplifying, it could be argued that if the price of a marketable security is expected to rise, the manager may be induced to invest in such a security at a relatively low price so as to be in a position to take advantage of an anticipated higher price. Thus, the *speculative motive* may be defined as the need to hold cash so as to be in a position to take advantage of temporary fluctuations in the prices of marketable securities.

## 7.4.2 The Costs of Holding Cash

Given that a hospital must have a cash balance, management must decide how much cash it should hold. When reaching such a decision, management should consider essentially two types of situations—short-costs and long-costs.

The first type arises when the cash balance is insufficient to meet current demands for cash. In such a situation, the hospital is said to incur a short-cost. The magnitude of short-costs usually varies with the frequency and extent of cash shortages. If cash shortages are small and relatively infrequent, the differences between the demand for and availability of cash usually can be met either through borrowing on an open line of credit or, if available, through the sale of marketable securities. On the other hand, if the shortages are large and frequent, they will result in a loss of purchase discounts, borrowing at high interest rates, a poor credit rating, and perhaps insolvency. Any of these consequences obviously are costly and should be avoided. Therefore, management should maintain a cash balance sufficient to satisfy not only the demands for cash that emanate from routine transactions but also the precautionary and speculative demands for cash.

As will be described in detail later, the presence of short-costs and the probability of incurring them should induce management to hold a relatively large cash balance. However, management also must be concerned with long-costs.

Long-costs can be defined as the costs incurred whenever a cash balance is maintained. When cash is allowed to remain idle, the hospital in effect is investing some of its funds in cash holdings as opposed to some other investment. This means that the hospital will incur an opportunity cost equal to the income that could have been earned had the funds been invested in a different way. The magnitude of long-costs varies directly with the rate of return available through alternate investment opportunities as well as the size of the cash investment.

## 7.5 ELEMENTS OF THE CASH BALANCE DECISION

This section addresses the factors that influence the decision on the size of the cash balance. The hospital's cash balance consists of several portions, each of which corresponds to one of the basic motives for holding cash (i.e., transaction, speculative, and precautionary demands). It is assumed that the speculative and precautionary demands are satisfied by a reserve held by the hospital. Conversely, the cash held to satisfy the transaction demand for cash is related to the hospital's provision of service. Even though cash may be held for any number of reasons, the focus here is on the cash balance, which is related to satisfying the transactions motive.

The major factors that influence the decision concerning the size of the cash balance are:

1. the behavior and magnitude of cash flows
2. the returns and the transaction costs associated with marketable securities
3. the time horizon
4. the size of the cash balance below which short-costs are incurred
5. the short-cost function
6. the long-cost function
7. the optimum cash balance that minimizes the cost of holding cash

The rest of this chapter examines the influence these factors exert on the decision as to the size of the cash balance held by the hospital.

## 7.5.1 The Nature of Cash Flows

The cash flows during a given period may be divided into two categories: (1) cash receipts and disbursements over which the administrator exerts no control and (2) transactions over which management does exert direct control. As an example of the first category, cash disbursements related to obligations incurred in previous periods must be honored by the hospital. Such cash outflows usually arise out of contractual obligations and it is assumed that these obligations will be honored even if the cash balance is equal to zero. The manager of a hospital reimbursed prospectively also is unable to exert control over a significant portion of the cash receipts. For example, once the amount of the periodic prepayment has been determined, the cash received from the third party payer (e.g., P.I.P. and payment from the provincial plan) is beyond the control of the administrator. Similarly, payments on accounts receivable generally are beyond management's control.

There are essentially two types of transactions over which management is able to exert direct control: (1) cash borrowing on a short-term basis and (2) the purchase or sale of marketable securities. If we now subsume the cash flows over which management is unable to exert direct control under "other transactions," it becomes clear that, apart from the reserves held by the hospital, each cash transaction belongs to one and only one of the following classes:

1. cash borrowing on a short-term basis
2. purchase or sale of marketable securities
3. other transactions

Thus far in this analysis, three distinct sets of cash transactions have emerged. The first set of transactions represents uncontrollable or passive transactions, while the two others are subject to the direct control of management. Figure 7-4 uses a Venn diagram to depict these three sets of cash transactions. In this diagram, each point represents a possible cash transaction into which the hospital

**Figure 7-4** Venn Diagram Depicting Cash Transactions

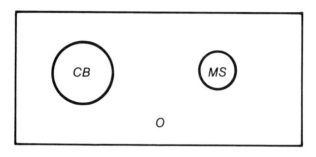

may enter and the entire figure represents all possible cash dealings that relate to the transaction motive for a specified period. In this diagram, *CB* represents the set of transactions associated with cash borrowing, *MS* the transactions involved with the acquisition and disposal of marketable securities, and *O* all other transactions over which management is unable to exert direct control.

As seen earlier, cash inflows may be characterized as either random or non-random. Here, this characterization is extended by identifying a second method of classifying cash transactions that involves the random and nonrandom nature not only of cash receipts but also of cash disbursements. A nonrandom cash flow is defined as one that is known with certainty. Such a cash flow assumes one and only one value. Examples of nonrandom cash transactions include cash flows that arise out of contractual obligations and, in the case of many hospitals that are reimbursed prospectively, cash flows intended to finance the operations of the institution on a current basis. It should be noted that cash flows that are not regarded as nonrandom must belong to the set of random cash transactions. A cash flow belonging to this set may assume more than one value.

Letting the letter *C* connote the set of cash flows that are known with certainty (i.e., nonrandom cash transactions) and *R* the set of cash flows not known with certainty (i.e., random cash flows), the sets of random and nonrandom cash flows may be depicted as in Figure 7-5. Superimposing Figure 7-5 on Figure 7-4 results in a complete characterization of the cash flows as defined by the six intersections of sets in Figure 7-6. It should be observed that the six possible intersections are obtained by combining *C* with *MS*, *CB*, and *O* and by combining *R* with *MS*, *CB*, and *O*. Such a portrayal indicates that each cash flow belongs to one and only one of the six intersections.

The following analysis assumes that there are no random transactions involving cash borrowing or the acquisition and disposal of marketable securities. On the basis of this assumption, the analysis is limited to the sets defined by the intersection of *C* with *CB*, *MS*, and *O* and by the intersection of *R* and *O*. Since the intersection of *C* and *CB* has been considered previously while that of *C*

**Figure 7-5** Random and Nonrandom Cash Flows

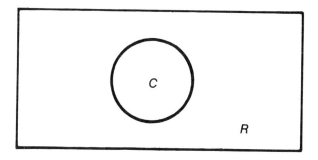

**Figure 7-6** Merging Sets of Cash Flows

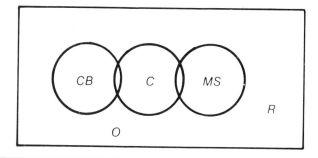

and *MS* is analyzed in the next chapter, the remainder of this chapter focuses on the set formed by the intersections of *C* and *O* and of *R* and *O*. Before turning to these intersections, the cash balance below which short-costs are incurred must be described.

### 7.5.2 The Minimum Cash Balance

The minimum cash balance is defined as the balance below which a short-cost is incurred. For most individuals, a critical minimum balance of zero is appropriate. In the case of a hospital, however, it may be desirable to establish a positive minimum balance. Several valid grounds for such a policy are identifiable.

First, from the perspective of the bank and other financial institutions, a substantial minimum balance is desirable because it provides the financial entity with resources that may be invested or loaned to other borrowers. Maintaining a large minimum cash balance not only provides the financial intermediary with the use of these resources but also improves the credit standing of the hospital. It is in this regard that it is to the hospital's advantage to maintain a large minimum balance when attempting to obtain cash from the bank on favorable terms.

Second, bankers and other financial entities frequently require borrowers to maintain a minimum cash balance stated in terms of a specified percentage of the outstanding principal. Usually, the percentage depends on the financial position of the borrower as well as on conditions prevailing in the money market.

A third reason for maintaining a minimum cash balance in excess of zero stems from an attitude toward risk and the fear of running out of cash. Of course, the shorter the planning horizon, the less the need for a cash reserve since precautionary actions may be taken as unfavorable developments occur. Here, management always must consider short-costs as well as long-costs in developing cash balance policies of this type.

Since management has developed a minimum cash balance, it is necessary to consider the two ways in which the institution may incur short-costs. The minimum balance may be violated by (1) allowing the cash balance to fall below the critical minimum, in which case the short-costs consist of interest charges on loans that may be required to reestablish the minimum balance, and (2) by postponing the payment of obligations that fall due during the period. The penalties the latter action imposes on the institution consist of discounts foregone as well as the costs associated with a deteriorating credit rating.

The next section considers the concept of a minimum cash balance under conditions of certainty, while the last section examines the expected long-cost and short-cost functions as well as the method of determining the optimum cash balance under conditions of uncertainty.

## 7.6 THE CASH BALANCE UNDER CONDITIONS OF CERTAINTY

Virtually all hospitals have cash flows that are nonrandom. When studying a problem with identifiable random attributes, it is useful to assume nonrandom behavior of the variables and obtain a solution to the simplified case. Such a procedure frequently will provide insights into the more complex situation. A consideration of a simple model also is of value since some of the tools and concepts developed here are helpful when considering a situation characterized by uncertainty.

In light of the discussion of Figure 7-6, the concern here is the intersection formed by the sets $C$ and $O$. This is because transactions concerning marketable securities and short-term borrowing originally were assumed to be nonrandom. Under the assumption of certainty, the intersections of sets $R$ and $O$ and of $R$ and $C$ are void of cash transactions.

In principle, the analysis of cash flows under conditions of certainty is similar to the treatment when developing the cash budget. Here, a schedule of cash receipts and disbursements is developed in whatever detail is required. In constructing such a schedule, it should be recognized that the cash budget coupled with an analysis of receivables, payables, and other sources of cash flows provide the basis for obtaining the required information. Once the schedule is prepared, the algebraic difference between cash inflows and cash outflows may be computed. This difference is referred to as the net cash flow. The net cash flow may be negative, positive, or zero. If it is positive, cash receipts exceed cash disbursements; if it is negative, cash disbursements exceed cash receipts; and if it is zero, cash receipts equal cash disbursements.

For each day in the planning period there need not be a perfect correspondence or synchronization between cash receipts and cash disbursements even though they are known with certainty. Indeed, the net cash flow may be positive for some days of the planning period and negative for other days.

The important point for management is that the sum of the net cash flow plus the beginning balance will yield an end-of-period cash balance that is greater than, equal to, or less than the minimum balance. As the end-of-period cash balance approaches the minimum balance, the probability of incurring short-costs rises. As mentioned earlier, these short-costs consist of discounts foregone, interest expenses associated with short-term borrowing, foregone interest income associated with selling marketable securities prematurely, and a deteriorating credit rating.

This discussion suggests that cash in excess of the minimum cash balance is a candidate for investment in marketable securities. Conversely, if the cash balance is less than the critical minimum, the difference must be financed through a manipulation of instrumental variables. This means that the imbalance between the cash balance and the critical minimum must be redressed through cash borrowing or through the sale of marketable securities.

The premature sale of marketable securities results in an opportunity cost equal to the interest income foregone as well as certain transaction costs (e.g., broker's fee). Thus, the conversion of marketable securities into cash results in costs that are equal to the sum of gross returns and the selling costs associated with disposing of securities.

This does not take into consideration the possibility of altering the operating budget to redress the imbalance between the cash and critical minimum balances. In general, the operating budget has been adopted and an alteration in the anticipated level of expenditure may have an adverse impact on the level and quality of patient care. To obtain better operating results, the chief financial officer and the fiscal services division should estimate those costs in advance and provide this information when budgeting decisions are reached. When such a procedure is implemented, management is afforded sufficient lead time to obtain adequate funding at least cost.

This point emphasizes the relationship between budgeting decisions and the type of data and analysis that are relevant when reaching such decisions. Here, the usefulness of the chief financial officer and the fiscal services division hinges on their ability to anticipate both the cash requirements and the costs of obtaining cash that are associated with various levels of hospital operations.

Thus far, for the sake of simplicity, this analysis has assumed that cash flows have been scheduled for only one period. The scheduling process, however, should extend—explicitly or implicitly—over all periods in the cash planning period. Such a procedure enables management to take advantage of expected changes either in borrowing conditions or in the prices of marketable securities.

Although many of the hospital's cash receipts and cash disbursements are known with certainty, many more must be regarded as random variables. To accommodate these random cash flows, a separate model is required. The next section introduces the element of chance, as expressed by the expected long-cost and short-cost functions, in deriving the optimum cash balance under conditions of uncertainty.

## 7.7  OPTIMUM CASH BALANCE AND UNCERTAINTY

This section focuses on determining the optimum cash balance under the assumption that random and nonrandom cash flows occur during the period. The optimum cash balance is defined as the balance that minimizes the cost of holding cash. In determining that level, management is faced with two facts: (1) excess cash balances result in long-costs that are equal to the rate of return that could have been earned by investing funds in an interest-bearing security; (2) inadequate cash balances result in the hospital's incurring short-costs that consist of the interest charges associated with short-term borrowing and/or a deteriorating credit rating.

Frequently, cash flows are not perfectly synchronized and, as a result, management from time to time may be in danger of incurring either long-costs or short-costs. If the initial cash holdings plus all cash inflows are less than the demand, the hospital is likely to incur short-costs. For example, suppose that the initial cash balance and the cash flows of the hospital are as follows:

|      |                      |          |
| ---- | -------------------- | -------- |
|      | Initial Cash Holdings | $10,000  |
| Plus | Cash Inflows         | 7,000    |
|      | Available Cash       | 17,000   |
| Less | Cash Demand          | 20,000   |
|      | Cash Shortage        | 3,000    |

Given the initial cash balance and the cash inflows of the period, the hospital will be unable to satisfy the total demand for cash. In the absence of cash borrowing or the disposal of marketable securities, the hospital's credit rating will suffer. If the shortage is financed by short-term borrowing, the hospital will encounter an out-of-pocket expenditure equal to the interest charges on the loan.

On the other hand, if the sum of the initial cash balance and the cash receipts of the period exceeds the demand for cash, the hospital is in danger of incurring long-costs. Suppose, for example, that the initial cash balance and the cash flows of the period are as follows:

|      |                      |          |
| ---- | -------------------- | -------- |
|      | Initial Cash Balance | $10,000  |
| Plus | Cash Inflows         | 20,000   |
| Less | Cash Demands         | 4,000    |
|      | Cash Surplus         | 26,000   |

In this case the hospital might incur long-costs equal to the rate of return it could have earned by investing the cash surplus in an interest-bearing security.

As might be surmised from this discussion, the potential for incurring these costs is related to the hospital's cash balance. More specifically, the relation between the cash balance and expected long-costs and short-costs may be summarized as follows:

1. as the cash balance increases, expected short-costs decrease; and
2. as the cash balance increases, expected long-costs increase.

To demonstrate that expected short-costs are related inversely to the cash balance and that expected long-costs are related positively to the cash balance, it is necessary to explain the long-cost and short-cost functions.

## 7.7.1 Expected Short-Cost Function

As noted earlier, short-costs are incurred whenever the hospital is forced to finance a cash shortage by obtaining a short-term loan. The need to finance a cash shortage usually arises during periods in which the net cash flow (cash inflows minus cash outflows) is negative. In determining the balance that minimizes the total cost of retaining cash, management must evaluate the expected short-costs associated with a series of strategies concerning the amount of cash the hospital will hold. Such an evaluation requires an estimation of the costs management expects if cash shortages occur during the period. Suppose that management is considering a number of different strategies designated by the subscripts $1, \cdots, j, \cdots, n$. Suppose that management also has identified a set of potential negative net cash flows represented by

$$NNCF = \{NNCF_1, \cdots, NNCF_i, \cdots, NNCF_{p-1}, NNCF_p, NNCF_{p+1}, \cdots,$$

$$NNCF_m, \cdots, NNCF_z\}$$

where

$$|NNCF_1| <, \cdots, < |NNCF_i| <, \cdots, < |NNCF_{p-1}| < |NNCF_p|$$

$$< |NNCF_{p+1}| <, \cdots, < |NNCF_m| <, \cdots, < |NNCF_z|$$

In the following, let $CB_j$ represent the cash balance associated with strategy $j$. Assuming that $|NNCF_m| > CB_j$, the expression

$$CS_{mj} = |NNCF_m| - CB_j \qquad (7.1.1)$$

represents the cash shortage that must be financed by a short-term loan. On the other hand, assuming that $CB_j > |NNCF_i|$, the expression

$$S_{ij} = CB_j - |NNCF_i| \qquad (7.1.2)$$

represents a surplus of cash that might be invested in an interest-earning security. In general, we may display the expression $y = CB_j - |NNCF|$ graphically as in Figure 7-7. In this figure, the cash shortage expressed by Equation 7.1.1 ($|NNCF_m| - CB_j$) is shown by line $cd$. Similarly, the cash surplus represented in Equation 7.1.2 ($CB_j - |NNCF_i|$) is shown by the height of line $ab$. The expression $y = CB_j - |NNCF|$ intersects the horizontal axis at the point $|NNCF_p|$. As a consequence, if management adopts strategy $j$ and the hospital realizes net cash flow $p$, neither long-costs nor short-costs are incurred since the cash balance is just equal to the absolute value of the negative cash flow. These observations suggest that negative net cash flows $NNCF_{p+1}, \cdots, NNCF_m, \cdots,$ $NNCF_z$ would result in a cash *shortage* if management adopted strategy $j$. On the other hand, negative net cash flows $NNCF_1, \cdots, NNCF_i, \cdots, NNCF_{p-1}$ would result in a cash *surplus*. As a result, even though the net cash flow is negative during a given period, it is possible for the hospital to incur long-costs. This possibility is considered later.

Referring to the set of negative net cash flows represented by $NNCF_{p+1}, \cdots,$ $NNCF_m, \cdots, NNCF_z$, we may calculate the expected short-costs associated with strategy $j$ by

$$E(SC_j) = \sum_{m=p+1}^{m=z} P(NNCF_m)[A + i\gamma T(|NNCF_m| - CB_j)] \qquad (7.2)$$

**Figure 7-7** Relationship between Negative Net Cash Flows, Cash Surpluses, and Cash Shortages

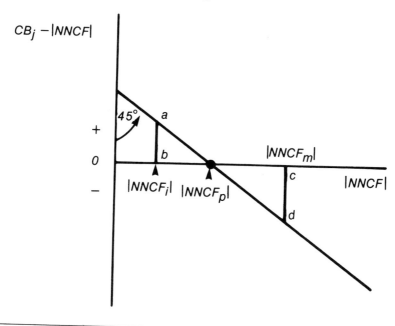

where, as before, $\left|NNCF_m\right| - CB_j > 0$. In this formulation, we let:

| | |
|---|---|
| $E(SC_j)$ | represent the expected short-costs associated with strategy $j$; |
| $P(NNCF_m)$ | represent the probability that negative cash flow $m$, for $m = p + 1, \cdots, z$, will occur; |
| $A$ | represent the fixed cost of obtaining a short-term loan; |
| $CB_j$ | represent the cash balance associated with strategy $j$; |
| $i$ | represent the interest rate associated with short-term borrowing; and |
| $\gamma T$ | represent the portion ($\gamma$) of the planning period ($T$) during which short-term financing is required. |

As seen earlier, the term $\left(\left|NNCF_m\right| - CB_j\right)$ represents the cash shortage that must be financed by short-term borrowing. Multiplying this value by the interest rate and the proportion of time during which funding is required, we find the interest expense the hospital will incur to finance the cash shortage $\left|NNCF_m\right| - CB_j$. Applying the probability $P(NNCF_m)$ to these charges, we obtain a statement of mathematical expectation that represents the expected short-costs associated with the negative net cash flow $m$ and the maintenance of the cash balance assumed under strategy $j$. Summing over all other relevant negative net cash flows results in the expected short-costs associated with maintaining the cash balance under strategy $j$.

As noted, the term $(|NNCF_m| - CB_j)$ represents the cash shortage that must be financed by a short-term loan. As the value of the cash balance increases, these results occur: (1) the amount of the cash shortage that must be financed through short-term credit decreases; (2) the interest rate charged by lenders may decline because of the hospital's more favorable credit rating; and (3) the percentage of the period during which cash shortages must be financed by short-term borrowing also is likely to decrease. These observations suggest that expected short-costs are inversely related to the cash balance, a relation portrayed in Figure 7-8.

## 7.7.2 Expected Long-Cost Function

As the hospital's cash balance increases, however, a point is reached at which the expected short-costs become negligible and further additions to the cash holdings will result in long-costs. As seen earlier, long-costs may be incurred not only during periods of positive net cash flows but also during periods in which the absolute value of the negative net cash flow is less than the cash balance. We consider first the long-costs that might be incurred during periods in which positive net cash flows are realized.

As before, we assume that the hospital wants to evaluate strategies $1, \cdots, j,$ $\cdots, n$ and that management has identified a set of positive net cash flows represented by

$$PNCF = \{PNCF_1, \cdots, PNCF_k, \cdots, PNCF_x\}$$

---

**Figure 7-8** Short-Cost Relation to Cash Balance

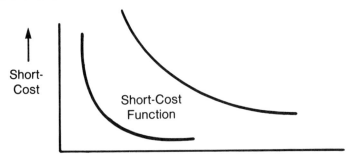

Short-Cost

Short-Cost Function

Cash Balance

where

$$PNCF_1 < \cdots < PNCF_k < \cdots < PNCF_x$$

Employing this notation, the expected long-costs associated with strategy $j$ are given by

$$E(LC_j) = \sum_{k=1}^{k=x} P(PNCF_k)[r\phi_k T(\beta_k PNCF_k)] + r\theta_j T(\psi_j CB_j) \qquad (7.3)$$

where

| | |
|---|---|
| $E(LC_j)$ | = the expected long-costs associated with strategy $j$; |
| $P(PNCF_k)$ | = the probability of realizing positive net cash flow $k$ during the period for $k = 1, \cdots, x$; |
| $r$ | = the rate of return that may be earned by investing excess funds in interest-bearing securities; |
| $\theta_j$ | = the proportion of the period $T$ that cash balance $CB_j$ is available for investment purposes; |
| $\phi_k$ | = the proportion of the period $T$ that positive net cash flow $k$ is available for investment purposes; |
| $\beta_k$ | = the proportion of positive net cash flow $k$ available for investment purposes; and |
| $\psi_j$ | = the portion of the cash balance $CB_j$ available for investment purposes. |

In this case, $\beta_k PNCF_k + \psi_j CB_j$ represents the amount of cash available for investment purposes during period $T$. The terms $\theta_j T$ and $\phi_k T$ represent the period of time during which cash balance $CB_j$ and positive net cash flow $k$ may be invested during the planning period, respectively. As a consequence, the introduction of $\theta_j$ and $\phi_k$ in Equation 7.3 explicitly recognizes the possibility that cash balance $CB_j$ and positive net cash flow $k$ may not be available for investment throughout the planning period. Similarly, the presence of $\beta_k$ in Equation 7.3 gives explicit recognition to the possibility that only a portion of positive net cash flow $k$ will be available for investment. For example, assume that $\phi_k$ = .30 and $\beta_k$ = .50. In such a situation, management could expect to invest 50 percent of positive net cash flow $k$ for 30 percent of the planning period. If either $\phi_k$ or $\beta_k$ is zero, the term $r\phi_k T(\beta_k PNCF_k)$ also is zero.

The sum of the cash balance and the positive cash flow represents the amount of cash available for investment. If this sum is multiplied by the rate of return $r$ and the period of time for which these funds may be invested, the result represents the opportunity costs incurred if a cash balance assumed by strategy $j$ is maintained and positive net cash flow $k$ is realized.

Consider next the long costs that may arise during periods in which the cash balance $CB_j$ exceeds the absolute value of a negative net cash flow. Figure 7-7 shows that cash balance $CB_j$ exceeds the absolute value of the negative net cash flows $NNCF_1, \cdots, NNCF_1, \cdots, NNCF_{p-1}$. As a result, the expected long-costs associated with this set of negative net cash flows are given by

$$E(LC_j^*) = \sum_{i=1}^{i=p-1} P(NNCF_i) \left[ r\alpha_i T(CB_j - |NNCF_i|) \right] \quad (7.4)$$

where

| | |
|---|---|
| $E(LC_j^*)$ | represents the expected long-costs of strategy $j$ and net negative cash flows; |
| $P(NNCF_i)$ | represents the probability of realizing negative net cash flow $i$ for $i = 1, \cdots, p - 1$; |
| $\alpha_i T$ | represents the proportion of the planning period for which $CB_j - |NNCF_i|$ is available for investment purposes. |

The sum of $E(LC_j)$ and $E(LC_j^*)$ represents the total expected long-costs associated with strategy $j$.

Since the terms $(\psi_j CB_j + \beta_k NNCF_k)$ and $(CB_j - |NNCF_i|)$ represent funds available for investment purposes, increasing the hospital's cash balance will increase expected long-costs. Similarly, as the cash balance grows, the proportion of time during which funds are available for investment also increases. These observations indicate that expected long-costs are related positively to the cash balance maintained by the hospital. This relation is seen in Figure 7-9.

### 7.7.3 The Optimum Cash Balance

If we sum the expected long-costs and short-costs of each strategy, we obtain the total costs the hospital is likely to incur if the cash balance assumed by the strategy is maintained. Thus, combining the functional relation in Figure 7-7 with the relationship in Figure 7-9, we express the total expected costs as a function of the cash balance. This is seen in Figure 7-10 where, to the left of $CB^*$, the vertical distance between the expected total cost function, $E(TC)$, and the expected short-cost function represents expected long-costs. To the right of $CB^*$ the vertical distance between the $E(TC)$ curve and the $E(LC)$ curve represents expected short-costs. Since management seeks to minimize the cost of holding cash, Figure 7-10 suggests that the cash balance designated by $CB^*$

**Figure 7-9** Long-Cost Relation to Cash Balance

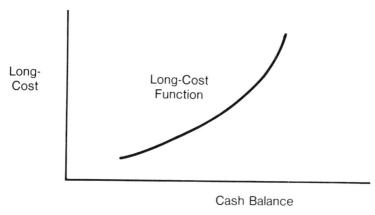

**Figure 7-10** Expected Costs and Cash Balance

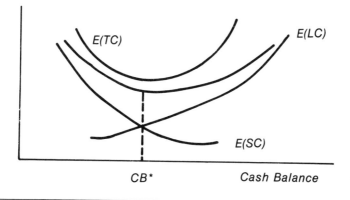

corresponds to the minimum point of the expected total cost curve. Thus, in minimizing the total cost of holding cash, management should maintain a cash balance of *CB\**.

The process by which the optimum cash balance may be determined can be illustrated most effectively by examining a hospital that is reimbursed prospectively as well as a hospital that is reimbursed retrospectively. Assume that the cash outflows of the two hospitals are identical and known with certainty. The cash disbursements of the two hospitals may be regarded as nonrandom cash transactions. The nonrandom cash outflows of these institutions for a single period are as follows:

| | |
|---|---|
| Nonrandom cash outflows: | |
| Wages and salaries | $170,000 |
| Accounts payable | 38,000 |
| Total | 208,000 |

With regard to the hospital reimbursed prospectively, assume that the cash inflows for the period consist of random and nonrandom components as follows:

| | | |
|---|---|---|
| Nonrandom cash inflow: | | |
| Prospective payment | $200,000 | |
| | | |
| Random cash inflows: | | |

| Level of Cash Inflow | Probability | Expected Cash Inflow |
|---|---|---|
| $2,000 | .2 | $400 |
| 4,000 | .3 | 1,200 |
| 6,000 | .2 | 1,200 |
| 10,000 | .2 | 2,000 |
| 12,000 | .1 | 1,200 |
| | | 6,000 |

The algebraic difference between the *nonrandom* cash inflow of $200,000 and
the *nonrandom* cash outflows of $208,000 is equal to −$8,000. Regarding the
random component of the hospital's cash receipts, it is assumed that an analysis
of the accounts receivable (Chapter 6) yielded the amounts and the probabilities
listed above. As can be verified, the random cash receipts are expected to equal
$6,000, which results in an anticipated negative cash flow for the period of
$2,000.

Consider next the impact of random cash receipts on the hospital's net cash
flow. In the absence of an adequate cash balance or random payments on outstanding accounts receivable, management will experience a cash shortage of
$8,000. The net cash flows pertaining to the example can be calculated by
subtracting the cash inflow from payments on receivables from the nonrandom
cash outflow of $8,000. As indicated, management expects to receive cash
payments on receivables of $2,000 with a probability of .2, $4,000 with a
probability of .3, $6,000 with a probability of .2, etc. If the hospital received
payments of $2,000 during the period, the net negative cash flow would be
$6,000 and the net negative cash flow $4,000 if cash payments on these accounts
amounted to $4,000. Similarly, a net positive cash flow of $2,000 would result
if cash payments of $10,000 were received. Since the likelihood of these pay-

ments is known, the net cash flows, and their corresponding probabilities are as follows:

| Net Cash Flow | Probability | Expected Net Cash Flow |
|---|---|---|
| −$6,000 | .2 | −$1,200 |
| −4,000 | .3 | −1,200 |
| −2,000 | .2 | −400 |
| 2,000 | .2 | 400 |
| 4,000 | .1 | 400 |
| | | −2,000 |

Thus, the expected negative cash flow is −$2,000, which agrees with the result obtained earlier.

With regard to the hospital reimbursed on a retrospective basis, assume that the cash inflows consist of random cash transactions having the following properties:

| Random Cash Inflow | Probability |
|---|---|
| $202,000 | .2 |
| 204,000 | .3 |
| 206,000 | .2 |
| 210,000 | .2 |
| 212,000 | .1 |

Since management knows with certainty that the hospital's cash distributions will equal $208,000, the net cash flows are as follows.

| Random Cash Inflow | − | Nonrandom Cash Outflow | = | Net Cash Flow | Probability |
|---|---|---|---|---|---|
| $202,000 | | $208,000 | | −$6,000 | .2 |
| 204,000 | | 208,000 | | −4,000 | .3 |
| 206,000 | | 208,000 | | −2,000 | .2 |
| 210,000 | | 208,000 | | 2,000 | .2 |
| 212,000 | | 208,000 | | 4,000 | .1 |

As these calculations indicate, the expected net cash flows of these two institutions are identical and may be represented by the following probability function

| Net Cash Flow | Probability |
|---|---|
| −$6,000 | .2 |
| −4,000 | .3 |
| −2,000 | .2 |
| 2,000 | .2 |
| 4,000 | .1 |

Having estimated the net cash flows for the two hospitals, it is necessary now to specify the long-costs and short-costs likely to occur. As mentioned earlier, long-costs may be represented by opportunity costs in the form of interest income that is foregone when excess cash remains idle. For illustration, suppose that a rate of return equal to 7 percent may be earned if the hospital invests excess cash in marketable securities. Thus, it is assumed that the value of the term $r$ in Equation 7.3 is 7 percent. Regarding the term $\theta_j T$, which represents the proportion of time that $CB_j$ may be invested, it is assumed for the sake of simplicity that the total cash balance of a given strategy is available for investment throughout the period and that positive cash flows occur at the end of the period ($\theta_j = \psi_j = 1$; $\phi_k = \beta_k = 0$). This assumption implies that the positive cash flow of the period is not available for investment purposes. Referring to Equation 7.4, we assume that $\alpha_i = 1$, which implies that $CB_j - |NNCF_i|$ for $i = 1, \cdots, p - 1$, is available for investment during the period.

Similarly, it is assumed that the short-costs consist of $150 plus 6 percent of any cash shortage. Short-costs are expressed in terms of a fixed component ($150) and a variable component (6 percent of any cash shortage). The fixed component corresponds to the term $A$ of Equation 7.2 while the variable component corresponds to the rate of interest $i$ that is charged on short-term borrowing. As suggested earlier, the fixed component represents the cost of a short-term loan and it is assumed that whenever the hospital seeks short-term financing, it must devote time and energy to obtaining the funds and that these costs are invariant with respect to the amount as well as to the maturity of the financing. Regarding the proportion of the time during which funds are required, it is assumed that the cash shortage exists throughout the period (i.e., the term $\gamma$ in Equation 7.2 is assumed to equal 1).

Suppose further that several different cash balances have been identified and that management wants to evaluate the relative costliness of each to determine which one minimizes the cost of holding cash. Letting $S_1, S_2, \cdots, S_6$ represent these different strategies, assume that

$$S_1 = \$1,000$$
$$S_2 = \$2,000$$
$$S_3 = \$3,000$$
$$S_4 = \$4,000$$

$$S_5 = \$5,000$$
$$S_6 = \$6,000$$

Thus, the task of management is to determine which of these strategies minimizes the cost of holding cash.

Table 7-2 shows the costs the hospital will incur if each of the strategies is implemented and if each of the possible net cash flows identified earlier occurs. The first two columns of this table represent the long-costs to the hospital if each of the identified positive cash flows occurs and if each of the cash balances is maintained. Since only the cash balance is available for investment when a positive cash flow occurs, the long-costs are obtained by multiplying the cash balance assumed under each of the strategies by the rate of return (7 percent) that could be earned. As an example, the long-cost associated with the strategy of maintaining a cash balance of $6,000 during a period in which a positive cash flow of $4,000 occurs is given by (.07)($6,000) = $420. The other values in the first three columns are calculated similarly. Concerning the calculation of short-costs in the table, consider the situation in which the hospital maintains a cash balance of $1,000 and a negative cash flow of $6,000 occurs. As seen in the table, the short-costs are calculated to be $450. This value is given by

$$\$150 + .06(\$6,000 - \$1,000) = \$450$$

The other short-costs in the table are calculated in similar fashion. Whenever the negative cash flow is equal to the cash balance (i.e., $CB_j = |NNCF_n|$), both long-costs and short-costs are zero.

Given the nature of the random component of the hospital's cash receipts, it is necessary to calculate the expected costliness of the various cash balance strategies that, in turn, provides the basis for identifying the optimum cash

**Table 7-2** Total Costs of Each Strategy and Net Cash Flow

| Cash Balance Strategy | Net Cash Flow $4,000 | $2,000 | -$2,000 | -$4,000 | -$6,000 |
|---|---|---|---|---|---|
| $1,000 | $70 | $70 | $210 | $330 | $450 |
| 2,000 | 140 | 140 | 0 | 270 | 390 |
| 3,000 | 210 | 210 | 70 | 210 | 330 |
| 4,000 | 280 | 280 | 140 | 0 | 270 |
| 5,000 | 350 | 350 | 210 | 70 | 210 |
| 6,000 | 420 | 420 | 280 | 140 | 0 |

Long-costs = 7 percent of any excess minimum cash balance.
Short-costs = $150 + 6 percent of any cash shortage.

balance. As seen in Table 7-3, the expected cost associated with the strategy of maintaining a cash balance of $1,000 is $252, which is calculated by

$$.1(\$70) + .2(\$70) + .2(\$210) + .3(\$330) + .2(\$450)$$

Here, the values .1, .2, .2, .3, and .2 correspond to the probabilities that each of the net cash flows will occur, while the values in the parentheses correspond to the costs if a cash balance of $1,000 is maintained and each of the net cash flows occurs.

In general, the values in the last column of Table 7-3 may be obtained by employing the expression

$$t' = p'A$$

where

$$p' = [\,.1 \quad .2 \quad .2 \quad .3 \quad .2\,]$$

and

$$A = \begin{bmatrix} \$70 & \$140 & \$210 & \$280 & \$350 & \$420 \\ 70 & 140 & 210 & 280 & 350 & 420 \\ 210 & 0 & 70 & 140 & 210 & 280 \\ 330 & 270 & 210 & 0 & 70 & 140 \\ 450 & 390 & 330 & 270 & 210 & 0 \end{bmatrix}$$

**Table 7-3** Expected Costs of Each Cash Strategy

| Cash Balance Strategy | Net Cash Flow $4,000 (.1) | $2,000 (.2) | $-2,000 (.2) | $-4,000 (.3) | $-6,000 (.2) | Total |
|---|---|---|---|---|---|---|
| $1,000 | $7 | $14 | $42 | $99 | $90 | $252 |
| 2,000 | 14 | 28 | 0 | 81 | 78 | 201 |
| 3,000 | 21 | 42 | 14 | 63 | 66 | 206 |
| 4,000 | 28 | 56 | 28 | 0 | 54 | 166 |
| 5,000 | 35 | 70 | 42 | 21 | 42 | 210 |
| 6,000 | 42 | 84 | 56 | 42 | 0 | 224 |

The product **p'A** results in a row vector, each element of which corresponds to the expected total cost of a cash balance strategy. Thus, we find that

$$\mathbf{p'A} = [\ \$252 \quad \$201 \quad \$206 \quad \$166 \quad \$210 \quad \$224\ ]$$

Once the expected total cost for each cash balance strategy has been computed, management should compare the expected values and select the least costly cash balance  In the example, a cash balance of $4,000 minimizes the total expected costs of holding cash; in the absence of additional information, this strategy may be identified as the optimum cash balance.

It should be emphasized, however, that the total expected costs should not constitute the only basis for determining the cash balance. Referring to the example, management should consider the implication of maintaining a cash balance of $4,000. It it were to adopt such a policy, there is a probability of .2 that the hospital will experience a negative cash flow of $6,000, which implies that cash demands will exceed the available cash balance. Here management must consider its willingness to accept the risk of incurring the indicated cash shortage as well as its willingness to borrow.

The point that must be emphasized is that the cash balance decision should be based on a number of factors. Perhaps the most important is the level that minimizes cost since it indicates not only the least costly strategy but also the costs of the other cash balance strategies. It also should be noted that the final decision should not be based on only one factor. Rather, management should base the decision on an evaluation of the hospital's financial position that includes, but is not limited to, the expected costs of the various cash balance strategies.

**REFERENCES**

Berman, H. J., and Weeks, L. *The Financial Management of Hospitals,* 3rd ed. Ann Arbor, Mich.: Health Administration Press, 1976, Ch. 13.

Horn, F. E. "Managing Cash." *Journal of Accountancy,* April 1964, pp. 56–62.

Keister, O. R. "Cash Management in Hospitals." *Hospital Financial Management,* vol. 23, no. 11, November 1969, pp. 8–11, 37.

Orgler, Y. E. *Cash Management: Methods and Models.* Belmont, Calif.: Wadsworth Publishing Co., Inc., 1970.

Porteus, E. L. "Equivalent Formulations of the Stochastic Cash Balance Problems." *Management Science,* November 1972, pp. 250–253.

Stone, B. K. "The Use of Forecasts and Smoothing in Control-Limit Models for Cash Management." *Financial Management,* Spring 1972, pp. 72–84.

# Chapter 8

# Management of Marketable Securities

## Objectives

After completing this chapter, you should be able to:

1. Identify and describe the investment alternatives available to the hospital.
2. Describe the process and techniques of evaluating bonds as potential investment instruments.
3. Describe the process and techniques of evaluating stocks as potential investment instruments.
4. Understand and use the single security model to determine the level of investment that maximizes expected net income.
5. Understand the basic factors that are considered in managing a hospital's portfolio.

As seen in the previous chapter, management may encounter periods during which the funds available to the institution are greater than the demand for cash. If management is to avoid the opportunity costs that arise when surplus cash is allowed to remain idle, excess funds should be invested in securities that earn revenue for the hospital.

The major purpose of this chapter is to introduce the basic principles of investment analysis and the management of marketable securities. Given that many texts and articles have been written on investment analysis, a comprehensive review of the techniques and procedures usually associated with the management of marketable securities is not possible here. Rather, the intent is to introduce the vocabulary of investment analysis, the process by which securities are evaluated, and the basic techniques commonly used in reaching investment decisions. This is predicated on the view that management should rely on the advice and counsel of a professional investment analyst, the accountant, and the chief financial officer when reaching investment decisions. To obtain the maximum benefit from such advice, however, the manager should have a basic understanding of the process as well as the principles and techniques commonly used when evaluating the investment alternatives available to the hospital.

Accordingly, this chapter is developed in four phases. The first phase reviews the investment alternatives available to the hospital and describes the characteristics of these investment opportunities. The second section discusses the process by which investment alternatives may be evaluated. Assuming that only one of the available opportunities provides administration with sufficient liquidity and safety of principal and earns a satisfactory rate of return, the third section analyzes a management model that may be used in determining the level of investment that maximizes expected net earnings. The last section relaxes this assumption and considers the more general problem that arises when the hospital holds a number of different securities.

## 8.1 INVESTMENT ALTERNATIVES

Numerous investment opportunities are available to the hospital. However, short-term marketable securities probably provide the most attractive investment. This is because they are an almost riskless investment that is highly marketable and is available in a number of different maturities. As is discussed later, factors such as safety of principal, liquidity, maturity date, and satisfactory rate of return should be considered when selecting securities. Before analyzing the factors that influence the investment decision, however, the basic investment alternatives available to management should be considered.

### 8.1.1 Government Treasury Bills

Treasury bills (T bills) represent an attractive investment because they are obligations of the government and, as such, are considered a very safe investment. In addition, Treasury bills are highly liquid, which means the hospital can convert them into cash if it encounters unforeseen contingencies. Thus, in addition to yielding a reasonable rate of return, Treasury bills combine security with marketability that, when coupled with the maturity of under one year, make them an attractive investment opportunity to the hospital.

### 8.1.2 Certificates of Deposit

Certificates of Deposit (CDs) are given to the hospital by the bank in exchange for a time deposit of money. The bank promises to return the principal and interest to the holder of the Certificate of Deposit on a specified date. The certificate thus is transferable and may be exchanged or traded for cash prior to the maturity date. Certificates of Deposit usually have a maturity of 90 days, but maturities of up to a year are not uncommon.

### 8.1.3 Bonds

A portion of the hospital's investment portfolio is likely to consist of government and corporate bonds. This results from the emphasis that management places on the security of principal and stability of income. Bond prices usually exhibit relative stability while interest payments on bonds normally are received with certainty.

Both corporate and governmental bonds are available in varying terms and denominations. When the bond is issued, the nominal rate of interest, which is competitive in the capital market at the time of issue, is expressed as an annual percentage of face value even though interest usually is paid semiannually.

Corporate lawyers and financers have created a wide variety of bonds and, as a result, there is no single method by which these issues may be classified. However, it is common practice to classify them in terms of (1) the method of paying interest and principal and (2) the security or collateral pledged by the issuer.

When bonds are classified as to their collateral, they are either secured or unsecured. Unsecured bonds are called debentures and depend for security on the general credit standing of the issuer. A secured bond usually is accompanied by a mortgage or a lien on the assets of the issuer. Such bonds usually are classified in accordance with the type of asset pledged as security. Some of the more common categories are equipment trust bonds, real estate mortgage bonds, and collateral trust bonds. Equipment trust bonds are issued by railroads and are accompanied by a mortgage on rolling stock. Real estate mortgage bonds usually are secured by a mortgage on a portion or all of the issuer's plant and equipment. Collateral trust bonds are secured by stocks, bonds, and other negotiable instruments that are deposited with a trustee.

Bonds also may be classified as to the method of paying interest and principal. When bonds are classified by method of making payments, they may be serial bonds or sinking fund bonds. With serial bonds, a portion of the issue becomes due and payable over a period of years. For example, a company may issue a 10-year $500,000 serial bond, which means that $50,000 of the bonds become due and payable each year until the issue has been paid off. Sinking fund bonds provide in their deed of trust that money will be accumulated in a sinking fund that then is used to pay off the bonds at maturity.

When bonds are classified by method of payment, they are either registered or coupon bonds. Registered bonds require that the issuing corporation maintain a current list of bondholders and the periodic interest payments are received by bondholders of record. Registered bonds provide some protection from loss or theft. Coupon bonds are accompanied by coupons that the bondholder detaches and submits to the company for payment. Frequently, the ownership of coupon bonds is not registered and payment is made to the bearer of the bond.

### 8.1.4 Stocks

The investment of hospital resources in corporate stocks involves a degree of risk with regard to price declines, but can provide large returns in the form of dividends and appreciation if managed intelligently. When a corporation offers only one kind of stock, it is called common stock; if it issues more than one kind or class of stock, one generally is known as common stock, the other as preferred stock. As the name implies, preferred stock frequently is more desirable than common stock. For example, if the corporation declares dividends, the owners of preferred stock must be paid before owners of common stock. Preferred stockholders also may have first call on the assets of the company in the event of corporate liquidation. On the other hand, the annual dividends paid on preferred stock typically are fixed in amount regardless of the company's profits while common stock dividends tend to vary directly with profits. Preferred stock prices are likely to be less variable than those of common stock, which may fluctuate widely and provide greater potential for gain through appreciation.

Even though the dividends on most preferred stock are limited to a fixed amount or percentage of face value, some preferred stocks have the right, in certain circumstances, to dividends that exceed that basic percentage or amount. Such issues are called participating preferred stocks. These stocks may be fully participating or the participation may be limited to a fixed amount. For example, if a corporation issues fully participating, 5 percent, $100 par value preferred stock and $80 par value common stock, the owners of the preferred shares have a preference to a dividend of 5 percent or a $5 per share each year. Then, each year after the common stockholders have been paid 5 percent or $4 per share, the preferred stockholders have a right to participate fully with common shareholders in any additional dividends.

As mentioned, the participation of preferred stockholders may be limited. For example, a $100 par value, 6 percent preferred stock may be issued with a right to participate in dividends up to 8 percent of its par value. Such shares have preference to dividends of 6 percent each year, plus the right to participate in additional dividends until holders have received $8 per share.

This discussion is not intended to summarize the entire spectrum of investment opportunities available to the hospital. Rather, it is intended to describe investment alternatives that are perhaps most appropriate from management's view of the relation between risk and potential return. Investors generally demand increased returns as compensation for assuming an increased risk. As indicated above, debt issues of the federal government are considered to be a safe investment alternative, which means that the risk of default is negligible. The relation between risk and return for bonds, preferred stock, and common stock is:

|  | Bonds | Preferred Stock | Common Stock |
|---|---|---|---|
| Risk | Low | Medium | High |
| Yield/Cost | Low | Medium | High |

Bonds are the least risky, followed by preferred stock, and finally by common stock. Conversely, the potential for large gains is associated with common stock, followed by preferred stock, then bonds.

The evaluation of bonds, debentures, and corporate short-term debt is a time-consuming and specialized task. However, independent agencies such as Moody's Investors Service, Inc., and Standard & Poor's Corporation provide rating information on the quality of a wide range of investment opportunities. Various keys and symbols are employed to summarize this information, with Moody's letter system being one of the most widely used. Table 8-1 provides a brief summary of this rating system.

## 8.2 THE EVALUATION OF BONDS

One of the major factors in most investment decisions is the trade-off between risk and return. While individuals vary, most administrators have proved to be averse to risk. Since bonds are a relatively secure investment alternative, this section considers the techniques by which bond issues may be evaluated. Corporate stocks, which are a less secure investment, and the process of stock analysis and selection, are examined in the next section.

**Table 8-1** Summary of Moody's Rating System

| Symbol | Meaning |
|---|---|
| $A_{aa}$ | Best quality (smallest degree of investment risk) |
| $A_a$ | High quality (margin of protection less than $A_{aa}$) |
| A | Higher medium grade (present position adequate but future impairment possible) |
| $B_{aa}$ | Lower medium grade (protection elements lacking) |
| $B_a$ | Speculative elements present (protection of interest and principal payments moderate) |
| B | Lacks characteristics of desirable investment |
| $C_{aa}$ | Poor standing and may be in danger of default |
| $C_a$ | Speculative, often in default |
| C | Lowest grade |

As noted earlier, bonds are debt instruments that entitle the owner to interest payments that were competitive in capital markets at the time of issue. The face value of the bond specifies the obligation of the issuer at maturity, while the maturity date indicates when the obligation must be paid. Owners of bonds may sell them at current market prices to other investors.

The market price of a bond is a function not only of its face value, maturity, and nominal rate of interest (i.e., the interest rate paid by the issuer), but also of prevailing market conditions, including the current interest rates paid on other investments. For example, consider a bond with a face value of $1,000, a maturity of 10 years hence, and a nominal interest rate of 7 percent. Suppose that since these bonds were issued, interest rates have increased and investors are confronted with investment alternatives that pay 11 percent. This implies that if the holder is to dispose of such an instrument, the price of the bond must be reduced to the point at which the effective interest rate becomes competitive.

Consequently, if the nominal rate of interest is less than the market rate of interest, the bond will sell only at a discount (i.e., at a price less than the face value) that makes the effective yield competitive with the interest paid on similar securities. Conversely, if the nominal rate of interest exceeds the market rate, competitive bidding will raise the bond's price and cause it to sell at a premium (a price in excess of its face value). In such a situation, the bond price will increase until the effective yield is equal to the interest rates associated with similar investment opportunities. The purpose of this section, then, is to examine the techniques by which the market value and the effective yield of bonds may be calculated. First, however, it is necessary to review compound interest and the discounting process.

At the heart of any investment decision is the consideration of cash flows expected during several different periods in the future. Given the existence of interest, money has a time value and like amounts received in different periods are not equivalent. For example, suppose that the interest rate is 6 percent and we are offered $100 today or $100 one year hence. Given such a choice, the prudent financial decision is to select the offer of $100 today since interest of $6 could be earned during the year. As a result, the $100 received today is not equivalent to $100 received one year from now.

This example provides the basis for illustrating the calculation of compound interest that, in turn, provides the basis for understanding the discounting process. As before, suppose that the interest earned on money deposited in a savings account is 6 percent compounded annually. Therefore, $100 invested today will be worth $106 ($100 × 1.06) at the end of the first year. If the original $100 and the $6 interest payment remain in the account for an additional year, 6 percent is paid on the $106 during the second year and the balance in the savings account will be $112.36 ($100 × $(1.06)^2$ = $106(1.06)) at the end of the second year.

In general, let $A$ represent the amount deposited at time 0 and $i$ represent the annual rate of interest that is compounded annually. If $B_t$ is the amount on deposit at time $t$, where $t$ is the number of years that have passed, we find

$$B = A(1 + i)$$

$$B_2 = A(1 + i)^2$$

$$\vdots$$

$$B_t = A(1 + i)^t$$

Thus, the final equation allows us to calculate the value of $A$ dollars invested today for any year in the future under the assumption that interest is compounded annually.

Suppose we reverse the process. Assume that we are offered a contract that promises to pay us $B_1$ dollars one year from now, $B_2$ dollars two years from now, and in general $B_t$ dollars $t$ years from now. Given that the annual interest rate is $i$ percent compounded once a year, how much is such a stream of income worth today? In other words, how much would we have to invest at $i$ percent interest to obtain the income stream $B_1$ in one year, $B_2$ in two years, and so on.

As we saw earlier, $A$ dollars invested today yield $B_1$ dollars in one year where $B_1 = A(1 + i)$. Therefore, to obtain $B_1$ dollars one year from now, we would have to invest

$$\frac{B_1}{(1 + i)}$$

dollars today. Similarly to obtain $B_2$ dollars two years from now, we would have to invest

$$\frac{B_2}{(1 + i)^2}$$

dollars today. In general, to obtain $B_t$ dollars in $t$ years from now we would have to invest

$$\frac{B_t}{(1 + i)^t}$$

dollars today. Thus, the amount that would have to be invested today to obtain the income stream $B_1$ in one year, $B_2$ in two years, $\cdots$, $B_t$ in $t$ years is given by

$$\frac{B_1}{(1 + i)} + \frac{B_2}{(1 + i)^2} + \cdots + \frac{B_t}{(1 + i)^t} \qquad (8.1)$$

This sum is referred to as the discounted present value (DPV) of the income stream $B_1, B_2, \cdots, B_t$. Letting $DPV$ denote discounted present value, we have

$$DPV = \frac{B_1}{(1 + i)} + \frac{B_2}{(1 + i)^2} + \cdots + \frac{B_t}{(1 + i)^t} \qquad (8.2)$$

The determination of bond yields is related to this concept of discounting. Specifically, the effective bond yield is determined by finding the discount rate, $r$, which equates the value of all future interest and principal payments with the market price of the bond. Future cash inflows consist of an annual dollar interest payment for a period of $t$ years and a lump sum payment equalling the face value of the bond at the end of year $t$ (repayment of principal at maturity). The formula for calculating bond yields is

$$MP = \frac{I}{(1 + r)} + \frac{I}{(1 + r)^2} + \cdots + \frac{I}{(1 + r)^t} + \frac{FV}{(1 + r)^t} \qquad (8.3)$$

where

$MP$ = current market price
$I$ = annual interest payment (i.e., $I = iFV$)
$FV$ = face value of the bond
$t$ = number of years to maturity

Here we assume that interest is paid annually, but this assumption will be relaxed later.

In summarizing Equation 8.3, the owner of the bond is entitled to annual interest payments of $iFV$ and a lump sum payment of $FV$ at maturity. These two components comprise the cash inflows to which the owner is entitled. The term $MP$ represents the current market price that corresponds to the initial outlay required to purchase the bond. Thus, given a knowledge of $MP$, $I$, and $FV$, the term $r$ is the discount rate that equates the initial cash outflow, represented by $MP$, with the stream of cash inflows represented by $I$ and $FV$ in Equation 8.3.

In most situations, the terms $MP$, $I$, and $FV$ are known and the task of the analyst is to calculate the discount rate $r$. When solving for $r$, however, we face a complex task since the powers to which the term $(1 + r)$ is raised preclude the development of a simple algebraic solution that leaves $r$ on one side of the equation and allows us to solve for this term directly. When calculating the value of $r$ that satisfies the expression, we might rely on a trial-and-error process, which means that we simply substitute different values for $r$ to see how close we come to making the right hand side of the expression equal the value of $MP$. Alternatively we may use bond yield tables or standard computer programs to calculate the value of $r$, which obviates the need for tedious calculations.

Once the discount rate has been computed using one of these techniques, management must employ these calculations in reaching an investment decision. The usual procedure is to compare the calculated value of $r$ with a desired rate of return, known as the cutoff, or with rates of return available on similar investment opportunities. If the calculated value of $r$ exceeds the desired rate of return or the best alternate rate of return, management is induced to purchase the bond. Conversely, if the calculated value of $r$ is less than the desired rate of return, the prudent financial decision is to abandon the bond as an investment outlet.

Equation 8.3 may be used in a variety of ways. If any three of the variables, $I, MP, r$, and $FV$ are known, we may use this expression to compute the value(s) of the fourth variable. In addition, Equation 8.3 may be modified to accommodate the more usual situation in which interest is paid more than once a year. If interest is paid $n$ times a year, Equation 8.3 should be modified as follows:

$$MP = \frac{I/n}{\left(1 + \dfrac{r}{n}\right)} + \frac{I/n}{\left(1 + \dfrac{r}{n}\right)^2} +$$

$$\cdots + \frac{I/n}{\left(1 + \dfrac{r}{n}\right)^{nt}} + \frac{FV}{\left(1 + \dfrac{r}{n}\right)^{nt}} \quad \textbf{(8.4)}$$

## 8.3 THE PROCESS OF STOCK SELECTION

This section focuses on the process and techniques by which stocks are analyzed and selected. The process of stock analysis may be divided into essentially three phases. The first phase consists of an examination of the company (or companies) in which the hospital might invest. The second phase is devoted to the development of projections concerning sales, costs, profits, dividends, and share prices. Once the historical performance of the company has been analyzed and the required projections have been developed, the third phase comes into play—using financial techniques such as the internal rate of return or present value analysis to reach an investment decision. The basic purpose of such an examination is to evaluate forecast share prices and cash dividends, the assessment of which is the major reason for investment analysis. This is because the analyst is concerned primarily with forecasting the total return to the investor—cash dividends and movements in share prices. With this objective in mind, the three phases and the techniques used in each are discussed next.

## 8.3.1 Historical Analysis

The purpose of the historical analysis is to provide the basis for developing forecasts of corporate profits, dividends, and share prices. When analyzing historical performance, the usual procedure is to prepare a summary of the company's business, its earnings record, and its net worth. Such a summary normally is developed from the company's financial statements, which usually provide the basis on which the analyst may estimate the firm's net worth, identify areas of managerial efficiency and weakness, and project ratios and trends.

The data in financial statements are used to derive certain ratios. Ratios are used as indicators of the company's asset structure, managerial performance, and operating efficiency. Ratio analysis also is used when making intercompany comparisons but these require that the firms being compared have similar accounting policies and similar businesses. Ratio analysis is a useful tool when evaluating a single company over a given time interval, providing that the firm's accounting principles and policies are consistent from one period to the next.

### 8.3.1.1 Profitability Ratios

Perhaps the most important factors used by the investment analyst are the profitability ratios that are summarized in Table 8-2. When considered jointly, these ratios provide an indication of the company's efficiency of operation.

For example, when the gross and net profit margins are considered together, the investment analyst may obtain valuable information concerning the company's internal operations. Suppose that the gross profit margin remained constant for several years while the net profit margin declined. The analyst would conclude that the firm had experienced higher expenses relative to sales, or a higher tax rate. These factors would be examined in more detail to determine the cause of the problem. On the other hand, if the gross profit margin fell, it would be concluded that the cost of goods relative to sales had increased. Such a situation could be a result of lower prices or of a reduced operating efficiency in relation to volume. If expenses remained constant in relation to sales, it would be concluded that the decline in the profit margin was attributable to the higher cost of goods sold relative to sales.

Although there are a number of combinations of changes in both gross and net profit margins, these examples illustrate the usefulness of these ratios to the investment analyst. When these ratios, coupled with items of expenditures expressed as a percentage of sales, are examined over time, the analyst may identify areas of deterioration or improvement.

**Table 8-2** Summary of Profitability Ratios

| Profitability Ratio | Definition | Comment |
|---|---|---|
| Gross profit margin | $$\frac{\text{Sales} - \text{Cost of goods sold}}{\text{Sales}}$$ | Demonstrates that the higher the gross profit margin, the less susceptible the firm is to increases in costs |
| Net profit margin | $$\frac{\text{Net profits after taxes}}{\text{Sales}}$$ | Indicates the relative efficiency of the firm after taking into account all expenses and taxes |
| Rate of return on common stock equity | $$\frac{\text{Net profits after taxes} - \text{Preferred stock dividends}}{\text{Net worth} - \text{Par value of preferred stock}}$$ | Indicates the earning power of the stockholders' investment as stated in terms of book value |
| Return on assets | $$\frac{\text{Net profit after taxes}}{\text{Total tangible assets}}$$ | Measures profitability relative to investment |
| Net operating rate of return | $$\frac{\text{Earnings before interest \& taxes}}{\text{Total tangible assets}}$$ | Reflects profitability and is independent of the way the firm is financed |

Consider next the rate of return on common stock equity. In Table 8-2 (third item), the numerator represents the funds available for payment to shareholders and, since net worth is equated with the stockholders' equity, the denominator measures the holders' book investment. Such a ratio provides the analyst with an indication of the earning power of the stockholders' investment as stated in terms of book value and is used frequently when comparing two or more companies in the same industry. Net worth also may be expressed in terms of market value rather than book value. When the market value of the firm's net worth is used in the denominator of the ratio, the price/earnings ratio of the stock is obtained.

It should be noted that the return on assets ratio summarized in the table is somewhat inappropriate when comparing two or more companies that are financed differently. This is because net profits are determined after payments are made to creditors and, since the funds they provide represent a source of financing the company's assets, the return on asset ratio may distort the relative profitability of a concern. As a consequence, when financing charges are significant, it is desirable to use the net operating rate of return rather than the return on assets ratio for comparative purposes.

The profitability ratios described here are of considerable value when comparing one company with similar firms. Only when these ratios are used in a comparative analysis can the investment analyst determine whether the profits of a company are good or bad and why. Obviously, absolute values are helpful in making these determinations, but it is relative performance that is most important.

### 8.3.1.2 Liquidity Ratios

The liquidity ratios summarized in Table 8-3 usually are used to evaluate a company's ability to satisfy currently maturing obligations. The importance and interpretation of the ratios for the most part are intuitively obvious, but several of the measures deserve additional comment.

Unlike the current ratio, inventories are excluded from the numerator of the quick ratio. Since inventories are the least liquid of the firm's current assets, the quick ratio is a more severe test of its ability to satisfy currently maturing obligations.

In addition to the use of the current and the quick ratios in assessing the relation between current assets and liabilities, the analyst frequently will examine the liquidity of the company's investment in inventories and outstanding receivables. Receivables, for example, may be far from current and, if a sizable portion of the company's receivables are overdue, its liquidity may be overstated.

When evaluating the liquidity of receivables, the investment analyst can use the average collection period ratio. This ratio measures the average number of days that receivables are outstanding and should be analyzed in relation to the

**Table 8-3** Summary of Liquidity Ratios

| Liquidity Ratio | Definition | Comment |
|---|---|---|
| Current ratio | $\dfrac{\text{Current assets}}{\text{Current liabilities}}$ | Demonstrates that the higher the current ratio, the greater the ability of the firm to meet its current liabilities |
| Quick ratio | $\dfrac{\text{Current assets} - \text{Inventories}}{\text{Current liabilities}}$ | Concentrates on liquid assets relative to current liabilities |
| Average collection period ratio | $\dfrac{\text{Receivables} \times \text{Days in year}}{\text{Annual credit sales}}$ | Indicates average number of days that receivables are outstanding |
| Inventory turnover ratio | $\dfrac{\text{Cost of goods sold}}{\text{Average inventory}}$ | Measures the rapidity with which inventories are transformed into receivables through sales |

terms of trade credit extended by the company. For example, suppose that the average collection period is 50 days and the credit terms extended by the firm are 2/10/30. A comparison of the average collection period with the terms of credit indicates that a fair proportion of the receivables is past due beyond the net period. On the other hand, if the trade credit terms are 2/10/60, the average receivable is collected before the end of the net period.

A comparison of the average collection period and credit terms of a given company with those of other companies in the same industry also can help the analyst evaluate the firm's investment in receivables. For example, a very low average collection period may suggest an overly restrictive policy that may serve to reduce both sales and profits. Conversely, a very high average collection period may indicate the credit policy is too liberal, and many receivables may be past due and uncollectable. In such a case, a liberal credit policy may result in excessive bad debt expenses, which obviously reduce profits, and may increase the need to finance a large investment in receivables, which also tends to reduce profits below levels that would be obtainable otherwise.

The investment analyst also will use the inventory turnover ratio to examine the liquidity of the firm's inventory holdings. This ratio, similar to the others described in the table, must be evaluated in terms of past and expected ratios and in relation to inventory turnover ratios of similar firms.

In general, a high inventory turnover ratio suggests that inventories are managed efficiently. However, a very high ratio may mean that inventories are maintained at a low level, resulting in frequent shortages. On the other hand, a low inventory turnover ratio may indicate that materials are slow-moving and that a portion of them may be obsolete. Obsolescence may require substantial write-downs, which can reduce the usefulness of inventory holdings in satisfying the company's current obligations.

### 8.3.1.3 Earnings Per Share

One of the major ratios analysts use to measure the performance of a company or to make interfirm comparisons is the earnings per share (EPS) ratio. This ratio is computed by

$$EPS = \frac{\text{Earnings after Taxes}}{\text{Number of Outstanding Shares}}$$

The earnings available to stockholders appear in the numerator, the number of outstanding shares in the denominator. A fairly accurate picture of a company's earnings may be obtained when the ratio of earnings to shares are analyzed over a number of years or compared with the earnings per share ratios of similar firms.

## 8.3.2 The Forecasting Phase

The second phase of the evaluation process involves the development of projections on dividends and share prices that, in turn, provide the basis for estimating the cash flows the investor might receive. At the risk of oversimplifying, we might posit that

Investment decision   $= f$ (expected dividends, expected share prices)
Expected share prices $= g$ (expected dividends, expected profits)
Expected dividends    $= h$ (expected profits)
Expected profits      $= k$ (expected revenues, expected costs)

In this formulation, expected dividends and share prices are related to the anticipated profitability of the company, which in turn is determined by expected sales and costs. Since stock market yields are associated closely with percentage movements in corporate profits, the estimation of corporate profitability is of vital importance and constitutes the major work of the investment analyst.

The techniques of forecasting the profitability of a company include: (1) basic projections of earnings per share, (2) an analysis of business activity and the firm's cost structure, (3) the use of industrial and economic statistics as indicators of the concern's performance, (4) the use of econometric and simulation models, and (5) the use of probability forecasting techniques that produce a range of projections. Thus, a primary task of the investment analyst is to forecast individual items that influence profitability and to develop economic projections that relate to the company's future performance.

Expected profitability of the company depends on projected sales and costs. Factors used in the process of developing projected sales, costs, and profitability, and a simplified approach to translating expected profits into projections on dividend payments, are discussed next.

### 8.3.2.1 Projecting Sales

When projecting sales, the analyst considers such factors as existing and potential demand for each product sold or manufactured by the company, business cycles and economic trends as they pertain to the earnings potential, and the absolute and percentage changes in sales during the recent past. When interpreting projected figures, the analyst must consider trade cycles, so it is necessary to ascertain the location of the company in the present cycle and to estimate the direction as well as relevant rates of change.

When estimating sales, the analyst also examines such factors as the existence of long-term contracts, geographic location, foreign exchange rates, and the monetary and fiscal policies of government. Long-term contracts obviously exert an influence on projected sales and profits. A company with a large portion of assets invested in a foreign country may risk expropriation. As might be suspected, concern over foreign exchange rates is greatest when evaluating a multinational company since it influences the firm's ability to trade in markets abroad.

### 8.3.2.2 Projecting Costs

After projecting a company's sales, the analyst's next step is to forecast the costs of generating the expected volume of sales. Typically, this requires analysis of the firm's cost structure. The investment analyst develops a breakdown of costs in terms of variable, semivariable, and fixed cost components. Fixed costs include depreciation charges, certain administrative expenditures, computer facilities, and rental payments on long-term leases. Variable costs usually include purchases of raw materials, labor, and power required to operate capital equipment. Each of these factors contributes directly to the cost of goods sold. Finally, semivariable costs usually change in relation to turnover.

### 8.3.2.3 Projecting Profits

At this stage of the evaluation process, the analyst may project corporate profitability from the forecast cost and sales data. When summarizing projected profits to develop intracompany and intercompany comparisons, the analyst frequently uses the profit margin ratios described earlier. Projections of these ratios are important because, even though sales figures may remain static when price levels and costs are relatively stable, gross profit margins sometimes vary considerably. Such variations frequently are related to a change in the product mix of the goods sold by the company. For example, even though total revenue remains the same as in the previous year, the concern may have sold a larger quantity of products that have a higher profit margin and a smaller quantity of goods with a lower profit margin. Similarly, the addition of a new product may produce increased sales that, in turn, may influence profits.

### 8.3.2.4 Projecting Dividends

Given an estimate of the company's profits, the analyst is then in a position to project dividends. Dividend forecasts are required since they are an important factor in the determination of share prices. In addition, many hospitals rely on the regular receipt of dividend payments to defray recurring expenditures and, as a result, base investment decisions on dividend performance.

Companies usually raise dividends only when they believe that the increase can be sustained. As a result, a large increase in a company's profits does not necessarily signal a rise in the dividend rate; similarly, a drop in profits need not necessarily be accompanied by a reduction in dividends.

When projecting dividend payments, the analyst usually assumes that the ratio of dividends to earnings is constant. When using a constant payout ratio, the analyst must consider other factors that influence the decision to declare a dividend: the liquidity of the company and the need to retain earnings that may be used to replace or expand capital assets. Given the rapid increase in the prices of capital equipment, company management must disburse considerably more money to replace old equipment with new units of similar capacity. To protect its net worth per share, the company may be forced to maintain or lower the payout ratio, even though profits have increased.

### 8.3.3  The Analysis Phase

At this point in the evaluation, the investment analyst has examined the company's past performance and has developed future earnings and dividend potential. The analyst then examines the implications of these data in terms of share prices and dividends. The primary concern is to project the total return to shareholders, in this case the hospital; this return normally consists of cash dividends and changes in share prices.

When a share of stock is purchased, the investor expects to receive cash dividends as well as, later, a cash inflow if the security is sold. The decision to invest in a stock usually is predicated on the belief that future cash inflows will exceed the purchase cost by an amount that provides a satisfactory return to the hospital.

#### 8.3.3.1  Present Value

As mentioned, the purchase of a share of stock represents a capital expenditure that entitles the owner of the security to a stream of future dividends and to a cash payment when the stock is sold. When reaching an investment decision, hospital management should compare the cash disbursement required to purchase the stock with the present value of the expected stream of cash receipts.

Since the cash outlay required to buy the stock already is expressed in present value terms, management's task is to determine the present value of the expected flow of cash receipts. Using the discounting process introduced earlier, the present value of these receipts is given by

$$PV = \frac{D_1}{(1 + i)} + \frac{D_2}{(1 + i)^2} + \cdots + \frac{D_t}{(1 + i)^t} + \frac{P_t}{(1 + i)^t} \qquad (8.5)$$

where

$D_1, D_2, \cdots, D_t$ = dividend payments in year 1, 2, $\cdots$, $t$;

$P_t$ = estimated cash proceeds resulting from the sale of the security;

$i$ = a discount rate expressed in terms of a percent per year.

The discount rate used in Equation 8.5 to reduce future cash inflows to their present value equivalents is referred to as the time value of money. The magnitude of this value is related to

1. the inconvenience of being unable to spend invested funds
2. the productive value of money
3. inflation which makes goods and services more expensive to buy

The time value of money usually is referred to as a risk-free interest rate. A number of surrogates are used for such a rate; among the more important are the yields on guaranteed government bonds, bank rates, and long-term and short-term loan rates. As a practical matter, however, the average yield on guaranteed government securities may be recommended in most cases. The discount rate used when expressing future cash receipts in terms of their present value equivalents also should reflect an adequate or satisfactory rate of return subject to the risk that management assumes when investing in the stock.

Once computed, the present value of future cash receipts is compared with the current market value of the share. If the expected cash inflow, as expressed in present value equivalents, is greater than the cash outflow, as expressed by the current value of the share, a reasonable financial decision is to purchase the stock. Conversely, if the present value of expected cash inflows is less than the cash outlay, hospital management probably should not buy the stock.

### 8.3.3.2 Internal Rate of Return

In addition to calculating the present value, the investor may use the internal rate of return method when assessing the desirability of the stock purchase. The internal rate of return method may be used in calculating the return on investment that is given by

$$P_0 = \frac{D_1}{(1 + r)} + \frac{D_2}{(1 + r)^2} + \cdots + \frac{D_t}{(1 + r)^t} + \frac{P_t}{(1 + r)^t} \quad \textbf{(8.6)}$$

where

$P_0$ = the market price paid for the share at time zero;

$D_1, D_2, \cdots, D_t$ = dividends for each year;

$P_t$ = sale proceeds of a share at year $t$;

$r$ = yield (the return on investment expressed as a percent).

As Equation 8.6 shows, the variable $r$ is the unknown for which a solution is sought. Thus, the value of $r$ is calculated from the formula and represents the return to the investor as expressed in terms of a percentage per year. If the calculated value of $r$ is less than the minimum rate of return that the hospital regards as acceptable, the security should not be purchased. Conversely, if the internal rate of return is equal to or greater than the minimum rate of return regarded as acceptable, the prudent financial decision is to buy the stock.

### 8.3.3.3 Intrinsic Value

An alternate technique frequently used when assessing a share is to compute the intrinsic or true value of the stock. This requires the derivation of the absolute price or range of prices for a share by discounting future dividends. The "true" or intrinsic value then is compared with the current market price; this comparison provides the basis for reaching investment decisions.

When using this method, the analyst relies on theoretical considerations that suggest that the true value of a share is the present value of all future dividends the shareholder may receive. Rather than forecasting terminal share prices, the analyst discounts all future dividends or dividend growth rates. It should be noted that share prices are determined by expectations concerning future dividend payments and, rather than attempting to estimate terminal share prices that may vary considerably, the analyst forecasts expected dividends since they usually are reasonably stable.

Although there are a number of variants associated with the intrinsic value technique, we consider only the formulation that is used most frequently. We find that the basic formula for the intrinsic value of a stock is similar to Equation 8.5, except that the terminal share price is not included in calculating the true value of the share. As a result, we express the intrinsic value ($IV$) of the stock by

$$IV = \frac{D_1}{(1 + i_1)} + \frac{D_2}{(1 + i_2)^2} + \cdots + \frac{D_t}{(1 + i_t)^t} \qquad (8.7)$$

where

$D_1, D_2, \cdots, D_t$ = dividend per share in the years, 1, 2, $\cdots$, $t$;
$i_1, i_2, \cdots, i_t$    = the discount rate that may vary from year to year.

As mentioned, the calculated value of $IV$ is compared with the current market price. If $IV$ exceeds the current market price, the hospital is induced to purchase the stock, while the obverse also is true.

The use of Equation 8.7 requires an estimate of all future dividends that the shareholder expects to receive. These forecasts usually are derived via the processes described earlier in this chapter. When estimating dividend payments over a long period, a detailed analysis of sales, cost structures, and resulting profits is not practical, so the analyst uses growth rates when forecasting future dividend payments. Consider a stock that (1) paid a current dividend of $\$D$, (2) is expected to grow at a compounded rate of $g$ percent per year, and (3) has a discount rate of $i$ for all years. The intrinsic value of such a stock is given by

$$IV = \frac{D}{(1 + i)} + \frac{D(1 + g)}{(1 + i)^2} + \frac{D(1 + g)^2}{(1 + i)^3} + \cdots \qquad \textbf{(8.8)}$$

It can be shown that Equation 8.8 reduces to

$$IV = \frac{D}{i - g} \quad \text{or} \quad i = \frac{D}{IV} + g \qquad \textbf{(8.9)}$$

Thus, given a constant growth rate $g$ and a constant discount rate $i$, Equation 8.9 suggests that the yield on a share is its current dividend yield plus the growth rate. This ''true'' yield then is compared with other investment alternatives when reaching decisions concerning stock selection.

### 8.3.3.4 Risk and Uncertainty

In addition to the time value of money, which is represented by the factor $i$ in Equations 8.5 and 8.9, investors expect to receive additional returns from equity investments. This is because the future returns are not known with certainty and, as a result, any forecast may prove to be inaccurate. By and large investors, and the hospital enterprise in particular, are risk averse and, given two similar returns, will prefer one that is guaranteed to one that is only a forecast. The risk associated with a return to the investor is related to an imperfect knowledge of all future dividends and share prices that, in part, are a function of forecast earnings and profits. Further, even though the intrinsic value forecast may be correct, it may take some time before the market recognizes the true value of the security. Consequently, if the hospital requires the invested funds for other purposes, it may be necessary to sell the stock at a low price. Equity investments are more risky to a hospital whose surplus funds may not be available for long periods.

The problem confronting the investment analyst is one of incorporating the risk factor when calculating the intrinsic value of the stock. The commonly used technique is to increase the discount rate so that it reflects a risk premium. An alternative is to develop a model based on subjective probabilities. Such models are designed to calculate expected payoffs that are derived by applying relevant subjective probabilities to differing assumptions concerning earnings and dividends. Given the results of such a model, the hospital then must decide which investment yields the best return for the degree of risk it is willing to accept.

## 8.4 A MANAGEMENT MODEL: THE CASE OF A SINGLE SECURITY

As noted, many investment alternatives are available to a hospital and one of management's primary tasks is to determine the proper quantity and composition of securities that will comprise its portfolio. Obviously, these decisions will depend in part on the results of the evaluation process described earlier.

For illustration, we assume here that the safety of principal and liquidity considerations dominate the hospital's investment policy and that there is a *single* investment opportunity that satisfies the need for quality, safety, and liquidity while providing a satisfactory return on excess funds. Thus, the hospital is assumed to allocate its funds into only one investment alternative. The main task is to consider the optimal level of investment in the marketable security.

### 8.4.1 The Basic Model

When determining the proper balance between cash holdings and the institution's investment in the security, management must

1. determine the desired cash balance it will maintain during the period,
2. estimate the probable cash flows for the period,
3. identify the various investment strategies that are to be evaluated,
4. determine the costs incurred when the security is bought and sold, and
5. estimate the value and amount of the security that must be sold at the end of the period as well as the amount which must be sold during the period in order to maintain the desired cash balance for each of the probable cash balances.

Given these estimates, the task of management is to project the net earnings associated with each of the investment strategies and to select the strategy it expects to earn the maximum return during the period.

In the following discussion, we assume that management has identified strategies $1, \cdots, j, \cdots, n$, each of which represents a different level of investment in the marketable security. The model by which management may identify the strategy that maximizes expected net earnings may be expressed in the form

$$e = g - (b + c) \qquad (8.10)$$

where

    **e** is a column vector of $n$ elements, each of which corresponds to the net earnings of one of the strategies;

    **g** is a column vector of $n$ elements, each of which represents the gross earnings of one of the strategies;

    **b** is a column vector of $n$ elements, each of which represents the buying costs associated with one of the strategies;

    **c** is a column vector of $n$ elements, each of which corresponds to the expected selling costs associated with one of the strategies.

The objective of this discussion is to develop the method of estimating or determining the values assumed by the elements of column vectors **g**, **b**, and **c**.

Consider first the gross earnings of each of the strategies. Letting $V_j$ represent the level of investment for strategy $j$ and $r$ correspond to the rate of return per period, we find that

$$
\mathbf{g} = \begin{bmatrix} V_1(r) \\ \vdots \\ V_j(r) \\ \vdots \\ V_n(r) \end{bmatrix} \qquad (8.11)
$$

As an example, suppose we decided to adopt strategy $j$, which involves an investment of \$100,000 during a period in which the rate of return is 8 percent. Under these assumptions, the gross earning from this strategy is given by

$$\$100,000(.08) = \$8,000$$

Similar calculations are required for each of the other elements of vector **g**.

Once the set of gross earnings has been calculated, management must estimate the costs it will incur under the assumption that each of the strategies will be adopted and implemented during the period. Recall that the elements of column vector **b** represent the buying costs of each of the strategies. In this case, we assume that the buying costs are composed of a fixed component and a variable component. The fixed component consists of the internal costs of such activities as recording the transaction in the books, making payments for the security, recording cash receipts and disbursements, and making provision for holding the security. In addition, the fixed cost component should reflect the time required for the controller or an assistant to arrange the security transaction.

The variable component is related to the charges assessed by brokers and other professional investment analysts whose services may be required by the hospital when securities are purchased. For the purposes of future illustration we assume that the commission for the purchase (and sale) of the shares is a known percentage of the dollar value of the securities involved.

We may summarize the foregoing discussion by letting

$FC$ = the internal fixed costs;
$\psi$ = the commission fee as expressed in terms of a percentage of the dollar value of the security purchased;
$V_j$ = the dollar value of security holdings associated with strategy $j$;
$V_o$ = the current level of investment in the security; and
$V_j - V_o$ = the dollar value of the increase in the hospital's holdings of the marketable security.

Using this notation, we find that the column vector **b** may be expressed in the form

$$\mathbf{b} = \begin{bmatrix} FC + \psi(V_1 - V_o) \\ \vdots \\ FC + \psi(V_j - V_o) \\ \vdots \\ FC + \psi(V_n - V_o) \end{bmatrix} \qquad (8.12)$$

Thus, buying costs are incurred only when management considers a strategy that involves the acquisition of additional securities and these costs are equal to the sum of the fixed cost component, represented by the term $FC$, and the variable cost component, $\psi(V_j - V_o)$.

Consider next the elements of the column vector **c**, which represents the selling costs for each of the strategies. When estimating selling costs, management must consider the interrelation between

1. the desired cash balance,
2. the probable cash balances of the period *without* the purchase or sale of the security,

3. the nccd to reduce the investment in the security so as to restore the minimum cash balance should the cash balance fall below the desired level, and

4. the timing of such sales.

The discussion that follows focuses on these interrelationships.

As explained in Chapter 7, management should determine the cash balance that minimizes the total cost of holding cash. In this chapter, it is assumed that the hospital has determined a proper level of transaction and precautionary balances. As noted earlier, the decision should reflect expected net cash flows, deviations from the expected net cash flows, the maturity dates of outstanding debts, and the preferences of management toward the risk of encountering a shortage of cash. On the basis of these factors, it is assumed that management has determined the cash balance it will maintain during the week. However, the cash balance can fall below this level temporarily. Should this occur, it is assumed that the resulting imbalance is redressed by selling marketable securities rather than by short-term borrowing.

This suggests that expected selling costs are composed of (1) internal fixed costs as well as a variable cost component represented by the product of the brokerage fee, $\psi$, and the value of the securities sold and (2) the opportunity costs incurred when securities are sold prior to the end of the period. As an example, suppose that management adopts strategy $j$ and is interested in the transaction costs of disposing of $\$K$ worth of the securities at the end of the period. In this case, we let

$e(T_{kj})$ represent the cost of disposing of $\$K$ worth of the security under the assumption that strategy $j$ is adopted;

$A_{kj}$ represent the event that, if strategy $j$ is adopted, securities amounting to $\$K$ will be sold at the end of the period in order to restore the desired cash balance;

$P(A_{kj})$ represent the probability that event $A_{kj}$ will occur;

$FC$ represent the fixed cost component of transaction costs; and

$\psi(K)$ represent the variable cost component of disposing of securities amounting to $\$K$.

Employing this notation we find that

$$e(T_{kj}) = P(A_{kj})[FC + \psi(K)] \tag{8.13}$$

represents the transaction component of the costs of disposing of securities of $\$K$ if strategy $j$ is adopted.

Consider next the opportunity costs of the premature disposal of all or a portion of the hospital's investment in order to maintain the desired cash balance.

As the total amount that must be sold at the end of the period to restore the desired cash balance increases, it seems reasonable to assume that the probability of selling a portion of this amount during the period also increases. When management is forced to sell a portion of the investment before the end of the period, the hospital incurs not only the fixed costs referred to earlier but also opportunity costs equal to the interest income that is foregone when securities are sold prematurely.

In the following discussion, we let

$e(S_j)$   represent the expected selling costs of strategy $j$;

$B_{ij}$   represent the event that, if strategy $j$ is adopted, securities amounting to $\$I$ will be sold before the end of the period;

$P(B_{ij}|A_{kj})$   represent the conditional probability of selling $\$I$ before the end of the period, given that securities of $\$K$ will be sold at the end of the period, for $I \leq K$;

$OC_i$   represent the opportunity costs when securities amounting to $\$I$ are sold prematurely.

Using this notation, we find that

$$e(S_j) = \Sigma\Sigma\{P(A_{kj})[(FC) + \psi(K)] + P(A_{kj})P(B_{ij}|A_{kj}) [FC + OC_i]\} \quad \textbf{(8.14)}$$

Although Equation 8.14 is simply an application of mathematical expectation, several of its terms deserve further comment. As will be recalled, fixed costs are incurred whenever the hospital buys or sells marketable securities; as a result, the term $FC$ must be included when calculating the costs of disposing of stocks during the period and at the end of the period.

As mentioned, the term $OC_i$ corresponds to the opportunity costs of selling securities prematurely. These costs may be estimated by

$$OC_i = r(bK) (aT) \quad \textbf{(8.15)}$$

where

$r$   is the rate of return per period;

$bK$   is the portion of the securities amounting to $\$K$ that must be sold before the end of the period (i.e., $0 \leq b \leq 1$);

$a$   is the percentage of the time remaining in the period after the securities are sold;

$aT$   is the amount of time remaining in the period after the securities are sold.

Consider next the term $P(A_{kj})P(B_{ij}|A_{kj})$, which appears in Equation 8.14. Concerning events $A$ and $B$, a fundamental postulate of probability allows us to assert that

$$P(B|A) = \frac{P(A \cap B)}{P(A)}$$

Multiplying both sides of this expression by $P(A)$ yields

$$P(A)P(B|A) = P(A \cap B)$$

which implies that the probability that events $A$ and $B$ will occur is equal to the probability of $A$ multiplied by the conditional probability of event $B$ given $A$. Making use of this fact, we may calculate the expected selling costs of strategy $j$ by

$$e(SC_j) = \Sigma\Sigma\{P(A_{kj}) [FC + \psi(K)] + P(A_{kj} \cap B_{ij}) [FC + OC_i]\} \quad \textbf{(8.16)}$$

We may use these results to estimate the values assumed by the elements of column vector $\mathbf{c}$. In this regard, we let

  **f**    represent a column vector, each element of which corresponds to internal fixed costs of arranging the security transaction;

  **v**    represent a column vector containing the variable cost component (i.e., $\psi(V_j - V_o)$);

  **w**  represent a column vector consisting of the opportunity costs of selling securities prematurely (i.e., $rbKaT$);

  **P**   represent a matrix consisting of the probabilities $P(A_{kj})$;

  **U**  represent a matrix consisting of the probabilities $P(A_{kj} \cap B_{ij})$.

Consequently, the column vector $\mathbf{c}$ is given by

$$\mathbf{c} = \mathbf{P}(\mathbf{f} + \mathbf{v}) + \mathbf{U}(\mathbf{f} + \mathbf{w}) \quad \textbf{(8.17)}$$

At this point, it should be noted that the product $\mathbf{P}(\mathbf{f} + \mathbf{v})$ results in a column vector and corresponds to the term $\Sigma\Sigma P(A_{kj}) [FC + \psi K]$ while the product $\mathbf{U}(\mathbf{f} + \mathbf{w})$ results in a column vector and corresponds to the term $\Sigma\Sigma P(A_{kj} \cap B_{ij}) \cdot [FC + OC_i]$.

In summary, the basic model presented in this section may be expressed in the form

$$e = g - (b + c)$$

Substituting $P(f + v) + U(f + w)$ for $c$, we find that

$$e = g - [b + P(f + v) + U(f + w)] \qquad (8.18)$$

When this method of evaluating a series of investment strategies is expressed in matrix notation, a computer program may be developed to examine the sensitivity of investment decisions to changing values of the parameters $r$, $\psi$ as well as the probability distributions represented by the matrices $P$ and $U$.

### 8.4.2 An Illustration

For illustration, assume that the planning horizon of the hospital is limited to a single period and that the controller analyzes the cash holdings as well as the institution's investment in the marketable security in relation to the cash projections for the coming week. It also is assumed that the yield on the marketable security is .10 percent per week and that the following strategies are being considered by management:

| Strategy | Level of Investment |
|----------|---------------------|
| $S_1$ | $700,000 |
| $S_2$ | 800,000 |
| $S_3$ | 900,000 |
| $S_4$ | 1,000,000 |
| $S_5$ | 1,100,000 |
| $S_6$ | 1,200,000 |

Given these strategies and a rate of return equal to .10 percent, we may use Equation 8.11 to calculate the gross earnings of each strategy as follows:

$$g = \begin{bmatrix} \$700,000 \ (.001) \\ 800,000 \ (.001) \\ 900,000 \ (.001) \\ 1,000,000 \ (.001) \\ 1,100,000 \ (.001) \\ 1,200,000 \ (.001) \end{bmatrix} = \begin{bmatrix} \$700 \\ 800 \\ 900 \\ 1,000 \\ 1,100 \\ 1,200 \end{bmatrix}$$

The first element of the column vector **g** corresponds to the gross earnings associated with strategy 1 (700,000 × .001), the second element represents the gross earnings of strategy 2 (800,000 × .001), and so on.

Next, we use Equation 8.12 to calculate the buying costs of each of the strategies. In this case, it is assumed that commission costs of buying and selling securities are .05 percent of the value of the transaction and that the fixed cost per transaction is $20. If the hospital holds securities of $700,000 at the beginning of the week, the increase in investment for each of the strategies may be calculated as follows:

| Strategy | $V_j$ | Less | $V_o$ | = | Amount Purchased |
|----------|-------|------|-------|---|------------------|
| $S_1$ | $700,000 | | $700,000 | | 0 |
| $S_2$ | 800,000 | | 700,000 | | 100,000 |
| $S_3$ | 900,000 | | 700,000 | | 200,000 |
| $S_4$ | 1,000,000 | | 700,000 | | 300,000 |
| $S_5$ | 1,100,000 | | 700,000 | | 400,000 |
| $S_6$ | 1,200,000 | | 700,000 | | 500,000 |

Using these results, we find that the buying cost of each strategy is given by

$$\mathbf{b} = \begin{bmatrix} 0 + .0005\ (\$0) \\ 20 + .0005\ (\$100,000) \\ 20 + .0005\ (\$200,000) \\ 20 + .0005\ (\$300,000) \\ 20 + .0005\ (\$400,000) \\ 20 + .0005\ (\$500,000) \end{bmatrix} = \begin{bmatrix} \$\ 0 \\ 70 \\ 120 \\ 170 \\ 220 \\ 270 \end{bmatrix}$$

By this point, we have computed the elements of the column vectors **g** and **b**. We now turn to the calculation of the elements of the column vector **c** that represent the expected selling costs of each strategy.

As noted in Chapter 7, management should determine the cash balance that minimizes the total cost of holding cash. Here, it is assumed that management has decided to hold a minimum cash balance of $500,000 during the week. However, it is possible for the cash balance to fall below this level temporarily. Should actual cash holdings drop below the desired balance, it is assumed that the imbalance will be redressed by selling marketable securities rather than by short-term borrowing.

The concern, then, is to determine the optimum balance between cash holdings and marketable securities on the basis of cash projections. Suppose that at
the beginning of the week the hospital has a cash balance of $580,000 and that
the probable ending cash balances for the coming week *without* the purchase or
sale of securities are estimated as follows:

| Cash Balance | Probability |
|---|---|
| $400,000 | .1 |
| 500,000 | .1 |
| 600,000 | .2 |
| 700,000 | .3 |
| 800,000 | .2 |
| 900,000 | .1 |

These estimates represent projections of potential cash holdings of the hospital
and are based on its past experience as well as a knowledge of variation in its
cash flows. On the basis of these projections, the probable cash balances associated with strategies that require the purchase of additional securities may be
derived. For example, suppose we are considering strategy $S_2$, which requires
the acquisition of an additional $100,000 worth of the security. The probable
cash balances that reflect the additional investment may be derived as follows:

| Cash Balance Without Purchase or Sale of Securities | Less | Change in Security Holdings | Equals | Adjusted Cash Balance |
|---|---|---|---|---|
| $400,000 | | $100,000 | | $300,000 |
| 500,000 | | 100,000 | | 400,000 |
| 600,000 | | 100,000 | | 500,000 |

When the probable cash balance is $400,000 and the investment in the security
is increased by $100,000, the adjusted cash balance is $300,000. As a consequence, there is a probability of .1 that management will be forced to sell
$200,000 in securities to restore the desired cash balance of $500,000. Similarly,
when the probable cash balance is $500,000 and the hospital increases the level
of investment in the security by $100,000, there is a probability of .1 that it
will sell $100,000 to restore the desired cash balance. As can be verified, the
amounts that must be sold and the corresponding probabilities associated with
the strategy that would increase the level of the hospital's investment by
$300,000 are as follows:

| Amount To Be Sold | Probability |
|---|---|
| $600,000 | .0 |
| 500,000 | .0 |

| | |
|---|---|
| 400,000 | .1 |
| 300,000 | .1 |
| 200,000 | .2 |
| 100,000 | .3 |

In this example, the amounts $600,000, $\cdots$, $100,000 correspond to the event $A_{kj}$ while the values .0, $\cdots$, .3 correspond to the probability $P(A_{kj})$. Extending this procedure for the strategies $S_1$, $S_2$, $S_3$, $S_4$, $S_5$, and $S_6$, we may derive the probabilities and the amounts to be sold under each of the investment alternatives in Table 8-4.

Consider next the disposal costs of selling various amounts of the marketable security. Recalling that internal fixed costs of $20 and brokerage fees of .05 percent of the market value are incurred when securities are sold, we find that

$$\$20 + .005(\$100,000) = \$70$$

represents the transaction costs of disposing of $100,000 in securities. The calculations and the resulting costs of disposing of investments amounting to $100,000, $\cdots$, $600,000 are presented in Table 8-5.

In addition to costs when securities are sold at the *end* of the period, it may be necessary to sell securities *before* the end of the period. In this case, the hospital incurs the fixed costs of $20 as well as lost interest income equal to $r(bK)(aT)$. For illustration, we assume that the probability of selling a portion of the securities prior to the end of the period increases as the total amount that must be sold grows. Referring to Equation 8.15, we assume that the term $b$ is equal to 1/2 or .5, which implies that one-half of the amount will be sold before the end of the week. Similarly, we assume that the term $a$ is equal to ¾ or .75, which implies that three-quarters of gross weekly earnings or .075 percent will be lost should the hospital sell the securities prematurely. These assumptions are summarized in Table 8-6.

Table 8-6 demonstrates that if $200,000 must be sold to restore the desired cash balance of $500,000, there is a probability of .10 that 1/2 of the amount will be sold prematurely. As a consequence, there is a fixed cost of $20 in

**Table 8-4** Probabilities and Amounts To Be Sold by Investment Strategy

| Strategy | Probability of Selling | | | | | |
|---|---|---|---|---|---|---|
| | $600,000 | $500,000 | $400,000 | $300,000 | $200,000 | $100,000 |
| $S_1$ | 0 | 0 | 0 | 0 | 0 | .1 |
| $S_2$ | 0 | 0 | 0 | 0 | .1 | .1 |
| $S_3$ | 0 | 0 | 0 | .1 | .1 | .2 |
| $S_4$ | 0 | 0 | .1 | .1 | .2 | .3 |
| $S_5$ | 0 | .1 | .1 | .2 | .3 | .2 |
| $S_6$ | .1 | .1 | .2 | .3 | .2 | .1 |

**Table 8-5** Total Selling Costs

| Amount | Fixed Costs | + | Variable Costs | = | Total Costs |
|---|---|---|---|---|---|
| (1) | (2) | | (3) | | (4) |
| $600,000 | $20 | | .0005 ($600,000) | | $320 |
| 500,000 | 20 | | .0005 ( 500,000) | | 270 |
| 400,000 | 20 | | .0005 ( 400,000) | | 220 |
| 300,000 | 20 | | .0005 ( 300,000) | | 170 |
| 200,000 | 20 | | .0005 ( 200,000) | | 120 |
| 100,000 | 20 | | .0005 ( 100,000) | | 70 |

**Table 8-6** Costs and Probabilities of Selling Securities Prematurely

| Amount to Be Sold ($A_{kj}$) (1) | Amount to be Sold Prematurely ($B_{ij}$) (2) | Fixed Costs (FC) (3) | Lost Interest Income ($OC_i$) (4) | Total (5) | $P(B_{ij}\|A_{kj})$ (6) |
|---|---|---|---|---|---|
| $600,000 | $300,000 | $20 | $225.00 | 245.00 | 1.00 |
| 500,000 | 250,000 | 20 | 187.50 | 207.50 | .60 |
| 400,000 | 200,000 | 20 | 150.00 | 170.00 | .50 |
| 300,000 | 150,000 | 20 | 112.50 | 132.50 | .30 |
| 200,000 | 100,000 | 20 | 75.00 | 95.00 | .10 |
| 100,000 | 50,000 | 20 | 37.50 | 57.50 | .00 |

addition to the lost interest income of $75 (i.e., $100,000 \times .00075$). The remaining values in this table were calculated in similar fashion.

Thus far in the discussion of column vector **c**, we have developed the information contained in the matrix **P** as well as the vectors **f**, **v**, and **w**. All that remains is to estimate the probabilities in the matrix **U**. As will be recalled the probability $P(A_{kj} \cap B_{ij})$ is obtained by the product of $P(A_{kj})$ and $P(B_{ij}|A_{kj})$. In this case, we may use the set of probabilities $P(B_{ij}|A_{kj})$ presented in the last column of Table 8-6 to form the diagonal matrix

$$\begin{bmatrix} 1.00 & 0 & 0 & 0 & 0 & 0 \\ 0 & .60 & 0 & 0 & 0 & 0 \\ 0 & 0 & .50 & 0 & 0 & 0 \\ 0 & 0 & 0 & .30 & 0 & 0 \\ 0 & 0 & 0 & 0 & .10 & 0 \\ 0 & 0 & 0 & 0 & 0 & .00 \end{bmatrix}$$

Similarly, we may employ the probabilities $P(A_{kj})$ to form the matrix

$$
\begin{bmatrix}
0 & 0 & 0 & 0 & 0 & .1 \\
0 & 0 & 0 & 0 & .1 & .1 \\
0 & 0 & 0 & .1 & .1 & .2 \\
0 & 0 & .1 & .1 & .2 & .3 \\
0 & .1 & .1 & .2 & .3 & .2 \\
.1 & .1 & .2 & .3 & .2 & .1
\end{bmatrix}
$$

the rows of which correspond to the columns of Table 8-4. As a result, the set of probabilities represented by $P(A_{kj} \cap B_{ij})$ is given by

$$
\begin{bmatrix}
1.00 & 0 & 0 & 0 & 0 & 0 \\
0 & .60 & 0 & 0 & 0 & 0 \\
0 & 0 & .50 & 0 & 0 & 0 \\
0 & 0 & 0 & .30 & 0 & 0 \\
0 & 0 & 0 & 0 & .10 & 0 \\
0 & 0 & 0 & 0 & 0 & .00
\end{bmatrix}
\begin{bmatrix}
0 & 0 & 0 & 0 & 0 & .1 \\
0 & 0 & 0 & 0 & .1 & .1 \\
0 & 0 & 0 & .1 & .1 & .2 \\
0 & 0 & .1 & .1 & .2 & .3 \\
0 & .1 & .1 & .2 & .3 & .2 \\
.1 & .1 & .2 & .3 & .2 & .1
\end{bmatrix}
$$

or

$$
\begin{bmatrix}
0 & 0 & 0 & 0 & 0 & .10 \\
0 & 0 & 0 & 0 & .06 & .06 \\
0 & 0 & 0 & .05 & .05 & .10 \\
0 & 0 & .03 & .03 & .06 & .09 \\
0 & .01 & .01 & .02 & .03 & .02 \\
0 & 0 & 0 & 0 & 0 & 0
\end{bmatrix}
$$

After rearranging these data slightly, the elements of the product matrix derived above might be summarized as seen in Table 8-7. Here, the rows of the product matrix correspond to the columns of Table 8-7.

We may now extract the data in Table 8-4 to form the matrix

$$
P = \begin{bmatrix}
0 & 0 & 0 & 0 & 0 & .1 \\
0 & 0 & 0 & 0 & .1 & .1 \\
0 & 0 & 0 & .1 & .1 & .2 \\
0 & 0 & .1 & .1 & .2 & .3 \\
0 & .1 & .1 & .2 & .3 & .2 \\
.1 & .1 & .2 & .3 & .2 & .1
\end{bmatrix}
$$

while the probabilities in Table 8-7 may be used to form the matrix

$$
U = \begin{bmatrix}
0 & 0 & 0 & 0 & 0 & 0 \\
0 & 0 & 0 & 0 & .01 & 0 \\
0 & 0 & 0 & .03 & .01 & 0 \\
0 & 0 & .05 & .03 & .02 & 0 \\
0 & .06 & .05 & .06 & .03 & 0 \\
.10 & .06 & .10 & .09 & .02 & 0
\end{bmatrix}
$$

**Table 8-7** Summary of the Probabilities $P(A_{kj} \cap B_{ij})$

| Strategy | Amount of the Sale at the End of the Period | | | | | |
| | $600,000 | $500,000 | $400,000 | $300,000 | $200,000 | $100,000 |
|---|---|---|---|---|---|---|
| $S_1$ | 0 | 0 | 0 | 0 | 0 | 0 |
| $S_2$ | 0 | 0 | 0 | 0 | .01 | 0 |
| $S_3$ | 0 | 0 | 0 | .03 | .01 | 0 |
| $S_4$ | 0 | 0 | .05 | .03 | .02 | 0 |
| $S_5$ | 0 | .06 | .05 | .06 | .03 | 0 |
| $S_6$ | .10 | .06 | .10 | .09 | .02 | 0 |

Similarly, referring to Column 4 of Table 8-5, we find that

$$\mathbf{f} + \mathbf{v} = \begin{bmatrix} \$320 \\ 270 \\ 220 \\ 170 \\ 120 \\ 70 \end{bmatrix}$$

while the elements of

$$\mathbf{f} + \mathbf{w} = \begin{bmatrix} \$245.00 \\ 207.50 \\ 170.00 \\ 132.50 \\ 95.00 \\ 57.50 \end{bmatrix}$$

are obtained from Column 5 of Table 8-6. In this example, then, we find that $\mathbf{c} = \mathbf{P}(\mathbf{f} + \mathbf{v}) + \mathbf{U}(\mathbf{f} + \mathbf{w})$ is given by

$$\begin{bmatrix} 0 & 0 & 0 & 0 & 0 & .1 \\ 0 & 0 & 0 & 0 & .1 & .1 \\ 0 & 0 & 0 & .1 & .1 & .2 \\ 0 & 0 & .1 & .1 & .2 & .3 \\ 0 & .1 & .1 & .2 & .3 & .2 \\ .1 & .1 & .2 & .3 & .2 & .1 \end{bmatrix} \begin{bmatrix} \$320.00 \\ 270.00 \\ 220.00 \\ 170.00 \\ 120.00 \\ 70.00 \end{bmatrix}$$

$$+ \begin{bmatrix} 0 & 0 & 0 & 0 & 0 & 0 \\ 0 & 0 & 0 & 0 & .01 & 0 \\ 0 & 0 & 0 & .03 & .01 & 0 \\ 0 & 0 & .05 & .03 & .02 & 0 \\ 0 & .06 & .05 & .06 & .03 & 0 \\ .10 & .06 & .10 & .09 & .02 & 0 \end{bmatrix} \begin{bmatrix} \$245.00 \\ 207.50 \\ 170.00 \\ 132.50 \\ 95.00 \\ 57.50 \end{bmatrix}$$

After performing the calculations indicated above, we find that

$$\mathbf{c} = \begin{bmatrix} \$7.00 \\ \$19.95 \\ \$47.93 \\ \$98.38 \\ \$164.75 \\ \$252.78 \end{bmatrix}$$

We may now complete the calculations required to identify the strategy that maximizes expected net earnings, $\mathbf{e}$, by recalling that

$$\mathbf{e} = \mathbf{g} - (\mathbf{b} + \mathbf{c})$$

In terms of our example, we find that

$$\mathbf{e} = \begin{bmatrix} \$700 \\ 800 \\ 900 \\ 1,000 \\ 1,100 \\ 1,200 \end{bmatrix} - \begin{bmatrix} \$ 0 + \$ 7.00 \\ 70 + 19.95 \\ 120 + 47.93 \\ 170 + 98.38 \\ 220 + 164.75 \\ 270 + 252.78 \end{bmatrix}$$

Thus, we find that the column vector containing the expected net earnings associated with each of the strategies is given by

$$
e = \begin{bmatrix} \$693.00 \\ 710.05 \\ 732.07* \\ 731.62 \\ 715.62 \\ 677.22 \end{bmatrix}
$$

This column vector suggests that strategy $S_3$ is expected to result in net earnings of \$732.07, which exceeds the expected net earnings of the other investment strategies. On the basis of these results, we could conclude that the optimum level of investment in the security for the week is \$900,000 and that this strategy yields an expected net income of \$732.07. Consequently, the hospital should invest an additional \$200,000 in the security. Should management invest \$1,000,000, the additional costs exceed the increment in interest income, so the hospital's investment should not be increased by more than \$200,000.

## 8.5 THE PORTFOLIO PROBLEM

In this section we relax the assumption that the hospital invests in only one marketable security and consider the more general problem of managing a portfolio that consists of a number of different shares or assets, as well as developing policies concerning the composition of the hospital's portfolio.

### 8.5.1 Reduction of Risk

One of the major reasons for holding several different shares or assets is to reduce the level of risk associated with equity returns. For example, assume that the hospital invests in only one company that has a 10 percent chance of going bankrupt. In this case, there is a probability of .10 that the hospital will lose all of its invested funds. On the other hand, if the institution puts half of its investable funds into the company and half into guaranteed government securities, the most it will lose due to bankruptcy is half of its investment. This example illustrates an important principle in managing the institution's portfolio: as long as the earning abilities of the stocks held by the hospital are not subject to the same set of external forces, diversification of the institution's portfolio serves to reduce risk.

When considering their portfolios, most hospital administrators are risk averse, which means that, for a given return, they prefer less risk. Here, risk refers to the uncertainty surrounding future returns. The main factors that influence the extent to which management is risk averse are as follows:

1. *The financial status of the institution:* Of considerable concern to management when reaching investment decisions is the amount of investable funds and the length of time they may be invested. In general, investments in stocks and other risky alternatives should be limited to institutions that can afford to invest funds for two or three years because even though stock market indexes often exhibit a tendency to rise, there have been periods in which investors have encountered negative returns. Thus, if the hospital is to realize earnings from the secular rise in stock market indexes, investable funds should be available for relatively long periods of time. Conversely, funds available for shorter periods probably should be invested in traditionally safe securities.

2. *Legal obligations:* Many hospitals receive endowments or other funds that have legal restrictions to which management must adhere. In some cases the restrictions specify the amount of risk that may be assumed when these funds are invested in securities. For example, the donor may specify that the hospital is not to invest more than 10 percent of the donated funds in a given security or that the funds are not to be invested in a security that has not paid dividends in, say, each of the last five years.

### 8.5.2 Marketability and Liquidity

In addition to the trade-off between risk and return, management also is constrained by marketability or liquidity considerations when developing policies on the composition of the hospital's portfolio. As mentioned, the marketability or liquidity of a security may be evaluated in terms of the ease with which it may be sold without loss of principal. There are several points that should be considered when evaluating marketability. The first factor involves the influence exerted on price by the volume of securities sold. The greater the dollar amount of a security that can be sold without significant price fluctuations, the more marketable it is. A second factor is the time required to convert the security into cash. The shorter this time, the more marketable the security.

Marketability or liquidity is of considerable importance to the hospital because many of its cash flows are uncertain and it may be forced to sell securities to meet unexpected or unpredicted demands for cash. If securities can be sold rapidly without a loss in principal, they obviously provide a better investment opportunity than less liquid alternatives.

### 8.5.3 Maturity

The maturity of a fixed-term security—whether it be a bond, a Treasury bill, or similar instrument—is important from the perspective of interest rate risk or the risk associated with fluctuations in the value of principal due to changes in the level of interest rates. In general, a rise in interest rates is accompanied by a decline in security prices. The risk of fluctuations in prices is related to the possibility that the security will be sold before maturity. It is for this reason that management should ensure that the portfolio consists of marketable securities that mature on different dates. A wide range of maturity dates provides management with the flexibility to match investment maturities with future cash needs. By synchronizing maturity dates and cash needs, management is in a better position to ensure that cash is used productively and that investment income is maximized.

### 8.5.4 An Investment Strategy

When considering the hospital's investment policy, this discussion suggests certain guidelines to follow when assessing the composition of the securities portfolio. First, with regard to the investment of operating surpluses, the decision on selecting securities should be based on maturity schedules, returns, risk, marketability, and the hospital's financial position. Second, concerning the maturity schedule, management should ensure that the fixed-term investments mature at different dates. Such a policy provides the flexibility to synchronize cash needs with the maturity schedule of securities, which reduces the interest rate risk.

Third, as was seen earlier, one of the major reasons for holding a number of different securities is to reduce the level of risk. Therefore, the hospital portfolio should be diversified if these risks are to be reduced. Fourth, since most administrators are risk averse when investing hospital funds, the portfolio should be composed primarily of traditionally safe securities. By diversification and minimizing the hospital's investment in securities that exhibit volatility, management further reduces the risks to which the hospital is exposed. It might even be argued that hospital management should limit the investment in the less secure instruments to risk capital, which may be defined as money the administration is willing to lose completely when seeking substantial gains through appreciation.

Fifth, the majority of the securities in the hospital's portfolio should be highly liquid. Adhering to such a guideline would enable management to convert a large portion of the holdings into cash to satisfy unforeseen contingencies.

As might be surmised from this discussion, the management of a portfolio is a complex and highly specialized task. In fact, a number of models that quantify the expected return and riskiness of portfolios have been developed in recent years; these models now constitute a theory of portfolio management. In general, the purpose of these models is to derive the best expected return, subject to specified levels of risk. However, there are a number of reasons for omitting analysis of these models here. A discussion of their specific details is beyond the scope of this text. These models also require an accurate measurement of the risk or uncertainty associated with *future* returns that is a difficult, if not impossible, task.

From a practical perspective, management encounters a number of problems in attempting to apply portfolio theory. An enormous amount of data must be either readily available to or derived by the investment analyst. This consideration, when coupled with the computational requirements, has reduced the application of the models in practical situations. For these reasons, then, a thorough discussion of portfolio theory is not presented here. However, readers are directed to the references at the end of this chapter.

One final word is worthy of note. Given that the management of a portfolio is a complex task, hospital administration should rely on the advice of the chief financial officer and of a professional investment analyst. The primary task of the general administrator is to ensure that the chief financial officer is performing the required functions properly and that the portfolio is being managed in accordance with the investment policies of the hospital.

---

**REFERENCES**

Bauman, W. S. "Investment Returns and Present Values." *Financial Analysts Journal,* vol. 25, no. 6, November-December 1969, pp. 107–120.

Baumol, W. J. "Mathematical Analysis of Portfolio Selection—Principles and Applications." *Financial Analysts Journal,* vol. 22, no. 5, September-October 1966, pp. 95–99.

Friend, I., and Blume, M. "Measurement of Portfolio Performance Under Uncertainty." *American Economic Review,* vol. 60, no. 4, September 1970, pp. 561–575.

Hirschleifer, J. "Investment Decision Under Uncertainty: Applications of the State-Preference Approach." *Quarterly Journal of Economics,* vol. 80, May 1966, pp. 252–277.

Hirschman, W. B., and Branweiler, J. "Investment Analysis: Coping with Change." *Harvard Business Review,* vol. 43, no. 3, May-June 1965, pp. 62–72.

Jacobs, D. P. "The Marketable Security Portfolio of Non-Financial Corporations: Investment Practices and Trends." *Journal of Finance,* vol. 15, September 1960, pp. 341–352.

Liff, B., and Policastro, P. "Excess Cash and Short-Term Investments = $." *Hospital Financial Management,* vol. 30, no. 3, March 1976, pp. 48–50.

Marglin, S. A. "The Social Rate of Discount and the Optimal Rate of Investments." *Quarterly Journal of Economics,* February 1963, pp. 95–112.

Markstein, D. L. "How to Make Short-Term Cash Work at Full-Time Rates." *Modern Hospital,* vol. 114, no. 1, January 1970, pp. 63, 64, 134.

Miles, J. E. "Formulas for Pricing Bonds and Their Impact on Prices." *Financial Analysts Journal,* vol. 25, no. 4, July-August 1969, pp. 151–161.

Packer, S. B. "Municipal Bond Rating." *Financial Analysts Journal,* vol. 24, no. 4, July-August 1968, pp. 93–97.

Snelling, R. E. "Short-Term Investment of Excess Cash." *Management Accounting,* January 1969.

Sharpe, W. F. "A Simplified Model for Portfolio Analysis." *Management Science,* January 1963, pp. 277–293.

————. "Risk Market Sensitivity and Diversification." *Financial Analysts Journal,* vol. 28, no. 1, January-February 1972, pp. 74–79.

Treynor, J. L. "How to Rate Management of Investment Funds." *Harvard Business Review,* vol. 41, no. 1, January-February 1963, pp. 63–75.

Wright, J. W. "Proper Investment of Endowment Funds." *Hospital Financial Management,* vol. 26, no. 8, August 1972, pp. 3–8.

# Chapter 9

# Inventory Management

## Objectives

After completing this chapter, you should be able to:

1. Describe the importance of inventory management.
2. Describe the functions of inventory management.
3. Understand and use the ABC system of classifying inventories.
4. Describe the system by which inventories are controlled.
5. Understand and describe the costs involved with inventory holdings.
6. Determine economic order quantities and reorder points under conditions of certainty.
7. Use a model of mathematical expectation to determine the reorder point under conditions of uncertainty.
8. Use the concept of buffer or safety stocks to determine the reorder point under conditions of uncertainty.

Thus far, the so-called "quick assets" that are composed of accounts receivable, cash, and marketable securities have been considered. This chapter turns to the management of inventories, which is the final component of the hospital's current assets to be studied in this text. It is convenient to develop this discussion in four phases:

1. the importance of inventories as well as the managerial functions that must be performed efficiently and effectively if the total cost of inventory holdings is to be minimized;
2. a method by which inventories may be classified for purposes of internal control;
3. the management of inventories under conditions of certainty;
4. the management of inventories under conditions of uncertainty.

## 9.1 THE IMPORTANCE OF INVENTORIES AND INVENTORY MANAGEMENT FUNCTIONS

To understand the importance of inventories, it is essential to distinguish between supply expenses and items held in inventory. Before consumable supplies are used in providing service, they are regarded as an inventory holding of the hospital and are reported in the balance sheet as a current asset. Once consumable supplies are employed to provide service, they may be viewed as a factor input whose use is reflected as one of the operating expenses reported in the hospital's income statement.

Given that consumable supplies are regarded as hospital assets until used in the production process, the control of inventories is a problem of working capital management. The inventory asset is a factor that can result in the hospital's incurring a significant opportunity cost equal to the revenue foregone when funds are invested in supplies. If not properly managed, the inventory asset also can result in unnecessary operating costs, so management must devote considerable time and effort to the administration of this cost element if operational goals are to be achieved.

### 9.1.1 The Importance of Inventories

Why are inventories held? In the case of a commercial company, three factors usually cited as justification are as follows. First, time usually is required to transform raw materials into finished goods. That production time forces the company to hold some inventories in the form of "goods in process." Second, the production process at many companies consists of several subprocesses, each of which must be coordinated to produce a final product. Unfortunately, the perfect synchronization of materials from one subprocess to another is difficult to achieve. Therefore, one or more of the subprocesses may remain idle for short periods in the absence of inventories. To prevent discontinuities or disruptions in the production process, extra stocks are maintained. The third factor is the inability to predict the demand for final goods or the volume of required raw materials with complete accuracy. To meet unexpected demands for final goods and services, buffer stocks of both finished goods and raw materials must be maintained.

Of these factors, only the uncertainty as to future demands for service appears to be germane to a hospital. The demand for hospital care and the resulting need for consumable supplies are difficult, if not impossible to predict with complete accuracy. In addition, the lifesaving nature of the hospital means that any disruption in the provision of care that results from a shortage of consumable supplies can be quite costly. Thus, management is faced with an uncertain demand for consumable supplies and a situation in which disruptions in care emanating from supply shortages can result in the loss of life. Consequently, hospital management must hold a buffer stock of inventory items to ensure that it can provide continuous needed services.

### 9.1.2 Inventory Management Functions

Since the hospital must hold inventories, it is necessary to review the managerial functions that must be performed if an adequate stock of supplies is to be available and disruptions in providing care are to be avoided. Inventory management may be defined as the development and administration of policies, systems, and procedures that minimize the total costs of inventory decisions. From this perspective, inventory management is broad in scope and affects many hospital functions. Inventory control involves maintaining inventory records and reports, administering the process by which consumable materials are acquired, and directing the physical and accounting control over inventory transactions.

Inventory control functions also may be defined to encompass the development of new or more sophisticated models by which inventory decisions may be reached and implemented. It should be noted, however, that sophisticated techniques do not necessarily lead to an increase in control; rather, they must be accompanied by several factors if the method's control potential is to be realized.

Perhaps the most important of these factors is an adequate data base and a reporting system capable of providing management with timely and accurate information. The effectiveness of any control system requires that information on the amount of inventory at the beginning of a period, the acquisition of supplies, and the use of supply items during the period is conveyed to management on a timely basis. In addition, for certain types of supply items, the information system should be capable of reporting the number of units on hand at any given moment. Thus a perpetual inventory system should be implemented for items over which management wishes to exert maximum control.

A second factor is the capability of the employees responsible for day-to-day operation of the program. Without a capable staff, the effectiveness of any inventory control system will be impaired seriously.

A third factor is that the inventory control system must be consistent with and contribute to the achievement of the hospital's major goals and objectives. Thus, one of the most important elements to consider when contemplating a control system is the relation of the nature and size of inventory holdings to the objectives and functions of the institution. For example, the composition and size of inventories held by a hospital that has as its primary objective the providing of emergency medical care is likely to differ from those of a hospital where psychiatric service is the major objective. Similarly, the inventory holdings of a small, short-term, acute general hospital will differ from those of a long-term convalescent hospital or a large teaching hospital.

The potential savings in any control system also should be considered before implementation. This requires an evaluation of the present system and identification of problem areas as well as the steps that must be taken to correct it. When considering improvements in an existing system or the implementation of a new control program, the potential savings should be compared with the incremental or marginal cost of introducing the proposed method. Obviously, if the potential savings exceed the incremental costs, as expressed in terms of their present value equivalents, management should introduce the new method. Alternatively, if the present value of the incremental costs exceeds the present value of the potential savings, management should abandon any change in approach.

As implied, whenever a hospital uses an inventory control system, it incurs certain operating expenses. The magnitude of the direct costs of an inventory system tend to vary directly with the degree of control exerted. If the hospital exerts maximum control over each inventory item held in stock, it is likely to incur unnecessary operating expenses. As a consequence, management should vary the control so as to reflect the relative importance of supply items. The following section examines one method by which supply items may be classified to achieve this objective.


## 9.2 THE ABC CLASSIFICATION SYSTEM

One of the most widely recognized concepts of inventory classification and control is the ABC system. Its objective is to vary the extent to which inventories are controlled in accordance with potential savings. For example, an item costing $500 has a much greater potential for savings than an item that costs $5. In the ABC approach, inventory items are grouped into three classes, A, B, and C, according to their relative importance. When this is done, appropriate control techniques are developed for each class of inventory. Items that fall into the A category require the use of precise control techniques, while those in the C category need only general control techniques. Obviously, items in the B category should be subjected to procedures more stringent than general control techniques but less stringent than the most precise methods.

From the perspective of the inventory control problem facing hospital management, the relative importance of each supply item may be defined in terms of

1. annual usage
2. unit cost

3. lifesaving properties
4. special storage problems

It should be noted that these four elements do not exhaust the number of possible criteria but probably represent the most important factors that should be considered in grouping the hospital's inventory items.

Consider first the annual usage criteria. The annual dollar usage of a given supply item is calculated by multiplying the number of units used each year by the unit cost. Inventory items then are ranked ordinally in terms of annual dollar usage. The ordinal listing should be accompanied by a column that shows the cumulative annual dollar usage. These data also should be expressed in relative terms. This procedure permits management to examine the distribution of annual usage and to ascertain the percentage of the annual dollar use represented by predetermined percentages of the supply items in the ordinal listing. Thus, management could assert that 10 percent of the top supply items represent, say, 60 percent of the total annual dollar usage of the hospital's supplies. If management had relied on the annual dollar usage as the sole criterion by which it classified inventories, the A category could be defined as consisting of the top 10 percent of the supply items. Suppose further that the next 10 percent of the items reflect an additional 30 percent of the annual dollar usage, which suggests that the B category could be defined to contain this set of items. The C category then would consist of the remaining supply items on the ordinal listing.

As noted, however, annual dollar usage is not the only dimension by which the relative importance of a supply item should be judged. When the three other dimensions are included in the process by which relative importance is determined, management should use a decision matrix similar to Table 9-1. In this

**Table 9-1** Decision Matrix for the ABC Classification

| Questions | Class of Yes Answer | Inventory Item 1 2 | 3 4 | 5 6 |
|---|---|---|---|---|
| 1. Is the annual usage $10,000 or more? | A | 0 0 | 0 0 | 1 0 |
| 2. Is the annual usage between $1,000 and $9,999? | B | 0 1 | 0 0 | 0 1 |
| 3. Is the annual usage less than $1,000? | C | 1 0 | 1 1 | 0 0 |
| 4. Is the unit cost $100 or more? | A | 0 0 | 0 0 | 1 0 |
| 5. Is the unit cost between $50 and $99? | B | 0 0 | 0 0 | 0 1 |
| 6. Is the unit cost less than $50? | C | 1 1 | 1 1 | 0 0 |
| 7. Are there special storage problems? | B | 1 0 | 0 0 | 1 0 |
| 8. Would a "stock-out" result in excessive costs (e.g., loss of life)? | A | 1 0 | 0 0 | 1 0 |
| Classification | | A B | C C | A B |

table, eight questions are asked of each supply item evaluated. The answers will depend on the specific item being analyzed.

A "yes" answer to any of the questions is indicated by a 1 and a "no" by a zero. The column next to the question provides the key to the classification by indicating the inventory class associated with a "yes" answer. For example, consider the first three questions in the table. If the annual dollar usage of the supply item is $10,000 or more, the item is considered an element of category A; if between $1,000 and $9,999, of category B; and if less than $1,000, of category C.

When there is more than one "yes" response for a given supply item, the item should be assigned to the highest category attained as indicated in the first of the six numbered columns. For example, the first supply item has an annual usage less than $1,000 (category C); a unit cost less than $50 (category C); and presents a special storage problem to management (category B). A shortage of this supply item would result in excessive cost and, as a consequence, it is classified in category A. An excellent example of a supply item similar to this profile is whole blood. From the perspective of the dollar outlay required to obtain whole blood, management probably would regard this type of inventory as an element of category C. However, given the special storage problems and the lifesaving qualities of whole blood, management must regard it as an element of category A and exert maximum control over the hospital supply.

In summary, the ABC classification provides the mechanism by which inventory items may be grouped so that the degree of control corresponds to the relative importance of the item. The next section examines the basic elements that should be present in the system.

## 9.3 THE CONTROL OF INVENTORY

The inventory control system of any hospital consists of requisitioning required goods, placing the purchase orders, receiving the merchandise, controlling the items until used, and dispensing them for use in providing health care services. A basic system of controlling inventory (Figure 9-1) is described here.

As suggested by the diagram, it is necessary to divide the responsibilities for requisitioning, purchasing, receiving, controlling, and dispensing inventories among several departments of the hospital. By way of illustration, assume that a department providing service finds that the floor stock is depleted below acceptable levels. When this occurs, the department head prepares a stock request in duplicate. The original is sent to central supply and the second copy is retained in departmental files.

When the stock request is received by central supply and an adequate supply of the item is on hand, the requisition is filled and the goods are forwarded to

**Figure 9-1** Basic Elements of an Inventory Control System

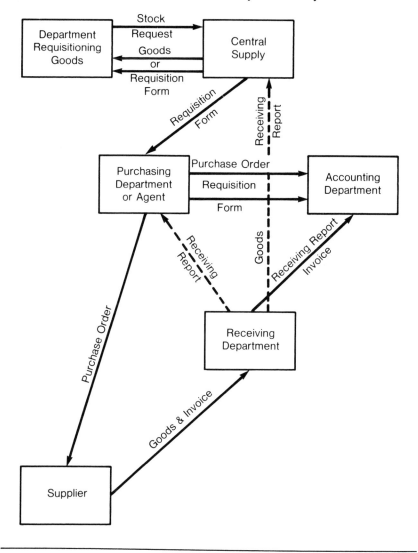

the requisitioner. The subsidiary inventory records maintained by central supply then should be revised by recording the number of units issued, the number of units remaining in stock, and the date of issue. These records should be verified by periodic inventory counts. A form summarizing the requisition should be sent to the accounting department, where it provides the basis for recording entries into inventory records and for charging the appropriate expense account.

If the requisition reduces the stock below the reorder point, which will be discussed later, the hospital's holdings of the inventory item should be replenished and an employee in central supply should complete a requisition form in triplicate. The first copy is sent to the purchasing department, or the purchasing agent in the case of a centralized purchasing arrangement; the second copy goes to the department requisitioning the goods; and the third copy is retained in the temporary files maintained by central supply.

Only the purchasing department or purchasing agent should be authorized to order goods. To understand the need for control over purchasing procedures, suppose that every employee of the hospital has and exercises the authority to purchase goods. Such a situation inevitably would lead to confusion as to what had been ordered, as well as duplications, shortages, and payment for goods not received. So, to repeat, to avoid such consequences, the responsibility and authority for ordering goods from suppliers must be assigned to a single agent or department. It is in this sense that the responsibility for controlling and dispensing stocks in-house rests with central supply and the authority to order goods from outside suppliers with the purchasing department. Once the purchasing department receives a requisition form from central supply, it prepares four or more copies of the purchase order. The copies are distributed as follows:

Copy 1 is sent to the supplier as a request for the required items and authority to ship the goods.
Copy 2 is forwarded, along with the requisition form, to the accounting department, where these documents may be compared.
Copy 3 is transmitted to central supply.
Copy 4 is retained on file by the purchasing department.

Upon receipt of the purchase order, the supplier ships the goods, along with an invoice, to the hospital. An invoice is an itemized statement of the goods shipped. Such a document is prepared by the supplier and always should accompany the shipment so that it may be used as the basis of comparison when the receiving department inspects the delivered goods.

Most large and medium hospitals maintain a special department that is assigned the responsibility of receiving and inspecting all incoming shipments. As each shipment is received, counted, or otherwise inspected, the receiving department prepares four or more copies of the receiving report that are distributed as follows:

Copy 1 is sent to the accounting department.
Copy 2 is transmitted to the purchasing department.
Copy 3 is forwarded to central supply.
Copy 4 is maintained on file in receiving.

The copies sent to purchasing and central supply serve as notification of the arrival of the goods. When the receiving report arrives in the accounting department, the following documents are available for inspection:

1. a stock request prepared by the requisitioner;
2. the supply requisition slip completed by central supply;
3. a purchase order that indicates the quantity, description, unit price, and total cost of goods ordered by the purchasing department;
4. an invoice that indicates the quantity, description, unit price, and the total cost of goods shipped;
5. receiving reports that list the quantity and condition of goods received.

Before approving the invoice for payment, the accounting department should check and compare the information recorded on all papers and should ensure that:

1. the items on the invoice agree with the requisition slip prepared by central supply;
2. the items on the invoice agree with the purchase order;
3. the items on the invoice agree with the receiving report;
4. the invoice prices are the agreed prices;
5. there are no mathematical errors;
6. the terms of trade credit are stated correctly.

After the invoice has been examined, the requisition forms, purchase order, and receiving report are attached to the invoice, which then is ready for final approval and payment.

A comment concerning the inventory accounting procedures management might use appears appropriate. When accounting for inventories, management may employ a periodic and/or a perpetual inventory system. Under the periodic system, there is no attempt to record the number of units available to the hospital on a day-to-day basis; rather, the actual stock on hand is determined by taking a physical inventory. Such a system may be appropriate for the less important items. For more important stock items such as blood, drugs, and oxygen, the perpetual inventory system is more appropriate and, for certain supply items such as drugs, is mandatory. The perpetual inventory system provides management with information regarding the day-to-day receipt and issuance of supplies as well as the number of units on hand at any moment. Thus, for items that management includes in the A category, the perpetual inventory system is appropriate.

Thus far in the analysis, systems of classifying and controlling inventories have been described. The remainder of this chapter examines the costs of inventories and the techniques that management may use when reaching decisions concerning the hospital's holdings.

## 9.4 COSTS OF INVENTORY

The costs associated with inventories are divisible into four major components: ordering cost, carrying cost, short-costs, and long-costs. Each of these components is described below.

### 9.4.1 Ordering Costs

The first major expense element associated with inventories is the costs of placing an order and is referred to as order costs. Order costs can be defined as the administrative and operating expenses of obtaining supplies. Examples of administrative functions that give rise to order costs include developing specifications, obtaining bids, analyzing bids, preparing purchase orders, receiving reports and invoices, validating related vouchers, and preparing checks to pay the account. Order costs can be large or small, depending on the nature of the purchased item. As an example, the costs of ordering a standardized item that is purchased routinely are likely to be small; conversely, if it is the first time the item has been bought and specifications must be developed, bids must be obtained, and so on, the order costs are likely to be relatively high.

As might be surmised, the cost of ordering supplies varies directly with the number of orders placed and inversely with the order size. As the number of orders per period increases, the total cost of placing orders also increases. Conversely, assuming that the number of units used during the period remains constant, an increase in the order size reduces the number of orders, which in turn reduces the total cost of placing orders for the period. Thus, the presence of order costs induces management to increase the size of the order, which reduces both the number of orders and the total order costs incurred during the period.

For purposes of future reference, the total cost of placing orders is symbolized by OC. Further, letting

$J$   = the average cost of placing a single order
$D_t$ = the total number of units purchased during the year
$Q$   = the order size

we find that $\dfrac{D_t}{Q}$ represents the number of orders placed during the period $t$ and that the total order costs for the period are given by

$$OC_t = J\left(\frac{D_t}{Q}\right)$$    (9.1)

### 9.4.2 Carrying Costs

Carrying costs refer to those incurred after stock has been acquired and consist essentially of two cost elements. The first element corresponds to the opportunity costs incurred when funds are invested in inventories, while the second is referred to as the storage costs of holding inventories.

The opportunity costs of holding inventories are equal to the income foregone when funds are invested in inventories rather than in other instruments. To estimate the opportunity costs of inventory holdings, it is necessary first to describe the basic inventory process. Here, it is assumed that the usage of inventory is known with certainty and constant over time. It also is assumed that the lead time (i.e., the time lapse between the placement and receipt of orders) is known and invariant. These assumptions are illustrated in Figure 9-2, where three inventory cycles are portrayed. In this figure, a quantity represented by $Q$ is ordered at the point $R$; this quantity is used at a known and steady rate over the three cycles designated $T_1$, $T_2$, and $T_3$. The average number of units of inventory held during a given period is found by dividing the sum of the beginning inventory ($Q$) and the ending inventory (zero) by two. Thus, the average number of items of inventory held during a representative period is $Q/2$.

Given that, on the average, $Q/2$ units of inventory will be held during a particular period, it is necessary to translate this physical quantity into monetary terms. If the purchase price $P$ is held constant, the dollar value of the average inventory holdings of the hospital is given by $P(Q/2)$. Letting $i$ represent the

---

**Figure 9-2** Three Inventory Cycles

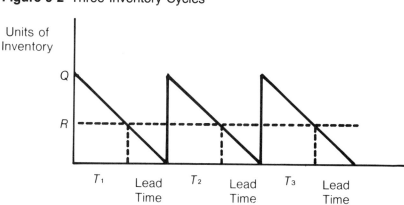

highest interest rate that the hospital could have obtained, we find that the income foregone when funds are invested in inventories, $FI$, is given by

$$FI = iP\left(\frac{Q}{2}\right) \tag{9.2}$$

Equation 9.2 suggests that the opportunity costs incurred by the hospital vary directly with the order size $Q$. That is, the higher the order quantity $Q$, the higher the opportunity costs, $FI$, of holding inventories. Thus, unlike the costs of ordering supplies, opportunity costs encourage management to *reduce* the order quantity.

As mentioned, the holding of inventories also involves a storage cost. That management must provide adequate protection and security for inventory goes without saying. To protect inventory, management must ensure that consumable supplies are properly stored, insured, and secured. Each of these considerations represents a cost that varies directly with the level of inventory held by the hospital. Thus, as the level of inventory holdings increases, total storage cost also will increase. If we let $G$ represent the storage cost per unit, total storage costs, $S$, are given by

$$S = G(Q/2) \tag{9.3}$$

Like opportunity costs, the presence of storage costs encourages management to *reduce* the order quantity size $Q$.

From the foregoing, it can be seen that the carrying costs, which we represent by $C$, is given by

$$C = FI + S \tag{9.4}$$

Substituting $iP(Q/2)$ for $FI$ and $G(Q/2)$ for $S$, we find

$$C = iP(Q/2) + G(Q/2)$$

$$= (iP + G)Q/2 \tag{9.5}$$

where $iP$ and $G$ are assumed to be constant. Thus, for purposes of future reference we define carrying costs, as

$$C = K(Q/2) \tag{9.6}$$

where

$$K = iP + G$$

This discussion suggests that ordering costs encourage management to *increase* the size of the order while carrying cost induces management to *reduce* the size of the order. In other words, the costs of ordering supplies suggest that the quantity should be as large as possible so as to reduce the number of orders and thereby reduce order costs. Conversely, the relation of opportunity cost and the storage cost to the level of inventory holdings suggests that the order quantity should be kept as small as possible if carrying costs are to be minimized. Hence, there is a conflict between the costs of acquisition and the costs of possession that must be resolved if management is to obtain a least cost solution.

In addition to these cost components, management may incur additional costs when either too much or too little inventory is held. The costs of holding unused and/or unnecessary quantities of inventory items are referred to as long-costs or overstocked costs. When too little inventory is held, management incurs short-costs or stock-out costs. Since long-costs and short-costs arise under conditions of uncertainty, these components are described next.

### 9.4.3 Long-Costs

Long-costs or overstocked costs are composed of two elements: a carrying cost component and a perishability component. With regard to the former, a surplus of inventory exists whenever goods are purchased for use in a particular period but are not used in that period. Management then is forced to hold the inventory items until they are used in providing patient care.

As an example of the unnecessary carrying costs of excessive inventories, assume that the beginning inventory of period 1 consists of 1,000 units of a particular supply item. Suppose further that during the period only 100 units of the supply item are used in providing patient care and that the remaining 900 units are not used until period 4. During this period, the 900 units were not required to assure continuous care and, as a consequence, the carrying costs of holding them were unnecessary.

Management also may incur a perishability cost when it holds excessive inventories. This component of long-cost is not relevant to all hospital stocks but should be discussed to provide a complete understanding of the long-costs that may arise. Of primary concern when considering this cost element are certain pharmaceutical stocks that can neither be used nor returned for credit after the expiration of specific periods of time. Suppose, for example, that the hospital is overstocked and unable to use drugs before their expiration date. In this case, the hospital incurs both the unnecessary carrying costs of holding excessive stock and a perishability cost equal to the full cost of the goods that must be discarded after expiration dates have passed.

### 9.4.4 Short-Costs

Short-costs involve holding an insufficient quantity of inventory. As mentioned, the hospital must obtain and have certain supplies available to avoid disruptions in the care process. It also will be recalled that if the institution is to operate efficiently, the quantity of inventory stocks must be related closely to the demand for hospital care. However, given the nature of the demand for care and the inability to predict the need for inventory with complete precision, the costs of failing to satisfy that demand for care can be costly. In the event that inventories are insufficient, management may be forced to:

1. place additional orders
2. exert additional efforts when the goods are received
3. go outside the normal delivery mechanism
4. arrange for special transportation in the event of an emergency in order to satisfy the demands for care

Each of these activities represents an out-of-pocket expenditure by the hospital that is reflected in unavoidable increased order and purchase costs if the production process is not to be disrupted.

The costs of insufficient inventories should be measured in both monetary and nonmonetary terms. When inventories are insufficient, it usually is not possible to provide care, which of course results in foregone income. In addition, an inadequate supply may result in nonpecuniary costs. It thus is necessary to measure the costs of inventory shortages in terms of such factors as prolonged illness, pain, and perhaps even death. Since no objective criteria exist for placing a value on these factors, the magnitude of these costs must be determined on a subjective basis.

Due to the nature of these nonpecuniary factors, a high value must be assigned to the costs associated with insufficient supplies. In fact, it could be argued that the costs of holding an insufficient inventory are of such a magnitude that management should ensure that a stock-out never occurs. However, from a practical point of view it is well known that resources are limited and as a result it is not possible to ensure absolutely that a stock-out will never occur.

In summary of this section, the total cost of holding inventories may be defined by

$$TC = J\left(\frac{D_t}{Q}\right) + K\left(\frac{Q}{2}\right) + LC + SC \qquad (9.7)$$

where

$$TC \quad = \text{total cost}$$
$$J\left(\frac{D_t}{Q}\right) = \text{ordering costs}$$
$$K\left(\frac{Q}{2}\right) = \text{carrying costs}$$
$$LC \quad = \text{long-costs}$$
$$SC \quad = \text{short-costs}$$

It should be noted that the long-costs and short-costs require a different management decision than the expense of carrying or ordering inventory. The long-cost and short-cost components of Equation 9.7 require that management reconcile the use of inventory with the level of inventory. On the other hand, the order and carrying cost components require management to balance the size of orders with their frequency. The manner in which long-costs and short-costs have been included in Equation 9.7 is a simplification of a more complex relationship. For example, rather than the simple additive relation in this equation, it is possible to argue that long-costs and short-costs are related to the size of the order as well as the derived demand for inventory.

Since costs are attached to inventories, the problem confronting management is to prescribe policies that result in a minimum $TC$. In describing techniques that may be used in developing such policies, the next section considers inventory control under conditions of certainty, and the chapter concludes with an examination of inventory management under conditions of uncertainty.

## 9.5 INVENTORY MANAGEMENT: CERTAINTY

In this section and the next, several methods are introduced that may be used to reach essentially two operating decisions. The first decision involves the determination of the optimum reorder point. The reorder point represents the level of inventory that signals the need to replenish existing stocks. Thus, when inventory is reduced to the reorder point, management should place an order to replenish depleted stocks. The second decision involves the determination of the order size.

Assume that an institution operates in a world of certainty where the demand for care and the demand for inventories are constant and known. Also assume that the placement of an order for supplies and the delivery of the supplies are not instantaneous. That is, there is a known and invariant time lag between ordering and receiving consumable supplies. This situation is illustrated in Figure 9-3 where the $t$'s correspond to the lead time or the lag between ordering and receiving supplies while $Q$ represents the amount ordered.

**Figure 9-3** Ordering and Receiving Supplies

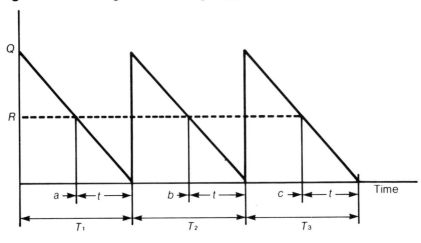

These assumptions imply that this quantity is used at a steady or constant rate during the period $T$. When inventory holdings reach a critical level, the quantity $Q$ is reordered and the process is replicated. Under these circumstances, management's major task is to determine the quantity of stock it should order and when it should place the orders.

On the basis of these assumptions, the long-cost and short-cost components in Equation 9.7 may be ignored since, in a world of certainty, the probability of the hospital's carrying excessive inventory or encountering a period in which inventory holdings are insufficient is zero. Thus, the expected stock-out and overstocked costs are zero, which means that the expression

$$TC^* = J\left(\frac{D_t}{Q}\right) + K\left(\frac{Q}{2}\right) \tag{9.8}$$

represents the total costs of holding inventories in a world of certainty.

As described earlier, order costs vary directly with the frequency of orders and inversely with their quantity. Conversely, carrying costs vary directly with the quantity and inversely with the frequency of orders. The relation between order costs, carrying costs, total costs, and the quantity ordered is seen in Figure 9-4. Here, the total cost function ($TC^*$) is obtained by computing the sum of the order costs and the carrying costs. At $Q^*$, the total costs are at a minimum. Thus, $Q^*$ corresponds to the point at which the marginal cost of rising expenses is equal to the marginal cost of decreasing expenses. In other words, $Q^*$ represents the point at which the slope of the increasing carrying cost function is equal to the slope of the decreasing order cost function. As a result, $Q^*$, which also is called the economic order quantity (EOQ), represents the optimum amount that management should order. The derivation of the EOQ is shown below.

Assuming a world of certainty, we saw that the total cost of inventories can be expressed in the form

$$TC^* = J\left(\frac{D_t}{Q}\right) + K\left(\frac{Q}{2}\right)$$

The optimum order quantity or the economic order quantity is found by differentiating this expression with respect to $Q$, setting the derivative to zero and solving for $Q$. Differentiating with respect to $Q$ yields

$$\frac{dTC^*}{dQ} = -\frac{JD_t}{Q^2} + \frac{K}{2}$$

Setting $\dfrac{dTC^*}{dQ}$ to zero, we have

$$-\frac{JD_t}{Q^2} + \frac{K}{2} = 0$$

and solving for $Q$ we find

$$\frac{JD_t}{Q^2} = \frac{K}{2}$$

$$Q^2 = \frac{2JD_t}{K}$$

$$Q^* = \sqrt{\frac{2JD_t}{K}} \qquad\qquad (9.9)$$

To illustrate the use of Equation 9.9, suppose that management possesses the following information:

$D_t$ = 10,000 units (usage per year)
$J$ = $5 (unit cost of placing an order)
$K$ = $10 (unit carrying cost)

When we substitute these values in Equation 9.9, the optimum order size is found to be

$$Q^* = \sqrt{\frac{2(5)\ (10,000)}{10}}$$

$$= \sqrt{10,000}$$

$$= 100 \text{ units}$$

These calculations suggest that an order size of 100 units will minimize the total cost of ordering and carrying inventory. Substituting $Q = 100$, $D_t = 10,000$, $J = \$5$, and $K = \$10$ into Equation 9.8 yields the minimum total cost of

$$TC_{100} = \$5\left(\frac{10,000}{100}\right) + 10\left(\frac{100}{2}\right)$$

$$= \$1,000$$

That an order quantity of 100 units results in minimum total cost of $1,000 is seen also in Table 9-2.

Having determined the order quantity that minimizes total cost, the management's next task is to determine when inventory should be reordered. Under the assumptions set forth earlier, the usage of inventory per day and the time interval between the placement and receipt of orders are known with certainty. Under conditions of certainty, then, the reorder point is equal to the number of units that will be used during the lead time. Thus, the reorder point is given by

$$R = \begin{matrix} \text{Known and} \\ \text{Invariant} \\ \text{Daily Usage} \end{matrix} \times \begin{matrix} \text{Lead} \\ \text{Time} \end{matrix}$$

The relation between the reorder point, daily usage, and the time interval between the placement and receipt of an order was seen in Figure 9-3. The $t$'s

---

**Table 9-2** Tabular Presentation of EOQ

| Order Quantity | Ordering Costs | Carrying Costs | Total |
|---|---|---|---|
| 25 | $2,000 | $125 | $2,125 |
| 50 | 1,000 | 250 | 1,250 |
| 75 | 667 | 375 | 1,042 |
| 100 | 500 | 500 | 1,000 |
| 125 | 400 | 625 | 1,025 |
| 150 | 333 | 750 | 1,083 |
| 175 | 286 | 875 | 1,161 |

**Figure 9-4** Ordering and Carrying Costs

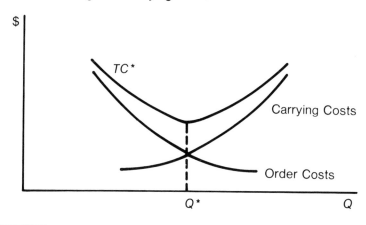

correspond to the lead time, while the absolute value of the slope of the line that depicts the relation between inventory holdings and time represents daily usage. Given a known and invariant lead time, the reorder dates are given by the points *a, b,* and *c,* while the level of inventory that signals the need to reorder is given by the point *R*.

If the hospital operates under conditions of certainty, the data required to develop a least cost solution to the problems of inventory management now are available. That is, the magnitude and timing of inventory reorders will be known with certainty by management. Unfortunately, however, hospitals do not operate in a world of certainty and this decision model is not completely realistic. As a result, the analysis must be expanded to accommodate the uncertainty regarding the derived demand for hospital inventories.

## 9.6 INVENTORY MANAGEMENT: UNCERTAINTY

To develop an inventory decision model that pertains to a world of uncertainty, it is necessary to consider the long-costs and short-costs that were ignored in the previous section. In a world of certainty, management knows that when the level of inventory reaches *R* it is time to reorder and that the goods will arrive just as the last unit in stock is being used in providing care. In the world of uncertainty, however, the actual demand for inventory during the lead time may differ from the expected or average usage per day. This may result in the hospital's being overstocked or, perhaps more importantly, understocked. The issue of concern to management is the variation in the demand for stocks during the lead time, since it is this variability that exposes the hospital to the danger of an inventory shortage.

### 9.6.1 The EOQ and Reorder Point: Uncertainty

As noted, short-costs should be measured in terms of the intangible costs of prolonged illness, pain, and death. Because of the nature of the intangible factors, a high value should be assigned to stock-out costs. Many administrators feel that the avoidance of insufficient stocks of certain types of inventory such as blood, oxygen, and certain drugs is critical. For these types of stock, management should maintain a buffer or safety stock.

To develop the notion of a buffer or safety stock, assume that we know only the probability distribution of demand during the period between the placement and receipt of orders but we do not know the actual demand during that period. Thus, when we establish the order point there is some probability that we will encounter a shortage of inventory, which may result in pain, suffering, and perhaps death.

The behavior of inventory under this assumption is illustrated in Figure 9-5. An order of size $Q$ is placed when inventory holdings reach a level represented by $R$ in Figure 9-5. Because of the uncertainties of demand for inventory, a shortage of consumable supplies can occur; such a situation is seen in the third cycle of the figure.

The hospital inventory now is divided into two components. The first component is operating or cycle stock and is defined as the portion of the inventory holdings that is a function of the order size $Q$. On the average, then, the operating stock will assume the value $Q/2$. The second component is called the buffer or safety stock. This refers to the difference between the reorder point $R$ and the average demand for inventory during the lead time symbolized by $\bar{Y}$.

---

**Figure 9-5** Inventory Behavior under Conditions of Uncertainty

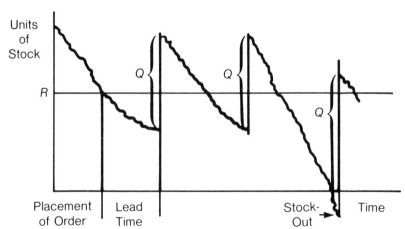

These two components are illustrated in Figure 9-6. As might be surmised, the larger is the safety stock, the lower is the probability that the hospital will encounter an inventory shortage. It follows, therefore, that the greater the safety stock, the higher the corresponding reorder point.

At this point in the analysis, it is useful to summarize briefly the interrelationships between the various costs, the reorder point, and the order size. First, if we decrease (increase) the order *point*, which implies that we place an order when a lower (higher) level of inventory is reached, the carrying costs associated with the safety stock decrease (increase) while the short-costs are likely to increase (decrease). Similarly, if the order *size* is decreased (increased), the carrying costs associated with the operating stock will decrease (increase) while the stock-out and ordering costs will increase (decrease).

These relationships suggest that a change in the order size will influence the frequency both of reaching the reorder point and of encountering an inventory shortage. Similarly, a change in the reorder point influences the probability of encountering a stock-out as well as the optimum number of times the order point should be encountered. As a result, the total cost of holding inventories is influenced by the order point and the order quantity.

As before, the objective of management should be to minimize the total costs incurred during a given period. In this situation, however, three types of cost must be considered: the cost of placing orders, the carrying costs, and the stock-out or short-cost expenses. As will be seen, the optimum order size will be a function of these three costs and inventory decisions will be related to the average demand for inventory during the lead time.

Similar to earlier examples, we assume that the lead time is known with certainty and is constant. Further, we assume that the demand for inventory is

**Figure 9-6** Two Components of Hospital Inventory

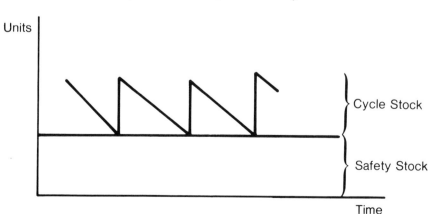

distributed normally and that the optimal reorder point $R$ is greater than the average demand during the lead time. The latter assumption requires that the difference given by $(R - \bar{Y})$ be positive. Finally, we assume that for certain categories of hospital inventory, the buffer or safety stock, on the average, is carried in inventory during the lead time. Our next task, then, is to determine how much to order, $Q$, and when to order, $R$.

In the following analysis, let:

$J$ = the cost of placing a single order
$K$ = carrying cost per unit
$S_u$ = unit cost of being out of stock
$D_t$ = average demand per period
$Q$ = order quantity
$Y$ = number of units used during the lead time
$\bar{Y}$ = average number of units used during the lead time
$\sigma_y$ = standard deviation of usage during the lead time

Concerning the optimum order size, we might calculate the economic order quantity by

$$Q^* = \sqrt{\frac{2JD_t}{K}}$$

which was developed earlier in this chapter. It will be recalled that the derivation of this formulation was based on the assumption that demand or usage was known with certainty; it is legitimate to examine the rationale for employing this equation in a situation in which the usage of inventory during the lead time is problematical.

The primary reason for using this equation in a world of uncertainty is that total cost is not particularly sensitive to errors in determining $Q$. Because of the square root, a substantial error in estimating demand results in a much smaller percent error in the order size as compared with the optimal order size. Consider the example in Table 9-2, where it was assumed that the annual demand was known to be 10,000 units. Had we erroneously thought the annual demand was 15,000 units, we would have obtained the following incorrect order quantity

$$Q^* = \sqrt{\frac{2(5)\ (15,000)}{10}} = \sqrt{15,000} = 123 \text{ units}$$

Because of the square root, a 50 percent error in estimating demand (15,000/10,000) results in a 23 percent error in the order size (123/100) as compared to the "correct" optimal order size of $Q = 100$. However, the error that results from using an incorrect order quantity should be evaluated in terms of its relative costliness. Substituting $Q = 123$ into the total cost function, we find that

$$TC_{123} = 10\left(\frac{123}{2}\right) + 5\left(\frac{10,000}{123}\right) = \$1,021.50$$

Comparing this cost with the total cost of the order quantity $Q = 100$ that was $1,000, we find that the percentage increase in cost, which is the penalty for using $Q = 123$, is only 21.50/1,000 or 2.15 percent. Thus, so long as the order quantity is estimated with reasonable precision, little benefit is gained by improving the accuracy of $Q$.

Once management has selected $Q$, it is important to take its value into account when determining the reorder point $R$. This is because the size of $Q$ directly influences the frequency with which orders are placed in a given period as well as the number of times the hospital is exposed to the risks of encountering a shortage of inventory.

Recall that the buffer or safety stock was defined as the difference between $R$ and $\bar{Y}$ where $R$ exceeds $\bar{Y}$. Applying marginal analysis, we may compare the expected marginal cost of increasing the reorder point by one unit with the expected marginal costs of *not* adding one more unit to $R$. It should be noted that the increment in costs of increasing $R$ by one unit is given by $K$, the carrying costs, since the additional unit normally will be added to the safety stock ($R - \bar{Y}$). On the other hand, the annual additional costs of not adding one more unit will equal the probability that the unit will be used during the period multiplied by the short-cost $S_u$, all of which is multiplied by the number of inventory cycles, $\frac{D_t}{Q}$. Therefore, we find

$$\Delta C = P(Y > R) \cdot S_u\left(\frac{D_t}{Q}\right) \qquad (9.10)$$

where

| | | |
|---|---|---|
| $\Delta C$ | = | marginal cost of not adding an incremental unit to $R$ |
| $P(Y > R)$ | = | probability that usage during the lead time will exceed the current value of $R$ |
| $S_u$ | = | unit stock-out cost |
| $\dfrac{D_t}{Q}$ | = | number of inventory cycles |

The marginal costs of adding or not adding the incremental unit to $R$ are seen in Figure 9-7. As the reorder point increases, the probability that the additional

**Figure 9-7** Marginal Costs and Incremental Units

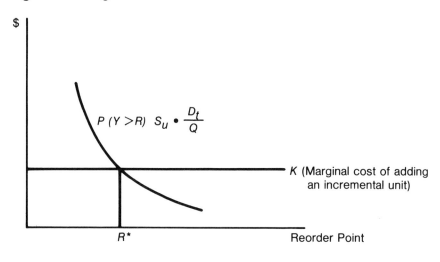

unit will be used decreases. As $R$ increases, $\Delta C$ declines until the additional cost of not adding the incremental unit equals the marginal cost of adding the incremental unit to $R$. The intersection of these two lines yields the optimum reorder point. Thus, at $R^*$ in Figure 9-7 we find

$$K = P(Y > R)\, S_u \left(\frac{D_t}{Q}\right)$$

Observing that

$$P(Y > R) = 1 - P(Y \leq R)$$

we find

$$K = [1 - P(Y \leq R)]\, S_u \left(\frac{D_t}{Q}\right)$$

Solving for $P(Y \leq R)$, the probability that usage during the lead time is less than or equal to the reorder point $R$, yields

$$P(Y \leq R) = 1 - \frac{KQ}{S_u D_t} \qquad\qquad \textbf{(9.11)}$$

When using Equation 9.11 to determine the optimal reorder point $R$, it is only necessary to:

1. determine $Q$ by employing Equation 9.9;
2. calculate the right hand side of Equation 9.11, which results in the probability that usage during the lead time will be equal to or less than $R$;
3. find the value of $Z$ for which the probability applies, assuming that usage during the lead time is distributed normally.

The term $P(Y \leqslant R)$ means that we establish $R$ so that there is a probability of $1 - \dfrac{KQ}{S_u D_t}$ that $Y$ will be less than or equal to $R$.

Assuming that usage during the lead time is distributed normally, we let $Z$ represent the number of standard deviations that corresponds to the probability $P(Y \leqslant R)$. This is seen in Figure 9-8. We then can determine the optimum reorder point $R$ as follows:

$$R = \bar{Y} + Z\sigma_y \qquad\qquad (9.12)$$

Thus, we find that the reorder point is equal to the average usage during the lead time plus the safety stock where the safety stock is $Z\sigma_y$.

To illustrate this technique, suppose that the following information is available to management:

$$
\begin{aligned}
D_t &= 1{,}000 \text{ units} \\
Q &= 100 \text{ units} \\
K &= \$10 \\
S_u &= \$50 \\
\bar{Y} &= 30 \text{ units} \\
\sigma_y &= 10 \text{ units}
\end{aligned}
$$

Substituting appropriately into Equation 9.11 we find that

$$P(Y \leqslant R) = 1 - \frac{\$10(100)}{\$50(1{,}000)} = .98$$

Therefore, the probability that the usage during the lead time will be less than or equal to $R$ is .98. Referring to the probability distribution function for the normal curve, we find that the corresponding $Z$ value is approximately 2.05 and the optimum reorder point is given by

**Figure 9-8** Determining the Optimum Reorder Point

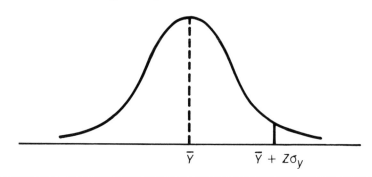

$$R = \bar{Y} + Z\sigma_y = 30 + 2.05(10)$$

$$\cong 51 \text{ units}$$

Thus, with a reorder point of 51 units, management is 98 percent certain that an inventory shortage will not occur during the lead time.

## 9.6.2 The Reorder Point: A Mathematical Expectation Model

Thus far, the long-costs to which we referred have been ignored. In arriving at a reorder point that minimizes the sum of expected long-costs and short-costs, management must obtain two types of information. The first type portrays the probable variation in demand that can be expected after the reorder point has been reached, while the second depicts the costs associated with being over-stocked and understocked.

Suppose that on the basis of historical data, management determines that the stock-out (understocked) cost is equal to $50 per unit and the overstocked cost is $5 per unit. Also assume that the probable variation in the demand for stock during the lead time has been developed and summarized as follows:

| Demand | Probability |
|--------|-------------|
| 10 | .10 |
| 11 | .15 |
| 12 | .30 |
| 13 | .25 |
| 14 | .10 |
| 15 | .10 |

On the basis of this information, management is in a position to calculate the expected costs of each reorder strategy and to determine which strategy results in the least cost solution.

The method of determining the least cost solution may be described as follows. The long-costs and short-costs of each strategy and each potential demand are determined in Table 9-3. As an example, the long-cost associated with the reorder strategy of 12 units and the potential demand of 10 units is found to be $10 (i.e., long-cost of $5 per unit × the surplus of 2 units). Similarly, the short-cost associated with the reorder strategy of 12 units and the potential demand of 15 units is $150 (i.e., the short-cost of $50 per unit × the shortage of 3 units).

The next step in determining the least cost solution is to calculate the total expected cost associated with each reorder strategy. Let

$$\mathbf{p}' = [.10 \quad .15 \quad .30 \quad .25 \quad .10 \quad .10]$$

and

$$\mathbf{Z} = \begin{bmatrix} \$\,0 & \$\,5 & \$10 & \$15 & \$20 & \$25 \\ 50 & 0 & 5 & 10 & 15 & 20 \\ 100 & 50 & 0 & 5 & 10 & 15 \\ 150 & 100 & 50 & 0 & 5 & 10 \\ 200 & 150 & 100 & 50 & 0 & 5 \\ 250 & 200 & 150 & 100 & 50 & 0 \end{bmatrix}$$

The expected total cost of each strategy is given by

$$\mathbf{t} = \mathbf{p}'\mathbf{Z}' = [\$120 \quad \$75.50 \quad \$39.25 \quad \$19.50 \quad \$13.50 \quad \$13.00]$$

where each element of the row vector represents the expected total cost of the corresponding reorder strategy. Thus, we find that the expected total cost of each reorder strategy is given by

| Reorder Strategy | Expected Total Cost |
|---|---|
| 10 | $120.00 |
| 11 | 75.50 |
| 12 | 39.25 |
| 13 | 19.50 |
| 14 | 13.50 |
| 15* | 13.00 |

**Table 9-3** Determining the Least Cost Solution

| Reorder Strategy | Potential Demand | | | | | |
|---|---|---|---|---|---|---|
| | 10 | 11 | 12 | 13 | 14 | 15 |
| 10 | $0 | $50 | $100 | $150 | $200 | $250 |
| 11 | 5 | 0 | 50 | 100 | 150 | 200 |
| 12 | 10 | 5 | 0 | 50 | 100 | 150 |
| 13 | 15 | 10 | 5 | 0 | 50 | 100 |
| 14 | 20 | 15 | 10 | 5 | 0 | 50 |
| 15 | 25 | 20 | 15 | 10 | 5 | 0 |

These data suggest that a reorder strategy of 15 units results in a least cost solution.

Given the least cost reorder point and the economic order quantity, management is now in a position to develop its inventory policy. The technique presented in this section provides management with the information required to develop policies concerning the reorder point while the economic order quantity provides the information for developing policies regarding the amount of inventory to be ordered.

REFERENCES

American Hospital Association. *Internal Control and Internal Auditing for Hospitals*. Chicago: American Hospital Association, 1969.

_____. *Readings in Material Management*. Chicago: American Hospital Association, 1973.

Ammer, D. S. *Purchasing and Materials Management for Health Care Institutions*. Lexington, Mass.: Lexington Books, 1975.

Baker, "How Imaginative Inventory Management Can Strengthen Internal Control." *Hospital Financial Management*, vol. 25, no. 2, February 1971.

Holmgren, J. H. *Purchasing for the Health Care Facility*. Springfield, Ill.: Charles C Thomas, 1975.

"Materials Management, Special Issue." *Hospitals*, JAHA, vol. 51, no. 12, June 16, 1977.

Nelson, R. J. "Effective Planning and Control of Inventory—A Management Approach." *Hospital Progress*, December 1968, p. 42.

Snyder, A. "Principles of Inventory Management." *Financial Executive*, April 1964, pp. 13–21.

# Part III
# Internal Control

# Chapter 10
# Cost Analysis

## Objectives

After completing this chapter, you should be able to:

1. Understand the importance and uses of cost analysis.
2. Identify the necessary prerequisites of cost analysis.
3. Perform cost analysis using:
   a. the direct apportionment method,
   b. the step-down method,
   c. the double distribution method.
4. Express the apportionment techniques in the notation of matrix algebra.

## 10.1 MANAGERIAL USES OF COST ANALYSIS

As noted earlier, the problem of containing costs is assuming an ever-increasing importance in Canada and the United States. If a hospital is to achieve the goal of providing required services at an acceptable level of quality and at minimum cost, it is imperative that management plan and control internal operations. The primary focus of this part of the book is on the process of internal control as well as techniques that may be applied to the problem of containing costs and ensuring that required services are provided to the patient population. More specifically, this chapter is devoted to cost finding or cost analysis, which is one of the techniques that should play an important role in achieving the goals of the hospital enterprise.

It is necessary first to recognize that cost analysis plays a dominant role in the process of determining the actual and expected full cost of providing services that earn revenue for the hospital. To understand the principles of cost finding, the hospital should be viewed as consisting of a set of general service or support centers and a set of patient service centers that provide the services that generate revenue. Cost finding is the process by which the costs of operating the general service centers of the hospital are allocated to the departments or functional units that provide direct patient care and, as a result, earn income for the institution.

The role played by cost finding in planning, monitoring, and controlling the operational activity of the hospital is shown in Figure 10-1. This figure demonstrates that cost analysis plays an important role in the process of developing the future plan of operations as expressed by the operating budget. In addition, cost-finding techniques may be used to develop indexes of actual operational activity that, when compared with the standard of performance as expressed by the budget, provide the basis for management to monitor, evaluate, and control the hospital's overall performance as well as the current operational results of its organizational units. The following discussion considers in detail the usefulness of cost finding in planning and controlling the performance of the hospital.

## 10.1.1 Planning Operational Activity

That the revenues generated by a hospital must at least equal the total economic costs of operation, including the cost of providing general support services and the replacement cost of capital, is well recognized in the health care industry. In assessing the extent to which the financial viability of the hospital will be preserved during the coming period, it is necessary to compare anticipated expenditures with expected revenues.

Figure 10-1, assumes that planned operating activity provides the basis for projecting the costs that are reflected in the expense budgets of the various departmental units or cost centers of the hospital. In this regard, the prospective development of the fee schedule must reflect not only the direct costs associated with those services that earn revenue but also the costs of providing general support services.

At this juncture in the planning process, cost-finding techniques may be used to determine the full costs (i.e., the direct cost plus an equitable share of the indirect costs of providing hospital care) of services that generate revenue. On the basis of the data generated by cost-finding techniques, management may develop the hospital's prospective fee schedule. The projected fee schedule, when coupled with the expected volume of services that earn income for the hospital, provides the basis for developing the revenue budget. Cost finding, then, provides the basis for developing the revenue budget of the hospital that, when compared with total anticipated expenditures, permits management to assess the extent to which the financial viability of the institution will be preserved during the coming period.

**Figure 10-1** The Role of Cost Analysis in Controlling and Evaluating Operations

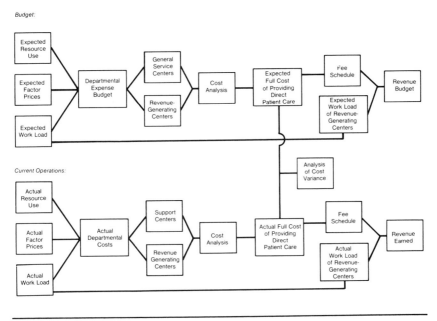

Cost finding is of value to management in other ways. For example, decisions regarding planned staffing patterns for various departments or responsibility centers comprising the hospital enterprise should be derived only with the full knowledge of the cost implications of alternate approaches and the real needs of the units concerned. Accurate cost analysis also is a prerequisite to effective personnel management as well as planning and presenting the views of management in the collective bargaining process.

## 10.1.2 Controlling Operational Activity

As implied in Figure 10-1, cost-finding techniques may be applied to the problem of controlling operational activity. In this case, cost analysis plays a central role in developing indexes or measures of actual operational results. As seen in the figure, cost finding provides the basis for determining the actual full cost of services that earn revenue for the hospital. Thus, cost finding allows management to compare the total costs and the revenues associated with providing direct patient care that, in turn, represents the basis for assessing the need to adjust the fee schedule of the hospital retrospectively. In addition, cost-finding techniques form the basis for comparing the anticipated full cost of providing direct patient care with the full costs actually incurred. Obviously, unfavorable variances frequently identify areas of operational activity in which remedial actions or policies are required to realign current performance.

Moreover, cost finding can help in the management of specific departments or functional units of the hospital. The purchasing department must concern itself with costs and inventory levels, the dietary department with controlling the unit cost of meals served. Similarly, the laundry and housekeeping departments must be concerned about the cost of performing their functions as compared with obtaining the same services from an external agency. Each of these department heads requires good information that can be derived through cost finding.

For these and other reasons, the effective management of the hospital enterprise requires an accurate appraisal of costs that may be obtained through cost-finding techniques.

## 10.2 NECESSARY PREREQUISITES

Four prerequisites which must be satisfied before cost-finding techniques may be used effectively: (1) a sound organization chart and a corresponding chart of accounts, (2) a classification of all cost centers, (3) an accurate accounting system, and (4) a comprehensive system by which nonfinancial information is gathered.

### 10.2.1 Organization Chart and Chart of Accounts

The organization chart and the chart of accounts provide the guidelines by which costs are allocated from the general service centers to the departments or functional areas providing direct patient care.

### 10.2.2 Classification of Cost Centers

The classification of all cost centers requires that departments or functional areas comprising the hospital be divided into two groups. The first group contains departments or units that provide support services such as plant operations, plant maintenance, laundry, housekeeping, and dietary. The second group is composed of departments that provide elements of care that are used in diagnosing, monitoring, and therapeutically managing the medical condition presented by the patient. Examples of departments in the second group are radiology, laboratory, operating room, nursing care units, and pharmacy. This classification is necessary so that all of the costs assigned to the general service centers may be apportioned to the departments that provide the services that earn revenue.

### 10.2.3 Accurate Accounting System

Once the cost centers have been identified, the accounting system must be capable of recording accurate cost data and assigning this information to the various general service and patient care centers. In this regard, it is necessary to review the System for Hospital Uniform Reporting (SHUR). Under the SHUR program, cost and utilization data must be classified on a functional cost center basis. Consequently, only expenses directly related to a given unit are charged to the unit. For example, under responsibility accounting, the entire expense associated with a nurse who is assigned to the intensive care unit is charged to that unit. On the other hand, under functional reporting, only expenses directly related to performing the functions of the ICU are charged to the unit. To illustrate the difference between responsibility and functional reporting, suppose that 20, 30, and 50 percent of the total number of hours worked by the nurse were devoted to performing functions assigned to central supply, the emergency room, and the intensive care unit, respectively. Under functional reporting, the expense associated with the nurse must be charged to central supply, the emergency room, and the intensive care unit in proportion to the amount of time devoted to the functions assigned to those units. More specifically, the SHUR program required the direct assignment of costs to the functional units of the hospital, costs such as building and fixture depreciation, movable equipment depreciation, salaries, related payroll benefits, medical supplies, drugs, plant maintenance, data processing, and central patient transportation.

### 10.2.4 Information System

The hospital must have information by which expenses that are shared or incurred by several departments are allocated so as to obtain accurate cost figures. To apportion these costs properly, the hospital must have a set of nonfinancial data that can be used to allocate costs among all centers. For each service department it is necessary to select a basic unit that best reflects the extent to which other departments consume its services. The nonfinancial information required of each center includes the square footage, number of employees, number of meals served, number of pounds of laundry used, and so on.

Assuming that these prerequisites are satisfied, several methods of cost analysis are available to the hospital: (1) direct apportionment, (2) the step-down method, and (3) the double-distribution technique. It also should be noted that the Canadian Hospital Association has suggested a method of cost allocation that uses the basic principles described below. However, since the method will not be considered here, the reader is directed to the supplement to the Canadian Hospital Accounting Manual cited at the end of the chapter.

A final introductory comment is worthy of note: Depending on the size of the institution, cost finding is a long and tedious process, particularly if all calculations are performed using a desk calculator. However, when the notation and operations of matrix algebra are used to express the cost-finding techniques, management may develop programs that permit the use of high-speed electronic computers to perform required calculations. As a result, to enhance the usefulness of cost-finding techniques in medium and large institutions, each of the cost-finding techniques is expressed in the notation of matrix algebra.

## 10.3 METHODS OF APPORTIONMENT

To illustrate the selected methods of cost apportionment, the data in Table 10-1 are assumed to be available to a hypothetical hospital. In the presentation that follows, it is assumed that the general service centers of the hospital are the dietary, housekeeping, and laundry departments while the revenue-generating or patient care centers are represented by the laboratory and radiology departments and a nursing unit.

The nonfinancial data in Columns (1), (2), and (3) represent the basis on which the costs of the general service centers are allocated to the revenue-generating or patient care centers. The examples in this chapter use the number of meals, square footage, and pounds of laundry to allocate the costs of the dietary, housekeeping, and laundry departments, respectively. Finally, it is as-

**Table 10-1**  Summary of Financial and Nonfinancial Information Required for Cost Finding

| | | Nonfinancial Data (Apportionment Basis) | | |
| | Pounds of Laundry | Square Feet | Number of Meals | Financial Data (Original Costs) |
| Department | (1) | (2) | (3) | (4) |
| --- | --- | --- | --- | --- |
| General Service Center | | | | |
| Dietary | 50,000 | 600 | 50 | $7,500 |
| Housekeeping | 40,000 | 200 | 30 | 6,000 |
| Laundry | 10,000 | 200 | 20 | 10,000 |
| Subtotal | 100,000 | 1,000 | 100 | 23,500 |
| | | | | |
| Revenue Generating Center | | | | |
| Laboratory | 5,000 | 800 | 15 | 40,000 |
| Radiology | 15,000 | 400 | 35 | 60,000 |
| Nursing unit | 180,000 | 2,000 | 950 | 220,000 |
| Subtotal | 200,000 | 3,200 | 1,000 | 320,000 |
| Total | 300,000 | 4,200 | 1,100 | 343,500 |

sumed that the following departmental codes have been assigned to the organizational units of the hypothetical hospital:

|  | Department | Code Number |
|---|---|---|
| General service centers: |  |  |
|  | Dietary | 1 |
|  | Housekeeping | 2 |
|  | Laundry | 3 |
| Revenue-generating centers: |  |  |
|  | Laboratory | 4 |
|  | Radiology | 5 |
|  | Nursing unit | 6 |

As mentioned, the objective of cost finding is to allocate the costs of the general service departments to the revenue-generating or patient care centers. Table 10-1 presents both the costs to be allocated and the costs assigned to the revenue-generating centers. The objective of the exercise, then, is to allocate to the revenue-generating centers the $23,500 assigned to the general service centers.

## 10.3.1 Direct Apportionment

When costs are distributed in accordance with the direct apportionment method, interdepartmental demands among the general service centers are ignored in the allocation process. As a result, the costs of the general service centers are apportioned directly to the patient service centers. Recalling that departmental codes 1, 2, and 3 correspond to general service centers, and departmental codes 4, 5, and 6 to the patient service centers, the direct apportionment method is depicted schematically in Figure 10-2. The total cost, $TC$, of each general service center is apportioned directly to the patient care centers. After the costs of the last department have been apportioned, the total expenses of the representative patient service center $j$ are found to be:

$$TC_j = D_j + AC_{1j} + AC_{2j} + AC_{3j}$$

where

$D_j$ = direct cost of center $j$;
$AC_{ij}$ = apportioned cost from center $i$ to center $j$ for $i = 1, 2, 3$

Recall that the basis for apportioning the cost of general service center $i$ is the relative use of its services by the other units to which the costs are to be

**Figure 10-2** Direct Apportionment Allocation

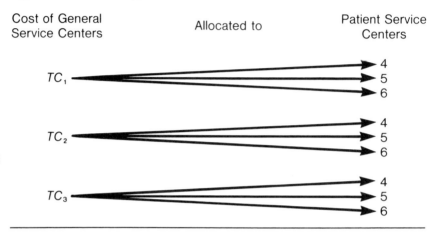

allocated. Consider, for example, the major function performed by the house-keeping department. The demand for its services might be expressed as a ratio of the square footage of the department to which costs are apportioned relative to the total square footage of all departments to which costs are allocated. Underlying this apportionment coefficient is the implicit assumption that the effort required of the housekeeping department to maintain a square foot in a given department is equivalent to the effort required to maintain a square foot in any other department. However, since the intensive care unit and operating room require more housekeeping effort per square foot than most nursing units, the measures of relative demand may not be proportional to the services actually provided and the surrogate for interdepartmental exchanges currently used may not be completely accurate.

Table 10-2 demonstrates the results of the cost allocation resulting from an application of the direct method to the hypothetical hospital. In this and the other examples in this chapter, the measures of relative demand represent the proportion of general services used by the department to which costs are allo-cated. For example, consider the apportionment coefficient by which the costs of the dietary department are allocated to the nursing unit. The nursing unit uses 95 percent of the meals provided to the revenue-generating centers. As a result, 95 percent of the costs assigned to the dietary department are allocated to the nursing unit. The denominator of the apportionment coefficient is composed of the total demand exerted on the general service centers by the centers (in this case the patient care units) to which the costs are apportioned. Accordingly, the numerator of the apportionment coefficient represents the demand for service exerted by the department to which costs are apportioned. The apportionment

**Table 10-2** Direct Apportionment Method

| Department from Which Costs Are Allocated | Cost to Be Allocated (1) | × | Apportionment Coefficient (2) | = | Apportioned Cost (3) | Department to Which Costs Are Allocated |
|---|---|---|---|---|---|---|
| Dietary | $7,500 | | 15/1000 = .015 | | $ 112.50 | Laboratory |
| | 7,500 | | 35/1000 = .035 | | 262.50 | Radiology |
| | 7,500 | | 950/1000 = .950 | | 7,125.00 | Nursing Unit |
| | | | | | 7,500.00 | |
| Housekeeping | 6,000 | | 800/3,200 = .250 | | 1,500.00 | Laboratory |
| | 6,000 | | 400/3,200 = .125 | | 750.00 | Radiology |
| | 6,000 | | 2,000/3,200 = .625 | | 3,750.00 | Nursing Unit |
| | | | | | 6,000.00 | |
| Laundry | 10,000 | | 5,000/200,000 = .025 | | 250.00 | Laboratory |
| | 10,000 | | 15,000/200,000 = .075 | | 750.00 | Radiology |
| | 10,000 | | 180,000/200,000 = .900 | | 9,000.00 | Nursing Unit |
| | | | | | 10,000.00 | |

is accomplished through the multiplication of each coefficient or fraction by the costs that are to be allocated.

Table 10-3 summarizes the results obtained from the direct method of apportionment. All of the costs of the general service centers have been allocated to patient service centers. For example, the apportionment indicates that the total cost of operating the laboratory is $41,862.50, which is the sum of the costs originally assigned to the unit and the $1,862.50 allocated from the general service centers to this unit.

The expression of the calculations required to perform cost analysis using the direct apportionment method can be simplified greatly using the notation and operations of matrix algebra. Letting $a_{ij}$ represent the apportionment coefficient

**Table 10-3** Summary of Direct Apportionment

| Patient Service Center | Cost Allocations | | | | |
|---|---|---|---|---|---|
| | Patient Service Cost Center (1) | Dietary (2) | Housekeeping (3) | Laundry (4) | Total (5) |
| Laboratory | $40,000.00 | $112.50 | $1,500.00 | $250.00 | $41,862.50 |
| Radiology | 60,000.00 | 262.50 | 750.00 | 750.00 | 61,762.50 |
| Nursing unit | 220,000.00 | 7,125.00 | 3,750.00 | 9,000.00 | 239,875.00 |
| | 320,000.00 | 7,500.00 | 6,000.00 | 10,000.00 | 343,500.00 |

by which the costs of center $i$ are allocated to center $j$, the results obtained from the direct method of apportionment may be expressed by a system of linear equations of the form:

$$t_4 = a_{14}c_1 + a_{24}c_2 + a_{34}c_3 + c_4$$

$$t_5 = a_{15}c_1 + a_{25}c_2 + a_{35}c_3 + c_5$$

$$t_6 = a_{16}c_1 + a_{26}c_2 + a_{36}c_3 + c_6$$

In this formulation, $c_1$, $c_2$, and $c_3$ represent the costs to be apportioned; $t_j$ corresponds to the total costs (original cost plus all cost allocations) of center $j$, while $c_4$, $c_5$, and $c_6$ correspond to the original cost assigned to the revenue-generating centers.

Now, let

$$\mathbf{t} = \begin{bmatrix} t_4 \\ t_5 \\ t_6 \end{bmatrix} ; \quad \mathbf{c}_1 = \begin{bmatrix} c_1 \\ c_2 \\ c_3 \end{bmatrix} ; \quad \mathbf{c}_2 = \begin{bmatrix} c_4 \\ c_5 \\ c_6 \end{bmatrix}$$

and

$$\mathbf{A} = \begin{bmatrix} a_{14} & a_{15} & a_{16} \\ a_{24} & a_{25} & a_{26} \\ a_{34} & a_{35} & a_{36} \end{bmatrix} \quad \text{such that} \quad \mathbf{A}' = \begin{bmatrix} a_{14} & a_{24} & a_{34} \\ a_{15} & a_{25} & a_{35} \\ a_{16} & a_{26} & a_{36} \end{bmatrix}$$

As a result, the system of equations introduced above may be expressed in the form

$$\mathbf{t} = \mathbf{A}'\mathbf{c}_1 + \mathbf{c}_2 \qquad (10.1)$$

Returning to our example, we find that

$$\mathbf{c}_1 = \begin{bmatrix} \$7,500 \\ 6,000 \\ 10,000 \end{bmatrix} ; \quad \mathbf{c}_2 = \begin{bmatrix} \$40,000 \\ 60,000 \\ 220,000 \end{bmatrix} \quad \text{and}$$

$$
\mathbf{A} = \begin{bmatrix} .015 & .035 & .950 \\ .250 & .125 & .625 \\ .025 & .075 & .900 \end{bmatrix}
$$

As a consequence, we may apply Equation 10.1 and obtain

$$
\mathbf{t} = \begin{bmatrix} .015 & .250 & .025 \\ .035 & .125 & .075 \\ .950 & .625 & .900 \end{bmatrix} \begin{bmatrix} \$7,500 \\ 6,000 \\ 10,000 \end{bmatrix} + \begin{bmatrix} \$40,000 \\ 60,000 \\ 220,000 \end{bmatrix}
$$

$$
= \begin{bmatrix} \$41,862.50 \\ 61,762.50 \\ 239,875.00 \end{bmatrix}
$$

Observe that these results agree with the calculations summarized in Table 10-3.

The major advantages of the direct apportionment method are its simplicity and the ease with which it is understood. Its major disadvantage is that it fails to reflect interdepartmental exchanges among the general service centers. For example, the laundry and housekeeping departments probably provide service to the dietary department. Since these departments are general service centers, however, there is no means by which these interdepartmental exchanges are reflected by the direct apportionment method. Consequently, this method is not recommended as the technique by which the hospital should analyze its costs. However, as will be seen later, this method plays a role in the double distribution method of cost analysis.

## 10.3.2 Step-Down Method

The major disadvantage of the direct method of apportionment is overcome somewhat by the step-down method of cost analysis. The step-down technique, or as it sometimes is called, the single distribution method is a more sophisticated approach to cost finding than direct apportionment since it provides for the allocation of the costs of general service centers to other general service centers and, in turn, to the patient service or final cost centers.

Under this method, the costs of the general service center serving the most departments (both general service and patient service centers) are allocated first.

The costs of the general service center serving the second largest number of departments are allocated next, and so on. In the event that two departments serve an equal number of departments, another criterion such as relative costliness should be used to determine the order of apportionment. For the sake of convenience, it is assumed here that the costs of the general service centers are apportioned in accordance with their departmental code numbers. The process by which these costs are apportioned under the step-down method is depicted schematically in Figure 10-3. The total cost of the first general service center is apportioned to each of the other general service centers and to each of the patient service centers. Next, the total cost of the second general service center *and* the apportionment from the first to the second general center are allocated to each of the remaining general service centers and to the patient service centers. The first general service center is "closed" and no allocation from other general service centers to this unit is permitted under the step-down method. Similarly, once the accumulated costs in the remaining centers are apportioned, these units are closed and no further apportionment is made to them. This process continues until the total costs accumulated in the last general service center have been apportioned directly to the patient service or final cost centers.

Table 10-4 shows the allocation of the costs resulting from the use of the single or step-down distribution method. Several comments on this method are in order. First, the values in the denominator of the apportionment coefficients reflect the total demand on the department whose costs are to be apportioned less the demand of the department on itself and the demand of the departments

**Figure 10-3** Step-Down Method of Allocation

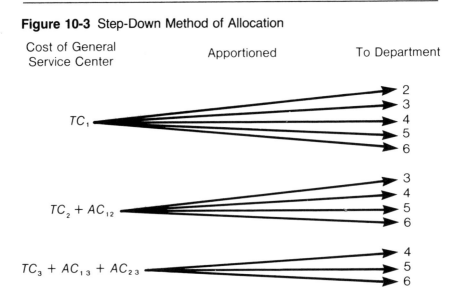

Cost of General Service Center     Apportioned     To Department

**Table 10-4** The Step-Down Method

| Costs Apportioned From | Initial Cost (1) | + | Previously Apportioned (2) | = | Cost to Be Apportioned (3) | × | Apportionment Coefficient (4) | = | Apportioned Cost (5) | Receiving Department (6) |
|---|---|---|---|---|---|---|---|---|---|---|
| Dietary | $7,500 | | 0 | | $7,500.00 | | 30/1,050 = .029 | | $217.50 | Housekeeping |
| | | | | | | | 20/1,050 = .019 | | 142.50 | Laundry |
| | | | | | | | 15/1,050 = .014 | | 105.00 | Laboratory |
| | | | | | | | 35/1,050 = .033 | | 247.50 | Radiology |
| | | | | | | | 950/1,050 = .905 | | 6,787.50 | Nursing unit |
| | | | | | | | | | 7,500.00 | |
| Housekeeping | 6,000 | | 217.50 | | 6,217.50 | | 200/3,400 = .059 | | 366.83 | Laundry |
| | | | | | | | 800/3,400 = .235 | | 1,461.11 | Laboratory |
| | | | | | | | 400/3,400 = .118 | | 733.67 | Radiology |
| | | | | | | | 2,000/3,400 = .588 | | 3,655.89 | Nursing unit |
| | | | | | | | | | 6,217.50 | |
| Laundry | 10,000 | | 509.33 | | 10,509.33 | | 5,000/200,000 = .025 | | 262.73 | Laboratory |
| | | | | | | | 15,000/200,000 = .075 | | 788.20 | Radiology |
| | | | | | | | 180,000/200,000 = .900 | | 9,458.40 | Nursing unit |
| | | | | | | | | | 10,509.33 | |

whose costs were apportioned previously. Second, the values in the column "costs to be apportioned" consist of two components: (1) the original costs of the department concerned and (2) the costs apportioned previously to the center from other general service units. For example, the costs to be apportioned from the laundry department ($10,509.33) are equal to the sum of its original cost ($10,000), the apportionment from radiology ($142.50), and the apportionment from housekeeping ($366.83).

The results obtained from an application of the step-down distribution to the hypothetical data are summarized in Table 10-5. As before, the total cost of operating the general service centers is allocated to the revenue-generating centers and, as a result, the sum of the total costs assigned to the final cost centers is equal to the full cost of hospital operations.

Similar to the discussion of the direct method of cost apportionment, the step-down technique may be expressed as a system of linear equations. The values in the column "costs to be apportioned" are composed of the direct costs of the department concerned plus the sum of the apportionments from departments whose costs were previously allocated. The interrelations among the general service centers assumed by the step-down method of cost apportionment may be represented by a system of linear equations of the form:

$$g_1 = (0)g_1 + (0)g_2 + (0)g_3 + c_1$$

$$g_2 = (a_{12})g_1 + (0)g_2 + (0)g_3 + c_2$$

$$g_3 = (a_{13})g_1 + (a_{23})g_2 + (0)g_3 + c_3$$

In this system, the $g$'s correspond to the costs that are allocated and $c_1$, $c_2$, and $c_3$ to the costs originally assigned to the general service centers. For example, in terms of the hypothetical hospital, the costs to be apportioned from the housekeeping department are given by

$$g_2 = (.029)\$7,500 + (0)\$6,217.50 + (0)\$10,509.33 + \$6,000 = \$6,217.50$$

**Table 10-5** Summary of Step-Down Method

| Patient Service Center | Original Cost (1) | Cost Allocations | | | |
| --- | --- | --- | --- | --- | --- |
| | | Dietary (2) | Housekeeping (3) | Laundry (4) | Total (5) |
| Laboratory | $40,000 | $105.00 | $1,461.11 | $262.73 | $41,828.84 |
| Radiology | 60,000 | 247.50 | 733.67 | 788.20 | 61,769.37 |
| Nursing unit | 220,000 | 6,787.50 | 3,655.89 | 9,458.40 | 239,901.79 |
| Total | 320,000 | 7,140.00 | 5,850.67 | 10,509.33 | 343,500.00 |

where the value .029 represents the apportionment coefficient $a_{12}$. Now let

$$\mathbf{g} = \begin{bmatrix} g_1 \\ g_2 \\ g_3 \end{bmatrix} \quad \text{and}$$

$$\mathbf{M} = \begin{bmatrix} 0 & a_{12} & a_{13} \\ 0 & 0 & a_{23} \\ 0 & 0 & 0 \end{bmatrix} \quad \text{such that} \quad \mathbf{M}' = \begin{bmatrix} 0 & 0 & 0 \\ a_{12} & 0 & 0 \\ a_{13} & a_{23} & 0 \end{bmatrix}$$

Employing this notation, we may express the interdepartmental exchanges among the general service centers in the form:

$$\mathbf{g} = \mathbf{M}'\mathbf{g} + \mathbf{c}_1$$

After a slight manipulation, we find that

$$\mathbf{g} - \mathbf{M}'\mathbf{g} = \mathbf{c}_1$$

and, as a result,

$$[\mathbf{I} - \mathbf{M}']\,\mathbf{g} = \mathbf{c}_1$$

Therefore, we find that the column vector $\mathbf{g}$ is given by

$$\mathbf{g} = [\mathbf{I} - \mathbf{M}']^{-1}\mathbf{c}_1 \qquad\qquad (10.2)$$

Returning to our numeric example, we defined the column vector $\mathbf{c}_1$ in our discussion of the direct method of cost allocation while Table 10-4 reveals that

$$\mathbf{M} = \begin{bmatrix} 0 & .029 & .019 \\ 0 & 0 & .059 \\ 0 & 0 & 0 \end{bmatrix}$$

Recalling that we require $(\mathbf{I} - \mathbf{M}')^{-1}$, the transpose of the matrix $\mathbf{M}$ is given by

$$\mathbf{M'} = \begin{bmatrix} 0 & 0 & 0 \\ .029 & 0 & 0 \\ .019 & .059 & 0 \end{bmatrix}$$

which implies that

$$\mathbf{I} - \mathbf{M'} = \begin{bmatrix} 1 & 0 & 0 \\ 0 & 1 & 0 \\ 0 & 0 & 1 \end{bmatrix} - \begin{bmatrix} 0 & 0 & 0 \\ .029 & 0 & 0 \\ .019 & .059 & 0 \end{bmatrix} = \begin{bmatrix} 1 & 0 & 0 \\ -.029 & 1 & 0 \\ -.019 & -.059 & 1 \end{bmatrix}$$

Referring to section 4.5, we see that the inverse of the matrix $\mathbf{A}$ is given by

$$[\mathbf{I} - \mathbf{M'}]^{-1} = \frac{1}{|\mathbf{I} - \mathbf{M'}|} \mathbf{G'}$$

where $\mathbf{G}$ is the corresponding matrix of cofactors. Returning to our example, the reader should verify that

$$|\mathbf{I} - \mathbf{M'}| = 1$$

while the matrix of cofactors is given by

$$\begin{bmatrix} 1 & .029 & .020711 \\ 0 & 1 & .059 \\ 0 & 0 & 1 \end{bmatrix}$$

Since $|\mathbf{I} - \mathbf{M'}| = 1$, we find that $(\mathbf{I} - \mathbf{M'})^{-1}$ is given by the transposed matrix of cofactors. As a consequence, the column vector $\mathbf{g}$ is found by

$$\mathbf{g} = \begin{bmatrix} 1 & 0 & 0 \\ .029 & 1 & 0 \\ .020711 & .059 & 1 \end{bmatrix} \begin{bmatrix} \$7,500 \\ 6,000 \\ 10,000 \end{bmatrix} = \begin{bmatrix} \$7,500.00 \\ 6,217.50 \\ 10,509.33 \end{bmatrix}$$

These results agree with the entries in Column (3) of Table 10-4.

After finding the column vector **g**, we may express the total costs of the patient service units, including the allocations from the general service centers, by the system of linear equations

$$t_4 = a_{14}g_1 + a_{24}g_2 + a_{34}g_3 + c_4$$

$$t_5 = a_{15}g_1 + a_{25}g_2 + a_{35}g_3 + c_5$$

$$t_6 = a_{16}g_1 + a_{26}g_2 + a_{36}g_3 + c_6$$

Letting

$$\mathbf{E'} = \begin{bmatrix} a_{14} & a_{24} & a_{34} \\ a_{15} & a_{25} & a_{35} \\ a_{16} & a_{26} & a_{36} \end{bmatrix}$$

we may express the system of equations in the form

$$\mathbf{t} = \mathbf{E'g} + \mathbf{c}_2$$

Substituting $[\mathbf{I} - \mathbf{M'}]^{-1}\mathbf{c}_1$ for **g**, we obtain

$$\mathbf{t} = \mathbf{E'}[\mathbf{I} - \mathbf{M'}]^{-1}\mathbf{c}_1 + \mathbf{c}_2 \qquad \text{(10.3)}$$

where **t** is a column vector containing the original costs of the patient care or final cost centers plus the cost allocations from the general service centers as calculated under the step-down distribution.

Returning to our numeric example, Table 10-4 reveals that

$$\mathbf{E} = \begin{bmatrix} .014 & .033 & .905 \\ .235 & .118 & .588 \\ .025 & .075 & .900 \end{bmatrix}$$

As a consequence, the equation $\mathbf{t} = \mathbf{E'}[\mathbf{I} - \mathbf{M'}]^{-1}\mathbf{c}_1 + \mathbf{c}_2$ is given by

$$\mathbf{t} = \begin{bmatrix} .014 & .235 & .025 \\ .033 & .118 & .075 \\ .905 & .588 & .900 \end{bmatrix} \begin{bmatrix} \$7,500.00 \\ 6,217.50 \\ 10,509.33 \end{bmatrix}$$

$$+ \begin{bmatrix} \$40,000 \\ 60,000 \\ 220,000 \end{bmatrix} = \begin{bmatrix} \$41,828.84 \\ 61,769.37 \\ 239,901.79 \end{bmatrix}$$

It should be noted that the entries of the column vector $\mathbf{t}$ are identical to the first three values appearing in Column (5) of Table 10-5.

Although the step-down method allows for a partial reflection of interdepartmental exchanges among general service centers, it may be criticized for failing to allow fully for all exchanges among the general service centers. As an example, consider the dietary department which, as mentioned, uses the services of the housekeeping and laundry departments. The costs of the dietary department were apportioned before the costs of housekeeping and laundry were allocated. Since the dietary department was closed after its costs were apportioned, no cost allocations from housekeeping and laundry to dietary are permitted under the step-down method. Thus, even though the step-down method partially reflects interdepartmental demands among the general service units, it does not fully reflect such exchanges.

### 10.3.3 Double Distribution Method

The double distribution method uses two rounds of allocations, which tends to overcome some of the weaknesses inherent in the step-down method. In the first distribution, the costs of all general service units are allocated to all the other departments (both general service and patient service units) in accordance with the relative demand exerted on the department whose costs are allocated. After the first distribution has been completed, the costs allocated to the general service units from other general service centers are redistributed to the final cost centers using either the step-down or direct methods of apportionment. The first allocation of the double distribution method is presented schematically in Figure 10-4.

Once the costs of a given general service department have been apportioned, it is "reopened" and costs from other general service units are allocated to it. As a consequence, each of the general service units will have a positive balance at the end of the first distribution. These amounts reflect the interdepartmental

**Figure 10-4** Double Distribution: First Allocation

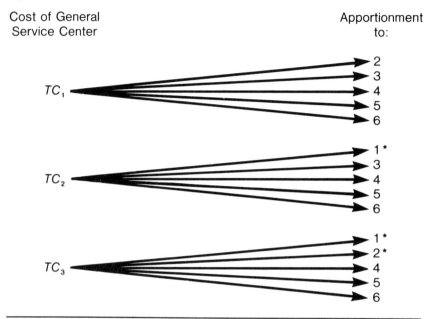

Cost of General
Service Center

Apportionment
to:

exchanges among the general service centers. As seen in Figure 10-5, the residual costs $(TC_i^*)$ remaining in general service department $i$ then are allocated to the final cost centers directly.

The results of the first allocation of the double distribution method (Table 10-6) show that the direct and indirect costs of all general service centers are distributed to the various cost centers by the agreed-upon basis of allocation. Since the double distribution method does not charge a department for the use of its own services, denominators of the apportionment coefficients in the example consist of the total demand on the department less the unit's use of its own service.

Several other differences between the step-down and double distribution methods are worthy of note. In the first apportionment of the double distribution method, the costs to be apportioned do *not* reflect previous allocations among general service units, as is the case under the step-down method. For example, housekeeping costs to be apportioned in the first distribution are $6,000 and not $6,217.50, as in the step-down method. As mentioned, once the costs of a general service center have been apportioned, the department is reopened and the costs of the other general service centers are allocated to that unit.

The results of the first allocation in the double distribution method are summarized in Table 10-7. The bottom row of the table reveals that each of the

**Figure 10-5** Double Distribution: Second Allocation

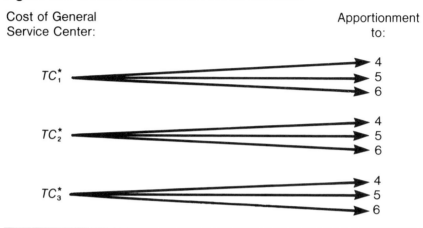

Cost of General
Service Center:

Apportionment
to:

general service centers has a positive balance at the end of the first distribution. This result reflects the interdepartmental demands among the general service centers. As noted, the positive balances associated with each of the general service centers may be allocated to final cost centers in the second distribution by the direct method of cost allocation. The results of the second distribution are shown in Table 10-8, where the values in Column (1) were obtained from the bottom row of Table 10-7. The apportionment coefficients are identical to those associated with the direct apportionment method in Table 10-2.

The results of the double distribution are summarized in Table 10-9. In this case, the upper half of the table corresponds to Table 10-7 and the summary of the second distribution was obtained from Table 10-8. As can be verified, the sum of the values in the bottom row of Table 10-9 represents the total cost of hospital operations.

As before, we use the notation of matrix algebra to express the double distribution method of cost analysis. Under the double distribution method, only the original costs of each general service center are apportioned in the first allocation and the demands of a given general service center on itself are not reflected in the allocation process. The balances in the patient care centers after the first distribution may be expressed by a system of linear equations given by

$$t_4^* = a_{14}c_1 + a_{24}c_2 + a_{34}c_3 + c_4$$

$$t_5^* = a_{15}c_1 + a_{25}c_2 + a_{35}c_3 + c_5$$

$$t_6^* = a_{16}c_1 + a_{26}c_2 + a_{36}c_3 + c_6$$

**Table 10-6** The Double Distribution Method: The First Distribution

| Cost Apportioned from | Costs to Be Apportioned (1) | Apportionment Coefficient (2) | Apportioned Costs (3) | Receiving Department (4) |
|---|---|---|---|---|
| Dietary | $7,500 | 30/1,050 = .029 | $217.50 | Housekeeping |
| | | 20/1,050 = .019 | 142.50 | Laundry |
| | | 15/1,050 = .014 | 105.00 | Laboratory |
| | | 35/1,050 = .033 | 247.50 | Radiology |
| | | 950/1,050 = .905 | 6,787.50 | Nursing unit |
| | | | 7,500.00 | |
| Housekeeping | 6,000 | 600/4,000 = .150 | 900.00 | Dietary* |
| | | 200/4,000 = .050 | 300.00 | Laundry |
| | | 800/4,000 = .200 | 1,200.00 | Laboratory |
| | | 400/4,000 = .100 | 600.00 | Radiology |
| | | 2000/4,000 = .500 | 3,000.00 | Nursing unit |
| | | | 6,000.00 | |
| Laundry | 10,000 | 50,000/290,000 = .172 | 1,720.00 | Dietary* |
| | | 40,000/290,000 = .138 | 1,380.00 | Housekeeping* |
| | | 5,000/290,000 = .017 | 170.00 | Laboratory |
| | | 15,000/290,000 = .052 | 520.00 | Radiology |
| | | 180,000/290,000 = .621 | 6,210.00 | Nursing unit |
| | | | 10,000.00 | |

* Department is reopened after assigned costs have been apportioned.

**Table 10-7** Summary of the First Distribution

| Allocations to / from | Dietary | Housekeeping | Laundry | Laboratory | Radiology | Nursing Unit |
|---|---|---|---|---|---|---|
| Dietary | $0.00 | $217.50 | $142.50 | $105.00 | $247.50 | $6,787.50 |
| Housekeeping | 900.00 | 0.00 | 300.00 | 1,200.00 | 600.00 | 3,000.00 |
| Laundry | 1,720.00 | 1,380.00 | 0.00 | 170.00 | 520.00 | 6,210.00 |
| Residual costs | 2,620.00 | 1,597.50 | 442.50 | 1,475.00 | 1,367.50 | 15,997.50 |

We may express the system of linear equations in matrix notation by letting

$$\mathbf{t}^* = \begin{bmatrix} t_4^* \\ t_5^* \\ t_6^* \end{bmatrix}$$

**Table 10-8** The Double Distribution Method: The Second Distribution

| Costs Apportioned from | Costs to be Apportioned (1) | Apportionment Coefficient (2) | Apportioned Costs (3) | Receiving Department (4) |
|---|---|---|---|---|
| Dietary | $2,620.00 | .015 | $39.30 | Laboratory |
|  |  | .035 | 91.70 | Radiology |
|  |  | .950 | 2,489.00 | Nursing unit |
|  |  |  | 2,620.00 |  |
| Housekeeping | 1,597.50 | .250 | 399.37 | Laundry |
|  |  | .125 | 199.69 | Radiology |
|  |  | .625 | 998.44 | Nursing unit |
|  |  |  | 1,597.50 |  |
| Laundry | 442.50 | .025 | 11.06 | Laundry |
|  |  | .075 | 33.19 | Radiology |
|  |  | .900 | 398.25 | Nursing unit |
|  |  |  | 442.50 |  |

and

$$\mathbf{H} = [\mathbf{H_1}{:}\mathbf{H_2}] = \begin{bmatrix} 0 & a_{12} & a_{13} & a_{14} & a_{15} & a_{16} \\ a_{21} & 0 & a_{23} & a_{24} & a_{25} & a_{26} \\ a_{31} & a_{32} & 0 & a_{34} & a_{35} & a_{36} \end{bmatrix}$$

such that

$$\mathbf{H'} = \begin{bmatrix} 0 & a_{21} & a_{31} \\ a_{12} & 0 & a_{32} \\ a_{13} & a_{23} & 0 \\ a_{14} & a_{24} & a_{34} \\ a_{15} & a_{25} & a_{35} \\ a_{16} & a_{26} & a_{36} \end{bmatrix} = \begin{matrix} \mathbf{H'_1} \\ ---- \\ \mathbf{H'_2} \end{matrix}$$

**Table 10-9** Summary of the Double-Distribution Method

| Allocation to<br>From | Laboratory | Radiology | Nursing Unit | Total |
|---|---|---|---|---|
| *First Distribution (1)* | | | | |
| Dietary | $105.00 | $247.50 | $6,787.50 | $7,140.00 |
| Housekeeping | 1,200.00 | 600.00 | 3,000.00 | 4,800.00 |
| Laundry | 170.00 | 520.00 | 6,210.00 | 6,900.00 |
| Subtotal (1) | 1,475.00 | 1,367.50 | 15,997.50 | 18,840.00 |
| | | | | |
| *Second Distribution (2)* | | | | |
| Dietary | 39.30 | 91.70 | 2,489.00 | 2,620.00 |
| Housekeeping | 399.37 | 199.69 | 998.44 | 1,597.50 |
| Laundry | 11.06 | 33.19 | 398.25 | 442.50 |
| Subtotal (2) | 449.73 | 324.58 | 3,885.69 | 4,660.00 |
| Subtotal of (1) + (2) | 1,924.73 | 1,692.08 | 19,883.19 | 23,500.00 |
| | | | | |
| Original Cost | 40,000.00 | 60,000.00 | 220,000.00 | 320,000.00 |
| Total Cost | 41,924.73 | 61,692.08 | 239,883.19 | 343,500.00 |

Employing this notation we find that

$$\mathbf{t}^* = \mathbf{H}_2' \mathbf{c}_1 + \mathbf{c}_2 \qquad\qquad (10.4)$$

yields the balances appearing in the final cost centers after the first allocation of the double distribution method.

Returning to our numeric example, Table 10-6 reveals that

$$\mathbf{H} = \begin{bmatrix} 0 & .029 & .019 & .014 & .033 & .905 \\ .150 & 0 & .050 & .200 & .100 & .500 \\ .172 & .138 & 0 & .017 & .052 & .621 \end{bmatrix}$$

As can be verified, the transpose of the matrix $\mathbf{H}$ is given by

$$\mathbf{H}' = \begin{bmatrix} 0 & .150 & .172 \\ .029 & 0 & .138 \\ .019 & .050 & 0 \\ \hline .014 & .200 & .017 \\ .033 & .100 & .052 \\ .905 & .500 & .621 \end{bmatrix}$$

Employing Equation 10.4, we obtain the balances appearing in the final cost centers after the first distribution by

$$
t^* = \begin{bmatrix} .014 & .200 & .017 \\ .033 & .100 & .052 \\ .905 & .500 & .621 \end{bmatrix} \begin{bmatrix} \$7,500 \\ 6,000 \\ 10,000 \end{bmatrix} + \begin{bmatrix} \$40,000 \\ 60,000 \\ 220,000 \end{bmatrix} = \begin{bmatrix} \$41,475.00 \\ 61,367.50 \\ 235,997.50 \end{bmatrix}
$$

Consider next the residuals remaining in the general service centers after the first allocation of the double distribution method. In this case, the system of linear equations given by

$$r_1^* = 0(c_1) + a_{21}(c_2) + a_{31}(c_3)$$

$$r_2^* = a_{12}(c_1) + 0(c_2) + a_{32}(c_3)$$

$$r_3^* = a_{13}(c_1) + a_{23}(c_2) + 0(c_3)$$

expresses the interdepartmental exchanges among the general service centers. We may express the system of linear equations in matrix notation by the equation

$$r^* = H_1' c_1 \qquad\qquad (10.5)$$

where

$$
r^* = \begin{bmatrix} r_1^* \\ r_2^* \\ r_3^* \end{bmatrix}
$$

We may verify that Equation 10.5 yields the residuals remaining in the general service centers after the first allocation of the double distribution method by returning to our numeric example. In this case, we find that

$$
r^* = H_1' c_1 = \begin{bmatrix} 0 & .150 & .172 \\ .029 & 0 & .138 \\ .019 & .050 & 0 \end{bmatrix} \begin{bmatrix} \$7,500 \\ 6,000 \\ 10,000 \end{bmatrix} = \begin{bmatrix} \$2,620.00 \\ 1,597.50 \\ 442.50 \end{bmatrix}
$$

The elements of the column vector $r^*$ are identical to the first three values in the bottom row of Table 10-7.

As illustrated earlier, the residuals in the column vector $\mathbf{r^*}$ are apportioned to the final cost centers by the direct apportionment method. Representing the costs apportioned to the final cost centers in the second distribution by

$$\mathbf{t^{**}} = \begin{bmatrix} t_4^{**} \\ t_5^{**} \\ t_6^{**} \end{bmatrix}$$

we find that

$$\mathbf{t^{**}} = \mathbf{A'r^*} \qquad (10.6)$$

where the matrix $\mathbf{A'}$ was defined previously.

In terms of our example, an application of Equation 10.6 to our hypothetical data yields

$$\mathbf{t^{**}} = \begin{bmatrix} .015 & .250 & .025 \\ .035 & .125 & .075 \\ .950 & .625 & .900 \end{bmatrix} \begin{bmatrix} \$2{,}620.00 \\ 1{,}597.50 \\ 442.50 \end{bmatrix} = \begin{bmatrix} \$449.73 \\ 324.58 \\ 3{,}885.69 \end{bmatrix}$$

Notice that when we add $\mathbf{t^*}$ and $\mathbf{t^{**}}$ we obtain

$$\begin{bmatrix} \$449.73 \\ 324.58 \\ 3{,}885.69 \end{bmatrix} + \begin{bmatrix} \$41{,}475.00 \\ 61{,}367.50 \\ 235{,}997.50 \end{bmatrix} = \begin{bmatrix} \$41{,}924.73 \\ 61{,}692.08 \\ 239{,}883.19 \end{bmatrix}$$

Since these results are identical to the values in the bottom row of Table 10-9, we may assert that

$$\mathbf{t} = \mathbf{t^*} + \mathbf{t^{**}} = \mathbf{H_2'c_1} + \mathbf{c_2} + \mathbf{A'H_1'c_1} \qquad (10.7)$$

where $\mathbf{t}$ represents a column vector, the elements of which are the total costs (assigned costs plus all cost allocations) of the final cost centers.

### 10.3.4 A Comparison of the Methods

Table 10-10 is a summary of the results obtained when the three methods of cost finding were used to allocate to the final cost centers those costs that had been assigned to the general service centers. Several comments on the information in the table are worthy of note.

First, the values in the bottom row show that the sum of the costs assigned to the final cost centers by all three methods is $343,500, which is the total cost of hospital operations. However, a comparison of the costs assigned to each of the units reveals that the techniques of allocation give rise to slightly different results. As seen earlier, the results of the double distribution method are more accurate than those of either the direct apportionment method or the step-down technique. This is because the double distribution technique reflects the interaction among general service centers with greater precision than the two other methods. Similarly, the step-down method results in a more accurate allocation of costs than the direct apportionment technique.

These observations are of particular importance when developing the hospital's prospective fee schedule. As will be seen later, the costs assigned to the revenue generating center (original plus all allocations) represent the basis for determining the unit charges for the services provided by the center. Consequently, when traditional approaches are used to determine the fee schedule, the extent to which charges accurately reflect the costs of operation depend, in part, on the results of the apportionment process. In this regard, the step-down technique and the double distribution method have been approved by the American Hospital Association, the Hospital Financial Management Association, and the Department of Health and Human Services. Moreover, the double distribution method or step-down techniques must be used when determining the amount of reimbursement from Medicare and from many Blue Cross plans.

A final observation: the discussion of the methods of cost apportionment has focused on the different mathematical properties of the three techniques. It is important to note that the accuracy of the results obtained from the apportion-

**Table 10-10** A Summary of the Apportionment Methods

| Department | Method of Apportionment | | |
|---|---|---|---|
| | Direct Apportionment | Step-Down Method | Double Distribution |
| Laboratory | $41,862.50 | $41,828.84 | $41,924.73 |
| Radiology | 61,762.50 | 61,769.37 | 61,692.08 |
| Nursing unit | 239,875.00 | 239,901.79 | 239,883.19 |
| Total | 343,500.00 | 343,500.00 | 343,500.00 |

ment process depends not only on the method of allocating costs but also on the measures of relative demand used as apportionment coefficients. The accuracy of the apportionment coefficients cannot be overemphasized. Management must exercise caution when developing the measures of relative demand.

## 10.3.5 Alternate Organizational Structures

Throughout the discussion, the illustration of the cost-finding techniques has been simplified by assuming that the hospital is composed of three general service centers and three final cost centers. However, when performing cost analysis in a hospital consisting of many general service and final cost centers, it is necessary only to expand the number of rows and columns of the above matrices accordingly. For instance, suppose that the hospital is composed of five general service centers and five final cost centers. To accommodate such an organizational arrangement, we might modify the matrix **A** that was used in the direct method of cost finding as follows:

$$\mathbf{A} = \begin{bmatrix} a_{16} & a_{17} & a_{18} & a_{19} & a_{110} \\ a_{26} & a_{27} & a_{28} & a_{29} & a_{210} \\ a_{36} & a_{37} & a_{38} & a_{39} & a_{310} \\ a_{46} & a_{47} & a_{48} & a_{49} & a_{410} \\ a_{56} & a_{57} & a_{58} & a_{59} & a_{510} \end{bmatrix}$$

By virtue of the departmental exchanges among the general service centers, the matrix **M** is square, which implies that $(\mathbf{I} - \mathbf{M}')^{-1}$ exists. Further, given the interrelation between the general service and final cost centers, the matrices and vectors are conformable for multiplication. These observations allow us to assert that the techniques described in this chapter may be applied in an institution consisting of any number of general service or final cost centers.

## 10.3.6 Alternate Methods of Cost Analysis

In addition to the techniques described earlier, algebraic methods involving 10 to 12 distributions have been developed in an attempt to improve the accuracy of cost finding. These techniques are characterized by multiple allocations of cost among general service centers and to patient care centers. It should be noted, however, that the results of cost analysis change very little after the fourth or fifth distribution since the additional allocations exert only a marginal impact on the final cost data.

### 10.3.7 Computer Applications

To achieve the maximum use of the algebraic methods as well as the techniques described in this chapter, a high-speed electronic computer is required. Several systems that permit management to perform cost analysis with relative ease are available. Matrix algebra and electronic computers are complementary tools that management may use to perform cost analysis. The apportionment techniques described in this chapter have been expressed in the notation of matrix algebra. On the other hand, APL (A Programming Language) is a language that permits management to employ computers to perform matrix algebra operations. As a result, APL, when coupled with the equations derived earlier, may be used to develop a program that permits the use of a computer to perform cost analysis.

In addition, the use of electronic data processing equipment permits the development of simultaneous equation models that reflect the relationships among and between departments. These systems represent the most precise methods of cost analysis currently available.

---

**REFERENCES**

American Hospital Association. *Cost Finding and Rate Setting for Hospitals*. Chicago: American Hospital Association, 1968.

Canadian Hospital Association. *Supplement to the Canadian Hospital Accounting Manual*. Toronto: Livingston Printing Ltd., 1974.

Cardone, A. "Uniform Reporting," *Topics in Health Care Financing*, vol. 6, no. 2, Spring 1980.

# Chapter 11

# Introduction to Budgeting

## Objectives

After completing this chapter, you should be able to:

1. Describe the importance of budgeting in terms of such operational activities as:
   a. planning.
   b. controlling.
   c. organizing.
   d. coordinating.
2. Describe and understand:
   a. global budgeting.
   b. line item budgeting.
   c. responsibility budgeting.
   d. program budgeting.
   e. zero-base budgeting.
3. Use cost-benefit analysis when addressing the general problem of optimization.
4. Define and understand the importance of:
   a. comprehensive and partial budgets.
   b. fixed and flexible budgets.

## 11.1 THE IMPORTANCE OF BUDGETING

The budget plays a central role in determining the amount or rate of prospective reimbursement received from the provincial plan in Canada and from several Blue Cross plans in the United States, as was documented earlier. In addition, the budget can play a significant role in determining the amount of the

Periodic Interim Payments received from the Medicare program. As a consequence, budget preparation is a continuing concern to hospitals that are financed
or that receive a portion of their funding under a system of prospective reimbursement.

The budget and the process of developing it also are of generic importance
to the general problem of planning, monitoring, evaluating, and controlling a
hospital's internal operations. The budget is perhaps the most effective device
available to management for identifying areas of activity that provide the most
benefits to the community and for monitoring, controlling, and evaluating the
day-to-day activities and expenditures of the hospital enterprise.

Management continually faces a variety of alternate courses of action. Each
alternative is associated with certain costs and a related level of benefit that
accrues to the community. If the institution is to satisfy its service-oriented objectives, management should adopt courses of action that provide the maximum
amount of benefits for a given level of expenditure. Management also should
ensure that existing areas are operated so that the last dollar spent on each hospital activity yields the same margin of benefit to the community. Thus, when
rationing scarce resources among competing demands, management must place
a high priority on projects that yield the most potential and realized benefits.

Budgeting also is the process by which the use of real and financial resources
is planned and reconciled among competing demands to achieve the hospital's
objectives. Thus, the budget and the process of its preparation provide the tools
by which management may evaluate the rates at which existing programs are
operated as well as the mechanism by which potential programs and areas of
activities may be assessed in terms of their relative value to the community.

## 11.2 BUDGETING AND THE FUNCTIONS OF MANAGEMENT

The use of the budget in carrying out administrative responsibility can be
understood best by examining its interrelation with the functions of management.
As noted, management functions traditionally have been defined as planning,
organizing, coordinating, monitoring, and controlling the activities and expenditures of the enterprise. As will be seen, the budget and the budget preparation
process can help management discharge each of these functions.

### 11.2.1 Planning

A budget is simply the operational plan of an institution as expressed in
monetary units, a plan in which the hospital's objectives and the resources
required to achieve its goals are expressed in real or physical terms. The budget
and the process of preparing it represent one of the major vehicles by which

management charts the future course of the institution and expresses that course in both real and monetary terms.

Budgeting helps management discharge its planning responsibilities in at least two ways. First, the budget and its formulation provide management with an opportunity to plan the institution's operational activities. Systematic and comprehensive planning is a task that does not occupy the day-to-day attention of management frequently. Instead, operating exigencies and other daily pressures demand the immediate attention of the administrator and, as a result, a relatively low priority usually is assigned to the planning function. By raising the priority of this function, the budget formulation process forces management to devote both time and energy to developing a systematic plan at least once a year. Second, the budget helps management by providing a systematic structure within which to plan. A hospital's annual budget is composed of four separate but interrelated units: the expense budget, the revenue budget, the capital budget, and the cash budget. These four, in addition to their role in ensuring the financial viability of the institution, provide the framework for the planning process since they force management to evaluate alternate courses of action in terms of expense requirements, revenue-generating potential, capital requirements, and cash flows.

## 11.2.2 Control

Closely related to planning is the managerial responsibility of controlling operational activities to achieve the institution's goals. The budget represents the standard against which actual operations may be compared and alerts management by identifying areas requiring remedial action to realign actual and desired performance. The budget is the vehicle by which the day-to-day activities of the hospital are evaluated on a more or less continuous basis to ensure that the goals of the institution are being achieved.

To control the hospital enterprise effectively, management must develop a budget for each of its responsibility centers. A responsibility center may be defined as a unit or a series of units for which a single individual is assigned primary responsibility. Thus, when a budget is developed for each of the responsibility centers, the manager of the unit(s) comprising the center is provided with a standard by which to compare actual operating results.

Obviously, more than just the development of a budget for each responsibility center is required if management is to have efficient and effective control. Therefore, as will be described in detail later, the control system also must have a reporting mechanism that routinely provides managers with information depicting the operational performance of the unit(s) for which they are responsible and by which they can monitor and control their units.

The budget also assists management in the performance of the control function by indirection, which may be expressed in terms of the budget's impact on managers' cost consciousness. The time and energy devoted to budget preparation, coupled with the very presence of the budget document, tend to raise the cost consciousness of the entire organization as well as increase the sensitivity of all levels of management to the relationship between actual and desired performance. By linking the budget preparation process, the resulting performance expectations, and the reporting system to the individual who is responsible for a unit or series of units, the need to control costs and to adhere to the budget is increased further. It is in this sense, then, that the budget not only provides the guidelines by which performance is controlled but also shapes the results of operational activity.

### 11.2.3 Coordination

As mentioned, budgeting plays a key role in coordinating revenues and expenditures to ensure the financial viability of the hospital enterprise. The budget development process also is valuable in coordinating hospital operations.

Implicit in the development of any budget is a specification of the institution's goals as well as their communication to the operating units. The achievement of the corporate goals requires the coordinated efforts of the units comprising the hospital enterprise; the process of establishing these common goals provides a frame of reference within which management should coordinate the operational activity areas. By requiring an examination of the goals and plans of each responsibility center, the budgeting process provides management with an opportunity to ensure that all aspects of hospital activity are coordinated.

The budget preparation process also is a valuable tool in reaching decisions on the coordination and allocation of scarce resources among competing demands. For example, suppose that management has specified the hospital objectives in operational terms such as providing a given number of days of care. Suppose further that management has determined the work load or rate of activity required of each unit to achieve the common goal. The specification of the rates of activity required of each responsibility center provides the basis for allocating and coordinating available resources. Thus, by focusing on the interrelations among responsibility centers as well as the coordination of their operational activities, the budgeting process provides the basis for allocating resources.

### 11.2.4 Organizing

As noted, a major management function involves the organization of the resources used in operational areas. Budgeting constitutes a major management tool for discharging this responsibility effectively. Effective budget preparation and the internal control system both require an organizational structure that clearly specifies the lines of responsibility and authority as well as the corresponding centers in which costs are incurred. By developing the budget in terms of clearly defined cost centers for which a given individual is responsible, the hospital can ensure that differences between actual and planned performance will be redressed by appropriate corrective action.

By providing the potential for improved operational control, budgeting can induce management to achieve an organizational structure characterized by clear lines of authority and responsibility. In addition, budgeting provides a periodic opportunity to review hospital activity and to correct elements of the organizational structure in which those lines of responsibility are not clear.

The budgeting process also helps management in organizing the use of resources to obtain the greatest total benefit for the community. In achieving this goal, alternate projects, programs, and levels of activity must be evaluated in terms of their associated costs and potential benefits. Such an evaluation requires that management establish funding priorities so that projects or programs with the greatest potential benefit are funded first while those with the least potential benefits are funded last.

At an abstract level, the importance of allocating resources to activities or projects that have been ranked in terms of their relative potential benefits is understood easily. However, moving from a level of abstraction to operational implementation creates several problems. The approach is complicated by the large number of alternatives that must be evaluated and by the unique nature of potential outcomes obtainable from each alternative. As the next section demonstrates, zero-base budgeting represents one approach for evaluating alternative expenditure opportunities and establishing funding priorities.

## 11.3 TECHNIQUES OF BUDGETING

This section describes various budgeting approaches and examines the value of each to management. First, however, the concept of global budgeting as it has been implemented in Canada is discussed.

### 11.3.1 The Global Budget

When a hospital has established a level of approved experience, budgets are reviewed on a global basis. Under the global budgeting system, the Canadian government assigns each hospital a sum of money it may use in implementing budgeted projects or programs of activity. Even though the approved budget provides details concerning an expenditure program, management can modify it during the year so long as the total amount assigned to the hospital is not overspent and the institution's service responsibility to the community is satisfied. Hospitals are expected to provide a realistic and detailed budget that, when coupled with supplementary documentation, establishes their aims and objectives as well as the programs and activities required to attain those goals.

The method of determining the annual amount assigned to the hospital traditionally has involved an assessment of the previous year's costs and, assuming that no major changes in the institution's program are anticipated, these expenditures are adjusted to reflect economic conditions expected during the budget period.

## 11.3.2 Line Item Budgeting

A line item budget is a statement of expected costs for each of the major items of expenditure incurred by the *entire* organization. Under line item budgeting, cost estimates are developed for such expense items as wages and salaries (which usually are broken down into many categories), medical supplies, laboratory supplies, etc., by adjusting the current level of expenditure on each item to reflect anticipated economic conditions.

The objective of line item budgeting is to control items of expenditure and plan for their use. However, in addition, the approach does not require management to examine the interrelations among areas of operational activity and the relation of each area to the achievement of the institution's goals. As a result, control of expenditures, rather than of operational areas, becomes the objective.

Since the organizational entity, rather than the operational area, is the unit of analysis, line item budgeting does not lend itself to an examination of the costs and related benefits of various programs, projects, or rates of activity that are anticipated during the budget period. As a consequence, line item budgeting cannot be regarded as an effective approach to the allocation, coordination, and organization of resources to obtain the greatest benefit for the community.

## 11.3.3 Responsibility Budgeting

As mentioned, hospital control is most effective when a budget is prepared for each responsibility center. The responsibility budget focuses on a unit or series of units for which a specific individual is obligated. For example, a responsibility budget might be prepared for such units as the laboratory department, radiology, or a series of operational areas for which a given individual is responsible.

As a general rule, the use of each component of care is more difficult to measure than is the use of factor inputs. As a result, budgets usually are developed to gain control over the resources that the hospital uses. In most hospitals, the responsibility for ensuring that actual expenditures are not greater than anticipated spending resides with department heads. Responsibility budgeting provides the standard of comparison by which department heads can evaluate and control the operational performance of the unit or units that they direct. Responsibility budgeting is a far more effective control tool than line item budgeting, in which levels of expenditure by type of resource are estimated for the entire organization. Obviously, such an approach fails to specify the desired performance for each responsibility center of the hospital.

It should be noted that a responsibility budget is not an approach to resolving the problem of how to allocate available resources among programs. Given that the basic objective of responsibility budgeting is to organize financial information in a manner that reflects the hospital's organizational structure as well as its distribution of responsibility, it is an approach to organizing decisions concerning the allocation of resources. As noted, the unit of analysis in responsibility budgeting is the responsibility center, while the unit of analysis in decisions on the allocation of resources is the program or project area. Since responsibility centers are likely to cut across program areas, responsibility budgeting is not particularly useful in identifying the costs, outcomes, and trade-offs associated with program alternatives.

Responsibility budgeting has several advantages. First, such a budget structure obviously establishes the expectations and standards for a unit or series of units for which a given individual has operational responsibility. Consequently, it clearly identifies the standard to be pursued as well as the individual responsible for implementing corrective action to ensure that actual performance does not deviate from expected or desired performance. Second, such a budget structure provides the necessary linkage between the expression of standards or expectations and the accumulation and reporting of actual results. Both of these elements are required in the operational control of the responsibility center.

Finally, responsibility budgeting requires the direct participation of the individuals responsible for management of the operational units of the hospital. Such direct participation involves not only the specification of goals of the unit but also the means by which they are to be accomplished. It is through this involvement that the operational manager becomes committed to perform in accordance with the plans and goals expressed in the budget.

## 11.3.4 Program Budgeting

Program budgeting usually employs an identifiable program of activity such as outpatient care, renal dialysis, or day care surgery as the unit at issue. The focus of program budgeting is on achieving the common goals of the institution by ensuring that the allocation of resources and the activities of each program are coordinated and directed toward the corporate goals and objectives.

The primary purpose of program budgeting is to identify and evaluate the relative costs, benefits, and trade-offs of various spending programs. Such an evaluation provides the basis for allocating resources to best attain the goals. Figure 11-1 identifies the principle components of program budgeting. Under this system, total hospital activity is divided into a number of program areas that may consist of several subprograms and program elements. Once the operational activity has been expressed in terms of program areas, management must ensure that the goals of each program, subprogram, and program element are consistent with the common objectives of the hospital. Management must determine the rates or levels of activity in each of the programs, subprograms, and program elements that best contribute to the attainment of the institution's common goals. After determining the resources required to sustain the desired rate or level of activity in each area, management then must allocate available factors of production to best achieve the goals. Program budgeting, then, is a tool that helps management reach macro decisions that achieve a balance between the allocation of hospital resources and the goals of the institution.

As an example of one method of implementing program budgeting, suppose that a hospital that engages in no formal research or teaching activities is contemplating the use of program budgeting as a mechanism to reach macro level decisions on the allocation of resources. Suppose further that one of the hospital's primary objectives is to provide the services required in the management

**Figure 11-1** Components of Program Budgeting

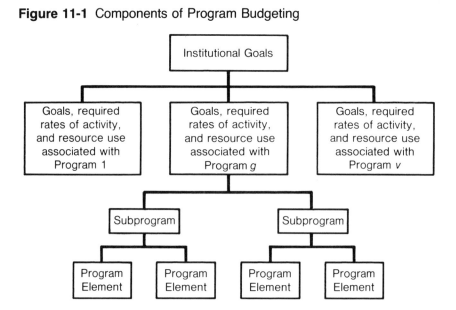

of the diseases or injuries that are presented by its patients. Having specified these major objectives, management must define the areas of program activity.

With the focus on the major objective of providing care at an acceptable level of quality, the quantity and composition of service used in diagnosing, monitoring, and therapeutically managing a given condition is determined, in varying degrees of precision, by medical knowledge and technology. In other words, medical knowledge and technology dictate, in varying degrees of precision, the quantity and composition of service the hospital should use in managing a given disease or injury. It seems reasonable, then, to define the program areas in terms of the diseases or injuries that the institution customarily manages. If this procedure were followed, a program area of activity could be defined as the process (i.e., provision of service) by which the expected number of cases of a given condition or a set of conditions is managed medically.

Most acute care hospitals provide service to patients who present a broad range of diseases and injuries. From a practical perspective, management might define program areas so that each encompasses a number of similar conditions. Program areas can be defined in terms of broad diagnostic categories similar to the 17 major groupings of disease or injury in the International Classification of Diseases, Adapted (ICDA). If management adopted this approach, it could define the objective of each program area as providing services required in diagnosing, monitoring, and therapeutically managing patients expected to be admitted with the diseases or injuries associated with its area of activity. This puts management in a position to ensure that the objective of each program area is consistent with and contributes to the attainment of the common goal of the institution. In fact, this suggests that, if the classification of program areas is both mutually exclusive and collectively exhaustive, the attainment of the objectives of all areas ensures that the goal of the institution will be reached.

Program areas of activity may be disaggregated further into subprogram areas that, in turn, may be divided into program elements. Suppose that management has defined program areas in terms of broad diagnostic categories, three of which respond to the needs of cancer, maternity, and heart disease patients. As an example of subprogram areas, consider the maternity program. As seen in Figure 11-2, four subprograms (prenatal care, family planning, delivery, and postnatal care) that are associated with this program may be identified. These may be expressed in terms of program elements required in performing the functions of the subprogram and the program area. For example, consider the subprogram concerned with providing the care required at the time the mother delivers. The activities required here obviously depend, to a significant extent, on the nature of the delivery, such as complicated or uncomplicated. The service bundle used during a normal delivery would be differentiated from the service mix required when performing a cesarean section. The basic purpose of defining subprograms in terms of program elements is to minimize the variation in the

**Figure 11-2** Three Diagnostic Subprogram Areas

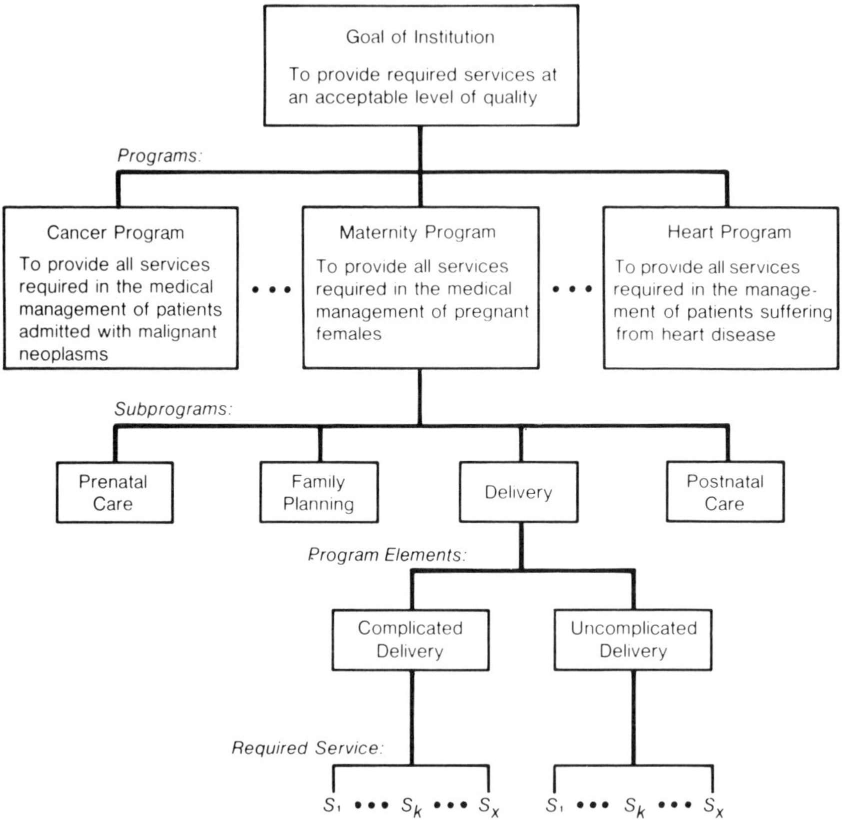

service bundle associated with a given element and to maximize the variation in the bundles associated with different program elements.

Once all programs, related subprograms, and program elements have been identified, management is in a position to estimate the quantity and composition of services associated with each program element. In Figure 11-2, the quantity and composition of service are represented by the set $(S_1, \cdots, S_k, \cdots, S_x)$. Suppose that the quantity of a service required in performing a subprogram's functions has been established. The quantity of this service required by all program elements obviously represents the requirements of the subprogram. Similarly, the service requirements of all subprograms of a given program area represent the needs of that program. Summing across all such programs results in an estimate of the total quantity of the service that will be required. Replicating this procedure for all services results in an estimate of the quantity and composition of activities that will be required to achieve the goals of the institution.

Once the quantity and composition of services necessary for attaining the goals of all program areas have been estimated, management can estimate the volume and mix that must be provided by each of the departmental or productive centers in the hospital's organizational chart. This is because each of the services $(S_1, \cdots, S_k, \cdots, S_x)$ that will be used in attaining program goals may be associated with an identifiable departmental or productive unit in the hospital.

Suppose that the set of services provided by the radiology department, $S_R$, may be written as

$$S_r = \{R_1, R_2, \cdots, R_i, \cdots, R_n\}$$

where each of the $R$s represents a specific type of radiological service. Also suppose that management identifies the program areas

$$P_1, P_2, \cdots, P_g, \cdots, P_v$$

which will require the use of service $R_i$. Finally, assume management has estimated that $r_{i1}$ units of service $R_i$ will be required to achieve the goals of program $P_1$, $r_{i2}$ units of $R_i$ to attain the goals of program $P_2$, etc. Letting $r_{ig}$ represent the volume of service $R_i$ required by program $P_g$, the rate at which this service must be provided to achieve the goals of all programs is given by

$$r_i^* = \sum_{g=1}^{v} r_{ig}$$

Replicating this procedure for all services provided by the radiology department results in the set

$$S_r^* = \{r_1^*, r_2^*, \cdots, r_i^*, \cdots, r_n^*\}$$

which represents the quantity and composition of radiological services needed to achieve the goals of all program areas. Also observe that $S_r^*$ corresponds to the work load of the radiology department and that this work load corresponds to the quantity and composition of radiological services that must be provided to achieve the goals of the various program areas as well as of the institution.

Given the set $S_r^*$, management can translate the rate at which each radiological service is to be provided into real and financial resource requirements. Such a translation provides the basis for determining:

1. the real and financial resource requirements of the radiology department;
2. the contribution of the radiology department to each program area as ex-

pressed in terms of the quantity and composition of services provided as well as the real and financial resources that will be consumed in supporting each area.

Assuming that departmental units also correspond to responsibility centers, the statement of resource requirements of providing the set $S_i^*$ constitutes the basis for developing a responsibility budget for the radiology department.

If this procedure is replicated for the other components of hospital care, management is in a position to

1. develop a responsibility budget for each responsibility center as expressed in terms of the quantity and composition of required services as well as the real and financial resources that will be needed if program and institutional goals are to be achieved;
2. monitor the activities of each productive or responsibility center to assure that the operation of organizational units of the hospital is consistent with and contributes to the attainment of program and institutional goals.

Thus, when program areas of activity are defined in terms of major groupings of disease or injury, the estimation of services required by the various programs provides a linkage between program budgeting and responsibility budgeting. The primary advantage of such an approach is that the budget of each responsibility center is based on the rate at which it must provide service in order to attain program goals. As a result, management may coordinate and evaluate both the productive units and the program areas of activity to achieve the common goals of the institution.

## 11.3.5 Zero-Base Budgeting

A major management task is to allocate resources to obtain the greatest benefit for the community. In maximizing the benefits obtained from a given set of resources, management must develop and evaluate various expenditure alternatives as well as establish funding priorities that identify projects that will yield the greatest benefits for the community.

Under the traditional budgeting process, managers who are responsible for established areas of activity usually are required to justify and defend only the *increase* in funding they request. The level of funding received earlier is accepted as being necessary and, as a result, the amount spent previously is approved implicitly.

Unlike the traditional approach, zero-base budgeting requires managers to defend the *entire* amount of funding they request for existing and potential areas of operation and to develop and evaluate expenditure alternatives. In such an evaluation, it is desirable to construct an ordinal ranking of alternate approaches that might be funded. An ordinal ranking is simply a list of projects arranged so that expenditure alternatives that yield the greatest benefits from a given set of resources appear at the head of the list.

Cost-benefit and cost-effectiveness analysis are techniques for developing the ordinal ranking. More specifically, cost-benefit analysis may be used to achieve the maximum monetary benefits, as measured in present value equivalents, that are obtainable from a given set of resources. Similarly, the objective of cost-effectiveness analysis is to obtain the maximum tangible outcomes, as measured in natural or epidemiological units, that are obtainable from a specified set of resources.

Zero-base budgeting consists of essentially two stages. The first involves the development of decision packages and data required for the analysis that is performed during the second phase. On the basis of that initial information, the second phase is devoted to an evaluation of the decision packages by constructing an ordinal ranking of expenditure alternatives. Management should use the results of the second stage of zero-base budgeting to construct the institution's funding priorities.

The first phase of zero-base budgeting requires:

1. an identification of the department or functional unit for which the analysis is performed;
2. an identification of the activity in the department or functional unit for which alternate approaches are developed (e.g., alternate methods of treatment of diabetes);
3. a statement of the objectives of the department or functional unit as related to the corporate goals of the institution;
4. a statement of the output, effectiveness, or benefits required to achieve stated goals;
5. a statement of alternate approaches to achieving those goals;
6. a statement of projections regarding the output, effectiveness, or benefits of each alternative developed;
7. a listing of projections concerning the real and financial resources required by each alternative.

The first phase of zero-base budgeting should be performed at the lowest practicable level of managerial responsibility in the organization. In particular, projections concerning the output, effectiveness, or benefits as well as the real resource requirements should be prepared by individuals who are intimately familiar with the functional unit as well as the technical aspects of the processes that will be used in generating the results of each alternative.

During the second phase, the alternatives developed in the first stage are evaluated and ranked ordinally by cost-benefit analysis, by cost-effectiveness analysis, or by relying on the subjective judgment of management. Expenditure alternatives should be ranked by the managers who were responsible for the development of projections concerning their effectiveness or benefits and corresponding resource requirements. In turn, managerial personnel at successively higher levels of responsibility should consolidate the alternatives and rankings received from subordinates and develop their own sets of priorities. Finally, senior management should consolidate these alternatives and rankings into a statement of priorities for the institution.

When allocating resources and developing ordinal rankings, management usually faces two types of problems. The first involves the allocation of resources and the development of ordinal rankings *within* a functional area, the second to the allocation of resources *among* or *between* functional areas. To reach decisions in a given functional area, management may use cost-effectiveness analysis; to make decisions on the allocation of resources among two or more functional areas or units, it may use cost-benefit analysis.

### 11.3.5.1  Cost-Effectiveness Analysis

Cost-effectiveness analysis is limited to situations in which management wants to compare different variations of a single alternative or different approaches to a common objective. It is important to remember that the effects of the different approaches may be unequal but they must be measurable in terms of the same outcomes.

The basic strategy of cost-effectiveness analysis is to compare the costs and outcomes associated with one or more alternatives (or multiple variations in a single alternative) with the status quo or the conventional method of operation. Suppose that the set of alternatives represented by $A_1, \cdots, A_j, \cdots, A_n$ were identified by management during the first phase of zero-base budgeting. The objective of the following analysis is to compare the cost and effectiveness of these alternatives with the cost-effectiveness of the status quo, represented by the letter $Z$. Cost-effectiveness analysis seeks to attain maximum tangible results, provided that budgetary limitations are not exceeded. Symbolically, the basic strategy of cost-effectiveness analysis is to maximize

$$\Sigma e_j x_j \qquad \text{for} \qquad j = 1, \cdots, n \qquad \qquad (11.1)$$

subject to the constraint

$$\Sigma C_j x_j \leq BC \qquad \qquad (11.2)$$

where

   $e_j$   represents the effectiveness of alternative $j$;

$x_j$   assumes the value of 1 or 0 depending on whether alternative $j$ is accepted or rejected;

$C_j$   is the cost of operating alternative $j$ as expressed in present value equivalents; and

$BC$   is the budget constraint (i.e., the sum of money available to the organizational unit for which the alternatives are evaluated).

As noted, the data required to perform cost-effectiveness analysis are obtained from the information developed during the first phase of zero-base budgeting. Assume that the planning horizon of the institution is five years and that the annual costs of operating alternative $j$ are limited to direct and indirect costs. Letting $DC_{jt}$ represent the direct costs of alternative $j$ in year $t$ and $IC_{jt}$ represent the corresponding indirect costs, the annual cost ($C_{jt}$) of operating alternative $j$ in year $t$ is given by

$$C_{jt} = DC_{jt} + IC_{jt} \tag{11.3}$$

When evaluating the relative cost of the various approaches, it is necessary to express anticipated expenditures in present value terms. To understand this point, suppose that by investing in a riskless security we are able to earn an annual rate of interest of 8 percent and that someone offers us either one dollar today or one dollar at the end of one year. Obviously, it is financially prudent to accept the dollar today, invest the money in the security, and, at the end of the year, collect $1.08. Other things held constant, suppose we are offered $1.00 today or $1.08 at the end of one year. In this case we are likely to be indifferent to the two offers since the present value of $1.08, which we will receive at the end of the year, is equal to the offer of $1.00 today. This may be seen by recalling that the present value of some future cash flow, $F$, is given by

$$PV = \frac{F}{(1 + i)^t} \tag{11.4}$$

where $i$ is the interest or discount rate per period and $t$ is the number of periods. In terms of our example, we find that

$$PV = \frac{\$1.08}{(1.08)^1} = \$1.00$$

This expression may be expanded to calculate the present value of a stream of cash flows occurring in different periods. By way of illustration, let us return to the problem of determining the present value of the costs associated with alternative $j$ that will occur during several periods in the future. In this situation, we find that

$$C_j = \sum_{t=1}^{t=5} \left[ \frac{C_{jt}}{(1 + i)^t} \right] \tag{11.5}$$

where $i$ is an appropriate discount rate. To illustrate the use of Equation 11.5, suppose that the values assumed by $C_{jt}$ for $t = 1, \cdots, 5$ are \$16,000, \$20,000, \$25,000, \$18,000, and \$12,000, respectively. Letting $i = .10$, we find that

$$C_j = \frac{\$16,000}{(1 + .10)} + \frac{\$20,000}{(1 + .10)^2} + \frac{\$25,000}{(1 + .10)^3} + \frac{\$18,000}{(1 + .10)^4} + \frac{\$12,000}{(1 + .10)^5}$$

$$= \$69,602.55$$

Once the costs of each alternative have been expressed in present value terms, the effectiveness of each alternative and the status quo should be measured in natural or epidemiological units such as the number of medical conditions discovered, lives saved, life years saved, units of service produced, and so on.

Assume that the analysis is limited to alternatives $A_1$, $A_2$, $A_3$, and $A_4$. Also suppose that the effectiveness of the four alternatives and the status quo is measured by the total number of lives saved in five years and that the following projections are available to management.

### Number of Lives Saved by Alternative

| Year | $A_1$ | $A_2$ | $A_3$ | $A_4$ | $Z$ |
|---|---|---|---|---|---|
| 1 | 220 | 220 | 20 | 180 | 50 |
| 2 | 230 | 250 | 20 | 170 | 50 |
| 3 | 240 | 270 | 10 | 190 | 50 |
| 4 | 250 | 280 | 10 | 160 | 50 |
| 5 | 260 | 240 | 20 | 150 | 50 |
| Total lives saved | 1,200 | 1,260 | 80 | 850 | 250 |

In addition, after applying Equation 11.5, suppose we are able to summarize our findings concerning the values of $E_j$ and $C_j$ as follows

| Alternative | $C_j$ | $E_j$ |
|---|---|---|
| $A_1$ | \$12,000 | 1,200 |
| $A_2$ | 13,000 | 1,260 |
| $A_3$ | 14,000 | 80 |
| $A_4$ | 6,000 | 850 |
| $Z$ | 4,000 | 250 |
| (Status quo) | | |

As seen in Figure 11-3, we may combine the estimates of $C_j$ and $E_j$ in a single graph that permits us to identify and eliminate dominated approaches. This figure reveals that alternative $A_3$ is less effective *and* costlier than the other approaches, so this alternative should be eliminated from consideration.

Once dominated alternatives have been identified and eliminated, the incremental costs and incremental effectiveness of the remaining approaches may be computed by

$$\Delta C_j = C_j - C_z$$

$$\Delta E_j = E_j - E_z$$

where $C_z$ and $E_z$ represent the costs and effectiveness of the status quo, respectively. Assume that, for various reasons, management is unable to exercise complete discretion and that the status quo represents a minimum requirement of the unit.

The next step in the analysis is to construct the ratios $\Delta E_j/\Delta C_j$, which provide the basis for developing the ordinal ranking of the alternatives as well as the

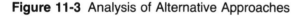

**Figure 11-3** Analysis of Alternative Approaches

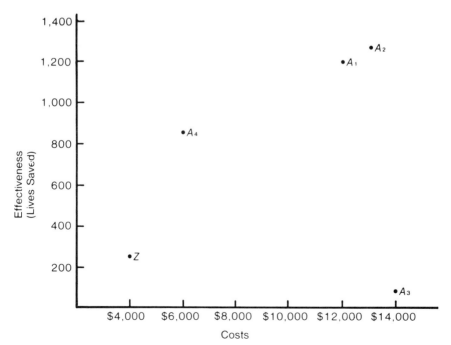

funding priority referred to earlier. As can be verified, the incremental cost-effectiveness ratios of alternatives $A_1$, $A_2$, and $A_4$ are as follows:

| Alternative | Incremental Costs | Incremental Effectiveness | $\Delta E_j/\Delta C_j$ | Funding Priority |
|---|---|---|---|---|
| $A_1$ | $8,000 | 950 | .119 | 2 |
| $A_2$ | 9,000 | 1,010 | .112 | 3 |
| $A_4$ | 2,000 | 600 | .300 | 1 |

These data suggest that, on the average, an additional dollar of expenditure on alternative $A_4$ results in the preservation of an additional .3 life. The incremental effectiveness-cost ratio of alternative $A_4$ is greater than those of the two other alternatives. As a result, the ordinal ranking indicates that alternative $A_4$ is the preferred approach.

Consider next a situation in which management is able to exercise complete discretion and one of the alternatives under consideration is closing the unit. If management elects to close the unit, the resulting costs and effectiveness both are zero. Consequently, when management has complete discretion, the various alternatives and the status quo should be compared with the option of closing the unit, which implies that the ratios $E_j/C_j$ replace the incremental cost-effectiveness analysis. In this situation, the set of ratios $E_j/C_j$ must be compared with a specified standard, $s^*$, and only those alternatives that satisfy the condition

$$E_j/C_j \geq s^*$$

should be considered by management.

### 11.3.5.2  Cost-Benefit Analysis

Cost-benefit analysis differs from cost-effectiveness analysis in that the output of each alternative is expressed in monetary units. Letting $B_j$ correspond to the present value equivalent of the total benefits of alternative $j$, we find that only those approaches that satisfy the conditions

$$B_j/C_j \geq 1 \quad \text{or} \quad B_j - C_j \geq 0$$

should be evaluated by management. Similar to the approach above, an ordinal ranking of the ratios $\Delta B_j/\Delta C_j$ represents the basis for constructing the funding priority for the unit. Extensive literature exists on the estimation of benefits and the references at the end of this chapter consider this important issue in detail. As a result, techniques of estimating benefits are not described here.

### 11.3.5.3 The General Problem of Optimization

Zero-base budgeting and cost-benefit analysis also may be applied to the general problem of optimization. Management must evaluate not only alternatives within functional units but also the rates at which the organizational units of the hospital are operated. Obviously, both considerations exert an impact on the allocation of resources among the various areas of activity.

Assume that the hospital is composed of departments $D_1$, $D_2$, and $D_3$, each of which must be operated to satisfy the service objectives of the institution. After using the analysis developed above, suppose further that alternative $A_1$ was selected for department $D_1$, $A_2$ for department $D_2$, and $A_3$ for department $D_3$. Management's objective in this case is to identify the financial resources required to sustain the rates of operation that provide the maximum benefits obtainable from a fixed budget of, say, \$490,000.

Assume that the data in Table 11-1 represent the present value equivalents of the costs and benefits of various rates of activity in each of the three departments. As will be demonstrated later, the rates of activity for which the general condition

$$\frac{\Delta B_1}{\Delta C_1} = \cdots = \frac{\Delta B_j}{\Delta C_j} = \cdots = \frac{\Delta B_n}{\Delta C_n}$$

is satisfied maximize the benefits to the community. As suggested above, we require the numerical values of $\Delta B_j$ and $\Delta C_j$, which, in terms of our example, are presented in Table 11-2. The incremental change in the benefits resulting from the second 1,000 units of service provided by department $D_1$ is \$45 (i.e., \$95 − \$50) while the corresponding increase in cost is \$5 (i.e., \$10 − \$5).

---

**Table 11-1** Summary of Costs and Benefits

| | Alternative (Department) | | | | | |
|---|---|---|---|---|---|---|
| | $A_1$ (D₁) | | $A_2$ (D₂) | | $A_3$ (D₃) | |
| Units of Service (in 1,000) | $B_1$ (in \$10,000) | $C_1$ (in \$10,000) | $B_2$ (in \$10,000) | $C_2$ (in \$10,000) | $B_3$ (in \$10,000) | $C_3$ (in \$10,000) |
| 1 | \$ 50 | \$ 5 | \$ 48 | \$ 6 | \$ 77 | \$ 7 |
| 2 | 95 | 10 | 90 | 12 | 147 | 14 |
| 3 | 135 | 15 | 126 | 18 | 210 | 21 |
| 4 | 170 | 20 | 156 | 24 | 266 | 28 |
| 5 | 200 | 25 | 180 | 30 | 315 | 35 |
| 6 | 220 | 30 | 192 | 36 | 350 | 42 |

**Table 11-2** Summary of Incremental Cost-Benefit Ratios

| Units of Service (in 1,000) | $A_1$ (D₁) | | | Alternative (Department) $A_2$ (D₂) | | | $A_3$ (D₃) | | |
|---|---|---|---|---|---|---|---|---|---|
| | $\Delta B_1$ (in $10,000) (1) | $\Delta C_1$ (in $10,000) (2) | $\frac{\Delta B_1}{\Delta C_1}$ (3) | $\Delta B_2$ (in $10,000) (4) | $\Delta C_2$ (in $10,000) (5) | $\frac{\Delta B_2}{\Delta C_2}$ (6) | $\Delta B_3$ (in $10,000) (7) | $\Delta C_3$ (in $10,000) (8) | $\frac{\Delta B_3}{\Delta C_3}$ (9) |
| 1 | $50 | $5 | 10 | $48 | $6 | 8 | $77 | $7 | 11 |
| 2 | 45 | 5 | 9 | 42 | 6 | 7 | 70 | 7 | 10 |
| 3 | 40 | 5 | 8 | 36 | 6 | 6 | 63 | 7 | 9 |
| 4 | 35 | 5 | 7 | 30 | 6 | 5 | 56 | 7 | 8 |
| 5 | 30 | 5 | 6 | 24 | 6 | 4 | 49 | 7 | 7 |
| 6 | 20 | 5 | 4 | 12 | 6 | 2 | 35 | 7 | 5 |

The other values assumed by the terms $\Delta B_j$ and $\Delta C_j$ were calculated in a similar fashion. The values in columns (3), (6), and (9) represent the set of ratios $\Delta B_j/\Delta C_j$.

These data now may be used to determine the financial resources required to sustain the rates of activity that maximize the benefits generated by hospital operations. Similar to the earlier analysis, management should allocate funds in accordance with the incremental benefits generated by each additional dollar of expenditure. Notice that the first 1,000 units of service provided by department $D_3$ generate an incremental benefit of $11 for each additional dollar spent. Since the incremental benefit-cost ratio of $11 exceeds the other values in columns (3) and (6), the prudent financial decision is to allocate the first $70,000 of the total budgetary allotment to department $D_3$.

Consider next the rates of activity and the corresponding incremental benefit-cost ratios that remain after allocating the first $70,000 to department $D_3$. The first 1,000 units of service provided by department $D_1$ and an additional 1,000 units provided by department $D_3$ both yield an incremental benefit of $10 for each additional dollar of expenditure. Since this ratio exceeds the incremental benefits associated with an additional dollar of expenditure in department $D_2$, management should increase the budgetary allotment to department $D_3$ by $70,000 and allocate $50,000 to department $D_1$. At this point, it should be verified that $190,000 of the total budgetary allotment of $490,000 has been allocated and that the financial resources required to produce 1,000 units of service in department $D_1$ and 2,000 units in department $D_3$ have been provided.

Assume that management continues to reach similar decisions until the budget limit of $490,000 is exhausted. As can be verified, providing 3,000 units of service in department $D_1$, 1,000 units in department $D_2$, and 4,000 units in department $D_3$ not only exhausts the budgetary allotment but also results in the equality

$$\frac{\Delta B_1}{\Delta C_1} = \frac{\Delta B_2}{\Delta C_2} = \frac{\Delta B_3}{\Delta C_3} = \$8$$

In terms of our example, the equality implies that the maximum benefits obtainable from the fixed budget of $490,000 amount to $4,490,000.

To demonstrate that this mix of services produces maximum benefits, suppose that the budget is *increased* from $490,000 to $500,000 and that management allocates available financial resources to provide 6,000 units of service in department $D_1$; 1,000 units in department $D_2$, and 2,000 units in department $D_3$. As should be verified, the total potential benefits resulting from these decisions amount to only $4,150,000. This suggests that, even though the total budget has been *increased*, the selection of a different mix of activity rates may result in a *lower* level of benefits than might have been obtained otherwise.

This discussion implicitly assumed that management could influence the number and type of patients treated as well as the quantity and composition of services provided. Given that 80 to 90 percent of all admissions are elective, it is quite possible for management to design a policy concerning admissions that is conducive to providing desired service mix.

It is important to note that the quantitative methods described must be tempered by practical considerations. For example, it is difficult, if not impossible, to develop a reasonable set of alternatives for the emergency room or the operating room, so a strict application of zero-based budgeting to the budgets for these units may not be appropriate. In addition, it is important to note that the subjective judgment of management should play an important role in developing the ordinal ranking of the alternatives. For example, certain intangibles are not quantifiable and, as such, cannot be considered in the formal analysis. Management thus is forced to evaluate intangibles subjectively. If used pragmatically, however, zero-base budgeting, cost-effectiveness analysis, and cost-benefit analysis are techniques that can improve the allocation of resources and increase the likelihood of providing maximum benefits to the community.

## 11.4  APPROACHES TO THE BUDGETING PROCESS

When considering the method of developing the budget, management may use one of two approaches:

1. It can employ a "vacuum" approach in which projects are reviewed and funded without reference to the common goals of the institution and the merits of other projects.
2. It can use a "universal" or "total entity" approach in which projects are reviewed and funded within the framework of the total overall objectives of the institution and in terms of the other projects and programs under consideration.

Obviously, the second of these two approaches is preferred since it is more likely to result in decisions that increase the chances of providing maximum total benefits to the community.

In implementing the universal approach, management should employ the program budgeting and zero-base budgeting techniques described earlier. As indicated, program budgeting is a managerial tool that may be used in reaching decisions on the allocation of resources among, rather than within, program areas. It is in this regard that program budgeting is useful in arriving at an allocation of resources consistent with the achievement of the common goals and objectives of the hospital enterprise. If used in a practical manner, without an overemphasis on quantifying all aspects of hospital activity and with an understanding of its limitations, program budgeting can be a useful technique for evaluating decisions concerning large resource expenditures.

Traditionally, an incremental approach that requires the justification and evaluation of additional budgetary requests has been used in resolving problems of resource allocation and the determination of allowable levels of expenditure. The incremental technique, however, fails to take advantage of the opportunity to review and justify all proposed expenditures and to evaluate trade-offs among alternatives so as to obtain the greatest total benefits. To overcome the basic weakness of the incremental approach, management should employ zero-base budgeting techniques in reaching decisions concerning resource allocation within program areas.

## 11.4.1 Comprehensive and Partial Budgets

A comprehensive budget is defined as one in which all aspects of operational activity are budgeted and the results are translated into monetary terms. Thus, all planned capital and operating costs as well as all revenues are projected and incorporated into a single budget document. For each dimension of operational activity, the estimated work load, resource requirements, and related financial implications are included.

In contrast, a limited or partial budget includes a single dimension or a series of dimensions of hospital activity. For example, a partial budget may include only salary and wage expenses or it may contain only capital expenditures. The partial budget, then, reflects only a single or several dimensions of activity and is not all-inclusive.

From a managerial perspective, it should be clear that a comprehensive budget is preferred to a limited or a partial budget. Only by developing a budget that encompasses the totality of activity can management adequately evaluate plans, objectives, and the extent to which planned activities are consistent with the achievement of the common objectives of the institution.

## 11.4.2 Fixed and Flexible Budgets

After considering all factors that may influence the demands on the hospital, management may estimate either a range of expected work loads or a single volume of service. If only a single volume of service is used, the resulting budget is said to be fixed. To the extent that the estimate of work load is accurate, a fixed budget is an accurate and reliable managerial tool.

Unfortunately, given the dynamic and stochastic nature of the demand for hospital services, it is not likely that a single estimate of activity will reflect the actual demand for care accurately. Given this environment, a fixed budget, though of value, is limited in terms of its ability to portray the cost implications of producing various levels of output. In light of these limitations, a flexible budget is preferred to a fixed budget.

A flexible budget is defined as a statement of expected financial performance that is adjusted to reflect potential variation in volume. A flexible budget, then, is nothing more than a series of fixed budgets covering a specified range of volume alternatives. Within the range of variations in volume, management should develop cost implications and budget alternatives only to the extent that variability in volume will influence budgetary expectations materially.

Theoretically, management should analyze the cost structure of each department to identify:

1. fixed costs (i.e., costs that remain constant irrespective of volume);
2. costs that do not vary in accordance with day-to-day volume but can vary in accordance with managerial decisions (closing a wing, nursing station, etc.);
3. costs that vary in accordance with the volume or rate of output.

Once these three categories of cost have been determined, management can estimate the extent to which total costs are expected to vary in accordance with differing levels or rates of production.

Suppose that the unit of analysis is the dietary department and that three estimates of output (meals) and their associated costs are as follows:

|  | Expected Meals | Expected Costs |
| --- | --- | --- |
| Minimum | 400,000 | $450,000 |
| Mean | 500,000 | 550,000 |
| Maximum | 600,000 | 650,000 |

In this example, we assume that

1. the fixed costs of the dietary department are $50,000;
2. the costs that vary with output are $1.00/meal; and
3. the hospital cannot eliminate the dietary department.

The relation between the total cost and the output of the dietary department may be expressed by

$$TC = \$50,000 + \$1.00\,M$$

where $TC$ represents total cost of the unit and the variable $M$ is the total number of meals produced. If 580,000 meals actually were produced at a total cost of

$750,000, management is alerted immediately to the fact that overspending of $120,000 has occurred and that corrective action may be required to restore the balance between actual and expected performance.

By beginning with the minimum level of expected output and proceeding to the maximum, management can evaluate alternate levels of volume and the extent to which actual costs incurred are consistent with budgetary expectations. Thus, when a flexible rather than a fixed budget is prepared, management is in a better position to evaluate and control the performance of the productive units comprising the hospital enterprise.

## REFERENCES

American Hospital Association. *Budgeting Procedures for Hospitals.* Chicago: American Hospital Association, 1971.

Anthony, R. N., and Herzlinger, R. E. *Management Control in Nonprofit Organizations.* Homewood, Ill.: Richard D. Irwin, 1975.

Anthony, R. N., and Reece, J. S. *Management Accounting: Text and Cases,* 5th ed. Homewood, Ill.: Richard D. Irwin, 1975, Ch. 20–22.

Bennett, J. E., and Krasny, J. "Functional Value Analysis: A Technique for Reducing Hospital Overhead Costs." *Topics in Health Care Financing,* vol. 3, no. 2, Summer 1977, pp. 35–54.

Berman, H. J., and Weeks, L. *Financial Management of Hospitals,* 3rd ed. Ann Arbor, Mich.: Health Administration Press, 1976, Ch. 15.

Burkhead, J., and Miner, J. *Public Expenditure.* Chicago: Aldine and Atherton, 1971, Ch. 6.

Cleverly, W. O. "One Step Further—The Multi-Variable Flexible Budget System." *Hospital Financial Management,* vol. 30, no. 4, April 1976, pp. 34–44.

_____. "Two Methods for a More Accurate Budget." *Hospital Financial Management,* vol. 26, no. 7, July 1972, pp. 5, 6, 39.

_____. "Input-Output Analysis and the Hospital Budgeting Process." *Health Services Research,* vol. 10, no. 1, Spring 1975, pp. 36–50.

Dillon, R. D. "Zero Base Budgeting: An Introduction." *Hospital Financial Management,* vol. 31, no. 11, November 1977, pp. 10–14.

Krouse, C. G. "A Model for Aggregate Financial Planning." *Management Science,* June 1972, pp. 555–566.

Newman, J. L. "Make Overhead Cuts That Last." *Harvard Business Review,* vol. 83, no. 3, May–June 1975, pp. 116–126.

Novick, D., ed. *Program Budgeting.* Cambridge, Mass.: Harvard University Press, 1965.

Pyhrr, P. A. *Zero-Based Budgeting.* New York: John Wiley & Sons, Inc., 1973.

# Chapter 12

# The Budgeting Process

## Objectives

After completing this chapter, you should be able to:

1. Describe the prerequisites to budgeting.
2. Understand the importance of basic terms such as:
   a. the background statement.
   b. assumptions.
   c. goals and policies.
   d. projections.
   e. financial and operating plans.
3. Understand and describe the various phases of budget preparation.

## 12.1 INTRODUCTION

The process by which the budget is prepared may be characterized by two separate but interrelated components. The first component focuses on the technical nature of budget preparation and is concerned with various methods by which it is developed. The second component is basically behavioral in nature and addresses the organizational and interpersonal aspects of the development of the budget as well as management of the budgeting process.

This chapter focuses only on the behavioral aspects of budget formulation, with an emphasis on the organization and management of the entire process. The technical aspects of the budgeting process are developed later.

## 12.2 THE PHASES OF BUDGET PREPARATION

The process by which the budget is prepared may be divided into essentially four phases (Figure 12-1). The first phase is basically a preparatory stage in

**Figure 12-1** The Phases of Budget Preparation

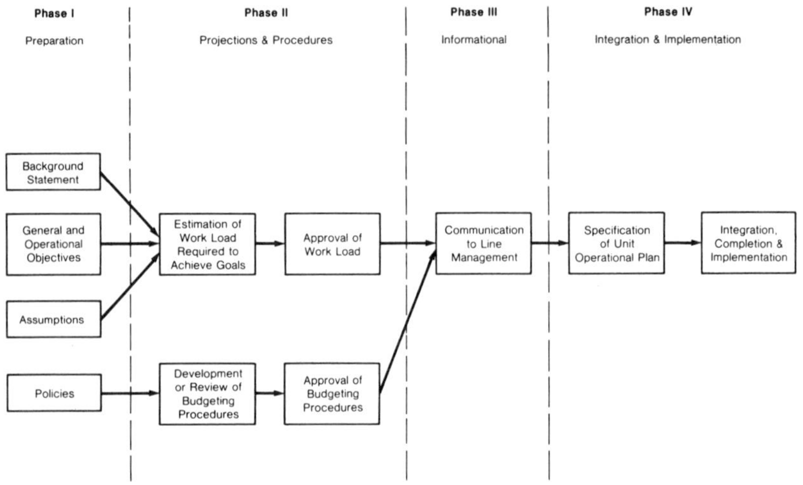

which senior management develops the foundation that provides the basis for the later stages of budget preparation. The second phase usually is devoted to the development or review of hospital budgeting procedures and the estimation of the work load required to achieve the goals of the institution during the budget period. The third phase involves informational and technical meetings during which line managers become actively involved in budget preparation. These meetings provide the basis for the fourth phase, during which line managers use the estimates of the work load required to achieve the institution's goals as well as the budgeting policies and procedures to develop an initial or tentative budget for the unit(s) for which they are responsible. The last step of the fourth phase is to submit the budget document to the appropriate authorities for approval. Once approved, the budget is implemented as a managerial tool in coordinating, monitoring, and controlling hospital activity. It should be noted that, even though budget preparation basically is a sequential process, several of the phases can be accomplished simultaneously; in this discussion, however, the phases are examined serially.

## 12.2.1 The First Phase

The first step in the systematic development of the budget is an analysis of the environment in which the hospital operates so as to specify the relationship between the institution and the system by which health care is delivered to the community. More specifically, when developing the background statement, management should examine the strengths and weaknesses of the institution in relation to the needs of the population served as well as in relation to the system of health care delivery. This evaluation provides the basis for an examination of the institution's role in providing health services as well as its capability to perform as an integral component of the delivery system. When evaluating health care delivery, it frequently is necessary to examine the current needs and the historical changes in the characteristics of the population at risk that have exerted an impact on the demand for services. By focusing on those needs and characteristics, management develops the foundation for analyzing factors that are likely to affect the use of service during the budget period and should be reflected in projections of the hospital's work load.

Once management has an understanding of the environment in which the hospital operates, it should formulate general objectives. A statement of the hospital's general objectives is required to give the budget a uniform direction. In the absence of clearly defined objectives, each responsibility center and/or program area may develop and pursue goals that, while not antithetical to the overall objectives of the institution, may not result in the best allocation and use of scarce resources.

The necessity of well-defined policies or guidelines for budget preparation is similar to the reasons advanced for the need to define general objectives. As suggested, the statement of objectives refers to the broad goals of the institution. On the other hand, when viewed from the perspective of budget preparation, policies have a much narrower focus that seeks to specify the procedures to be followed when preparing the budgets of the hospital's functional units.

After developing goals, policies, and the background statement, management should establish and test the assumptions or suppositions on which the budget will rest. The assumptions are management's projections on the state of the world or of the environment that is expected to prevail during the budget period. Usually, these assumptions are related to factors that influence the demand for hospital service, the use of resources in providing those services, and the prices of factor inputs that are likely to prevail during the budget period. Assumptions may be defined operationally as events or developments that may influence hospital activity but whose occurrence is beyond management control. Establishing and testing the assumptions on which the budget is based, therefore, is the first and perhaps the most fundamental element in the process of operational planning.

Since assumptions are projections or estimates of future events, they will be either right or wrong in the final analysis. To minimize the probability of basing the budget on a set of faulty assumptions, the projections as to conditions expected during the planning period should be evaluated carefully.

As might be surmised from this discussion, the assumptions on which the budget is based differ from the background statement and the statement of objectives. Recall that the set of assumptions represents management's predictions of future events and developments. As such, the assumptions represent the vehicle by which management formulates expectations concerning future events that emanate from the current environment as defined by the background statement. Assumptions also differ from objectives in that the former are, by definition, predictions concerning events over which the hospital is unable to exert control. Objectives, on the other hand, are controllable events or results that are desirable and obtainable through a set of purposeful and discretionary actions by the hospital.

However, even though there are important differences among objectives, assumptions, and the background statement, these elements are not independent; rather, their interrelations provide the basis for management to ensure their internal consistency. For example, the statement of objectives may prove to be inconsistent with management's best expectation concerning the environment during the planning period. In such a situation, a comparison of the expected operating environment with the statement of goals may force management to revise their expectations, the objectives of the institution, or both. Similarly, a set of assumptions may prove to be unreasonable when compared with the background statement. Thus, the interrelations among expectations, goals, and the background statement provide a useful system of checks and balances that should be present in any sound budgeting process.

A logical extension of these three elements is the establishment of program priorities and funding guidelines. As seen earlier, the development of program priorities involves program budgeting, while the establishment of funding guidelines is a far more complex task.

In establishing priorities, program budgeting has been described as a mechanism that may be used in assuring the coordination of the allocation of resources among areas of activity that are directed toward a common goal. Perhaps the simplest and most pragmatic way of applying the principles of program budgeting is to examine both the operating environment and the operational implications of management's projection of future events so as to identify program areas that should be given a high priority. From a theoretical perspective, existing and proposed programs should be ranked ordinally, using such quantitative techniques as cost-benefit or cost-effectiveness analysis. Such a ranking, when coupled with management's subjective evaluation, provides the basis for developing a set of program priorities.

On the other hand, without a funding guideline, the establishment of funding priorities is a useless exercise. Clearly, if funds are not available to support a program, its identification as a high priority is not meaningful. To avoid problems of false expectations, a funding guideline must accompany the ordinal ranking of the programs that actually will be supported.

When identifying program areas of activity that will receive financial support, it is necessary to develop a funding guideline that, in turn, is based on a multitude of factors. Among the more important of these factors are the current and expected financial position of the hospital, current and expected surpluses, and the possibility of obtaining additional funds through the issuance of long-term and short-term debt. Given the range of methods by which financial resources may be obtained, it is difficult, if not impossible, to formulate a set of generalizable rules for the development of funding guidelines.

The importance of these guidelines cannot be overemphasized. The development of a reasonable set of guidelines ensures that resources are not allocated to areas of low priority and that energies will not be misdirected by developing a plan that will not receive funding, thereby, avoiding the problems generated by false expectations. Moreover, funding guidelines provide a clear indication of the extent to which management's financial decisions are consistent with the hospital's goals.

The final step in the first phase of the budgeting process is to translate the statement of general objectives into a set of operational goals. In the absence of operational objectives, it is difficult, if not impossible, to evaluate the allocation of factors of production among programs and to examine the trade-offs between and within program areas. Without quantifiable or objective criteria, the budget, as an expression of the standards by which actual performance is compared and evaluated, is likely to fail as a tool that assists management in controlling the operational activities of the institution.

In specifying operational goals, management must ensure that they are realistic and attainable during the budget period. If, given the environment expected, the goals are unrealistic and unreachable, management may become discouraged and frustrated when they are not achieved. Consequently, unrealistic objectives may prove counterproductive to the efficient and effective use of the budget as a managerial tool.

It should be noted that the goals and objectives specified at this stage of the budgeting process correspond to the program level of activity. Their specification for hospital cost or responsibility centers should be developed later in the budgeting process by the individuals who are accountable for the operation of each center.

As has been discussed, the first phase of the budget process provides the basis for developing operational and financial plans and as such, is of considerable importance to the overall process. However, it must be noted that the first phase is not concerned with the means by which goals are to be achieved; rather, these and other related matters are treated in the remaining phases of budget preparation.

## 12.2.2 The Second Phase

On the basis of the information prepared in the first phase, management begins to develop the numerical data that provide the basis for the preparation of the operational plans by which the goals of the institution are to be achieved. Specifically, management must develop projections concerning the volume of output or the work load that will be required to achieve stated goals. By projecting this work load, management lays the foundation on which it can develop details of the operating plan and forecasts concerning the calculation of resource requirements. The projections should include the total number of patient days, the number of days of care in each nursing center, and the work load of each of the other responsibility centers. When the traditional approach to budget preparation is used, the work load projections of most responsibility centers require an estimate of patient days that is perhaps the most important forecast of all. The techniques by which these work loads might be estimated are analyzed later and are not considered in detail here.

However, the projections must be reviewed and approved by management during the second stage. Management must ensure that work load projections are accurate and reflect anticipated changes in such factors as the demographic characteristics of the population served, medical technology, the social and political environment, and historical trends and relationships. Management also must ensure that the projections are realistic and that the hospital is capable of providing the estimated volume of service.

At this stage of the process, stated goals and objectives, work load projections, and budgeting policies should be communicated to the hospital line managers. These managers also should be provided with historical volume and cost data, current employment and wage data, information on the use of consumable supplies, and a set of administrative forms on which to report the details of the operational plans for each unit.

## 12.2.3 The Third Phase

Once the information described above has been distributed to line managers, at least two general meetings plus several technical meetings between the budget officer and the head of each responsibility center usually are required.

The purpose of the first general meeting is to orient the line managers to the goals of the budgeting process and to the procedures that are to be followed when developing the operational plans of the units for which they are responsible. This meeting should be devoted to a review and an explanation of the information that was communicated earlier. It should include a review of the material developed during the first phase, an orientation of line management to the use of projected work loads, historical information, and the procedures to be followed in developing the budgets for each responsibility or cost center.

The second general meeting should address the technical aspect of developing the budget. Particular emphasis should be placed on an explanation of the mechanics of estimating the relationship between work load projections and resource requirements as well as their corresponding cost implications. Further, if the hospital uses zero-base budgeting the second meeting should specify the procedures to be followed when summarizing and reporting information on alternate courses of action and should discuss the more technical aspects of cost-benefit or cost-effectiveness analysis.

In addition to the two general meetings, a series of sessions between the budget officer and individual heads of departments or responsibility centers may be required. These meetings should be devoted to a discussion of technical matters that are unique to the preparation of the budget for the cost or responsibility center of the particular line manager.

### 12.2.4 The Fourth Phase

The fourth phase of the budgeting process differs significantly from previous stages. The first three phases are devoted to developing the basis for operational planning and budgeting. During the fourth phase, hospital line managers are responsible for the assimilation and transformation of the efforts expended in the first three phases into an initial or tentative operating plan for the centers for which they are accountable.

If the hospital uses zero-base budgeting, the fourth phase also covers the development of alternate courses of action and evaluates these approaches by cost-benefit or cost-effectiveness analysis. As will be recalled, these approaches must be consistent with the goals of the unit, which in turn must be consistent with the common objectives of the institution. The initial analysis of the alternate courses provides the basis for successively higher levels of management to reach decisions concerning the ordinal ranking of projects and the resulting allocation of resources.

To provide the information required to develop expectations of costs a unit will incur, line managers must identify the number, type, and (if appropriate) the expected hiring date of all personnel required to produce the required work load. In addition, line managers must estimate the quantity of supplies and other nonlabor resources they will need to produce the expected work load. Such a specification constitutes the tentative operational plan by which objectives are to be achieved.

The operational plan then must be transformed into monetary or financial terms. This involves at least two interrelated steps:

1. the expense budget of each responsibility center is developed by multiplying estimated resource requirements by the factor price that is expected to prevail during the budget period
2. the development of a revenue budget for each of the revenue generating centers

As noted, cost-finding techniques provide information for the development or revision of the hospital's fee schedule. The revenue budget for responsibility centers providing direct patient care then is derived by the product of appropriate elements of the fee schedule and the corresponding volume of service expected to be provided during the budget period. The transformation of the operational plan into revenue and expense budgets is basically a clerical function that should be performed by the fiscal services division or the controller's office.

The specification of the details for the operation of a given unit are best deferred until this stage of budget preparation. The deferral tends to eliminate wasted effort as well as to preserve the credibility of the budget document. If the estimates of resource requirements and their corresponding costs were developed earlier, line managers would be forced to devote substantial time and effort to specifying the details of projects that might not receive funding. In such a situation, line managers might become disenchanted with the budget process that could impair the ability of administration to chart the institution's cause. To avoid such consequences, a detailed specification of resource requirements and their related costs probably should be deferred until the initial decisions on project approval have been reached.

Once the operational plans of each department or responsibility center have been translated into financial or monetary terms, management is in a position to organize and integrate all plans into the total budget for the hospital—also a clerical or computational task that should be performed by the fiscal services division.

Once the revenue and expense budgets have been incorporated into a single document, this information must be integrated with projections on changes in the capital equipment and the physical plant expected during the planning period. Such an integration is necessary if management is to ensure that anticipated revenues are at least equal to expected expenses. As will be seen later, such a procedure also is required when evaluating the impact of expected rates of operation and changes in capital stock on the solvency of the hospital.

It is important to note that, at this stage of development, the revenue, expense, cash, and capital budgets must be regarded as initial or tentative documents. This is because, even though the expenses correspond to approved projects or programs, anticipated levels of expenditure have not been compared with expected revenues. If an imbalance is identified, it is necessary to adjust the expense and/or capital budget or to introduce revisions in the revenue budget.

If expected revenues are found to be less than expected expenditures, senior management must redress the imbalance. The rate structure used in developing the revenue budget should reflect all economic costs of operation and, if this condition is not satisfied, management should take steps to ensure that charges are based on the full costs of operation. If the imbalance remains, management must revise expense budgets by eliminating areas of activity or by reducing the expected rates at which selected components of hospital activity are operated. If an analysis of expected cash balances reveals that the financial solvency of the institution is likely to be jeopardized during the planning period, it may be necessary to cancel or postpone one or more of the anticipated capital acquisitions. Once the expected revenues and expenditures have been brought into balance and management believes that the hospital's financial solvency will be preserved, the budget is basically complete and ready for submission to the board of governors (or directors, or trustees) and other authorities for approval, after which it is implemented by management and is used to monitor and control hospital activities.

**REFERENCES**

American Hospital Association. *Budgeting Procedures for Hospitals*. Chicago: American Hospital Association, 1971.

Griffith, J. R. "Budgeting Process Integral to Effective Cost Control Systems." *Hospital Financial Management,* vol. 28, no. 7, July 1974, pp. 12–28.

——————. *Quantitative Techniques for Hospital Planning and Control*. Lexington, Mass.: Lexington Books, 1972.

Silvers, J. B., and Prahalad, C. K. *Financial Management of Health Institutions*. Flushing, N.Y.: Spectrum Publications, 1974.

# Chapter 13

# Traditional Budgeting Techniques

## Objectives

After completing this chapter, you should be able to:

1. Describe the components of the budget.
2. Understand the use of moving averages, exponential smoothing, and regression analysis in the estimation of work load.
3. Understand the process and techniques used in preparing:
   a. the wage and salary budget.
   b. the supply expense budget.
4. Understand the process and techniques used in preparing a revenue budget that reflects:
   a. standardized services.
   b. stay-specific services.
   c. services measured by hours of use.
   d. merchandising functions.
5. Describe the components of the capital budget.
6. Understand the process and techniques of preparing a cash budget.

This chapter shifts the emphasis of discussion from the behavioral and organizational dimensions of the budgeting process to the technical aspects of budget preparation—specifically, techniques that hospitals have used traditionally when formulating their budgets. First, however, it is necessary to specify further the components of the budget document.

## 13.1 COMPONENTS OF THE BUDGET

The hospital budget is composed of three separate but interrelated budgets that may be supplemented by other financial plans or estimates:

1. the *operating* budget, which consists of the accumulated estimates of revenues and expenditures for the budget period;
2. the *capital* or *plant* budget, which consists of financial data pertaining to fixed assets that are to be acquired during the budget period; and
3. the *cash* budget, which consists of accumulated estimates of cash or monetary flows to and from the institution during the budget period.

The operating budget is composed of two basic components: the revenue budget and the expense budget. The expense budget also has two parts—a salary and wage expense budget and a supply expense budget. As noted in Chapter 12, estimated resource requirements and expenses for personnel, supplies, and other items are collected by the responsibility center irrespective of whether the unit provides direct patient care such as nursing services, operative care, etc., or a basic support service such as plant maintenance, laundry, or housekeeping. As the name implies, the revenue budget expresses the income the hospital expects to earn through various aspects of operational activity.

In addition to the revenue expected from providing patient services, the revenue budget must reflect the other operating and nonoperating income anticipated during the budget period. As mentioned earlier, the revenue and expense budgets, as well as the resulting net income or loss, form the operating budget. It should be noted that, when calculating the anticipated surplus or deficit, it is necessary to estimate the deductions in revenue from bad debts, courtesy discounts, contractual agreements, and free or charity care. These adjustments permit management to develop a more accurate estimate of (1) the anticipated net income or loss of the period; and (2) the net realizable cash value of outstanding receivables. As will be seen later, the net realizable cash value of the institution's outstanding receivables plays an important role in the development of the cash budget.

The capital budget consists of estimates of the costs and sources of funding associated with replacement, improvement, and additions to the physical plant that are expected during the budget period. The cost of the estimated requirements as well as the anticipated date of acquisition should be reported for each responsibility center. The combining of individual reports provides information on anticipated acquisitions, their timing, priorities, and feasibility of procurement.

A cash budget is simply a forecast of working capital needs and consists of beginning cash balances, total cash inflows, total cash available, total cash outflows, and the ending cash balance. The cash budget plays a significant role in monitoring the ability of the institution to honor obligations expected to mature during the period. When developing the cash budget, it is important to include the cash inflows management expects to receive from all third party payers and patients as well as receipts related to other operating and the nonoperating revenues. Adding the cash inflows to the beginning cash balance yields the available cash for the period that, in turn, can be applied against anticipated cash outflows. Thus, one of the basic purposes of the cash budget is to ensure that an adequate cash balance is available to satisfy the hospital's obligations.

## 13.2 ESTIMATION OF WORK LOAD

The following discussion assumes that management has developed a statement of the hospital's operating environment, goals, and policies as well as a statement of assumptions and their operational implications. It also assumes that these factors have been reflected in the goals and objectives of each responsibility center. The purpose here, then, is to explore the traditional method of developing an operational plan and the translation of that plan into financial terms.

As mentioned, estimates of the work load or the anticipated volume provide the basis for developing the operational plan. The method by which any particular hospital projects its work load will vary from institution to institution. The basic approach that should be followed is to identify a model or technique that consistently generates accurate estimates. Using historical data, alternate techniques may be used to estimate work load requirements that, when compared with the actual volume, provide the basis for evaluating the various approaches. Since the technique for estimating the work load for the budget period is likely to vary from hospital to hospital, this discussion is designed to illustrate several approaches for developing volume projections.

Table 13-1 lists the work load elements that must be estimated for several major responsibility centers, and one or more forecasting techniques. The expected number of days of care plays a critical role in deriving most of the work load estimates and, as a result, the patient day forecast is one of the most important projections management can develop. A moving average coupled with the geometric mean, exponential smoothing, and regression analysis are identified as the principle techniques by which these forecasts may be developed.

### 13.2.1 The Moving Average and the Geometric Mean

For illustration, suppose that, on the basis of historical records, the hospital can generate the data shown in Table 13-2. The moving average is simply a technique for describing the overall movement in the use of care during previous time periods. Once the moving average has been constructed, the geometric mean may be used to estimate the average rate of change in the number of days of care provided previously; this, in turn, can be used to project the number of days of care that the hospital expects to provide during the budget period.

**Table 13-1** Work Load Elements and Methods of Work Load Forecasting

| Responsibility Center | Work Load Element | Technique |
|---|---|---|
| Hospital | Patient days | Geometric mean, exponential smoothing, regression analysis |
| Nursing unit | Patient days by month | Geometric mean or exponential smoothing |
| Dietary | Meals/month | Meals/patient day × number of patient days/month |
| Laundry | Pounds of laundry/month | Pounds/patient day × number of patient days/month |
| Radiology | Number of exposures/ month | Number of exposures/patient day × number of patient days/month |
| Laboratory | Number of procedures by major type of procedure/ month | Number of procedures by type of procedure/patient day × number of days per month |
| Housekeeping | Volume | Square feet |
| Outpatient visits | Number of visits/month | Moving average or regression analysis |

**Table 13-2** Hypothetical Number of Days of Care by Year and by Month

| | Year | | | | | | | |
|---|---|---|---|---|---|---|---|---|
| Month | 1973 | 1974 | 1975 | 1976 | 1977 | 1978 | 1979 | 1980 |
| January | 1,350 | 1,470 | 1,700 | 2,000 | 2,200 | 2,400 | 2,600 | 2,800 |
| February | 1,290 | 1,490 | 1,500 | 1,600 | 1,500 | 1,800 | 1,900 | 2,000 |
| March | 1,600 | 1,700 | 1,800 | 1,900 | 2,000 | 2,100 | 2,000 | 2,200 |
| April | 1,500 | 1,600 | 1,750 | 1,800 | 1,900 | 1,800 | 2,100 | 2,300 |
| May | 1,550 | 1,750 | 1,850 | 1,970 | 2,100 | 2,200 | 2,250 | 2,400 |
| June | 1,000 | 900 | 1,100 | 1,250 | 1,300 | 1,750 | 1,800 | 1,600 |
| July | 950 | 1,100 | 1,000 | 1,150 | 1,200 | 1,300 | 1,350 | 1,400 |
| August | 800 | 850 | 900 | 1,000 | 1,100 | 1,250 | 1,300 | 1,350 |
| September | 600 | 700 | 750 | 792 | 863 | 900 | 970 | 1,000 |
| October | 1,260 | 1,340 | 1,370 | 1,400 | 1,452 | 1,510 | 1,610 | 1,630 |
| November | 1,550 | 1,600 | 1,612 | 1,630 | 1,652 | 1,700 | 1,830 | 1,875 |
| December | 980 | 1,100 | 1,250 | 1,300 | 1,342 | 1,450 | 1,470 | 1,480 |
| Total | 14,430 | 15,600 | 16,582 | 17,792 | 18,609 | 20,160 | 21,180 | 22,035 |

A moving average is simply an artificial time series in which the value of each period is replaced by the mean of itself and the values corresponding to preceding and succeeding periods. For example, in estimating a three-point moving average, each of the values is replaced by the mean of itself and those of the immediately succeeding and preceding periods. Thus, if $x_t$ corresponds to the number of days of care rendered in period $t$, a three-point moving average for $n$ periods is computed by

$$\bar{x}_t = \frac{x_{t-1} + x_t + x_{t+1}}{3}$$

$$\bar{x}_{t+1} = \frac{x_t + x_{t+1} + x_{t+2}}{3}$$

.

.

.

$$\bar{x}_{t+n-1} = \frac{x_{t+n-2} + x_{t+n-1} + x_{t+n}}{3}$$

In a three-point moving average, no mean is calculated for the first and last years. Similarly, in a five-point moving average no mean is computed for the first and last two periods.

Returning to the example, consider first the construction of a three-point moving average for the total number of days of care provided annually during the eight-year period. The moving average for 1974 is computed by

$$\bar{x}_{1974} = \frac{14{,}430 + 15{,}600 + 16{,}582}{3} = \frac{46{,}612}{3} = 15{,}537$$

In similar fashion, the three-point moving average for 1975 is given by

$$\bar{x}_{1975} = \frac{15{,}600 + 16{,}582 + 17{,}792}{3} = \frac{49{,}974}{3} = 16{,}658$$

Similar values for the remaining years of the period are presented in Table 13-3.

The table also includes the percentage changes in the three-point moving averages. The values in the second column of the table may be computed by

$$1 + \%\Delta x = 1 + \frac{\bar{x}_{t+1} - \bar{x}_t}{\bar{x}_t} \tag{13.1}$$

To illustrate the use of Equation 13.1, consider the percentage change in the three-point moving average between 1975 and 1976. In this case, we find that

$$1 + \%\Delta x = 1 + \frac{17{,}661 - 16{,}658}{16{,}658} = 1.060$$

**Table 13-3**  Three-Point Moving Average of Total Days of Care and Percent Change in Moving Average for the Period 1970–1977

| Year | Three-Point Moving Average (1) | | Rates of Change (2) |
|---|---|---|---|
| 1973 | | | |
| 1974 | 15,537 | | |
| 1975 | 16,658 | > | 1.072 |
| 1976 | 17,661 | > | 1.060 |
| 1977 | 18,854 | > | 1.067 |
| 1978 | 19,983 | > | 1.059 |
| 1979 | 21,125 | > | 1.057 |
| 1980 | | | |

The other values in the second column of Table 13-3 were calculated in a similar fashion.

The growth of total patient days varies from year to year, and it might be asked which of these rates of change should be used in predicting the total number of days of patient care for the budget period. One solution is to compute the average rate of change for the entire period, which in turn may be used in forecasting the total patient days for the coming year. Such an average is given by the geometric mean. Given a set of numbers $y_1, y_2, \cdots, y_n$, the geometric mean may be found by

$$\log GM = \frac{\sum_{i=1}^{n} \log y_i}{n} \qquad (13.2)$$

which yields the logarithm of the geometric mean. The antilogarithm of log $GM$ gives the geometric mean. In terms of this example, we simply multiply each of the values in the second column of Table 13-3 by 100 and round for ease of calculation. The corresponding logarithms are available in any standard statistical text and are found to be

$$\log 107 = 2.0294$$
$$\log 106 = 2.0253$$
$$\log 107 = 2.0394$$
$$\log 106 = 2.0253$$
$$\log 106 = \underline{2.0253}$$
$$\sum_{i=1}^{n} \log y_i = 10.1347$$

Substituting into Equation 13.2 we find

$$\log GM = \frac{10.1347}{5} = 2.02694$$

The antilogarithm of 2.02694 is approximately 106.4. The results of these calculations indicate that the total number of patient days has increased on the average, by 6.4 percent per year for the last eight years.

At this point, management must evaluate the extent to which it is reasonable to expect the total number of patient days to increase by 6.4 percent during the budget period. This evaluation might involve several factors:

1. the most recent direction of change in the percentage increase or decrease in the patient load;
2. the capacity of the institution to accommodate the increase;
3. changes in medical technology that may alter admission rates as well as length of stay;
4. changes in the size and demographic characteristics of the population served that might alter admission rates and length of stay;
5. changes in the characteristics and components of the health delivery system (e.g., the construction of a new hospital or the closing of an old one);
6. changes in the socioeconomic and political environment.

Clearly, the list is not exhaustive but does indicate the types of factors that should be examined in evaluating the extent to which previous trends are likely to continue during the budget period. Obviously, such an evaluation may require an adjustment in the computed rate of growth so as to reflect accurately the operating environment expected during the budget period.

However, if it is found that the average rate of growth in patient days is expected to continue throughout the budget period, management need only apply the average rate of change to the current number of days of care to arrive at the expected number of patient days that will be provided during the budget period. Thus, the expected number of days of care, $E(PD)$, is given by

$$E(PD) = PD_t \cdot AGR$$

where $PD_t$ is the number of days of care provided during the current period and $AGR$ is the average growth rate. In terms of our example, we find that

$$E(PD) = 22{,}035 \times 1.064 \cong 23{,}445$$

days of care.

Although this analysis has been developed in terms of the total number of patient days of care per year, it is equally appropriate for estimating the number of days of care that will be provided each month of the budget period. In terms of our example, this analysis would simply be replicated for each of the rows in Table 13-2.

Once the patient day forecast has been completed, the estimates of the other elements of the hospital work load may be calculated. For example, consider the dietary department. As seen in Table 13-1, multiplying the number of meals per patient/day by the expected number of patient days results in an estimate of the number of meals likely to be planned, prepared, and served during the budget period. Similar techniques may be used for estimating the other elements of the hospital work load.

## 13.2.2  Exponential Smoothing

In recent years, increased effort has been devoted to the development of mechanical forecasting techniques that are easy to use and capable of providing projections on a routine and timely basis with a minimum of managerial attention. One of these methods is exponential smoothing.

When exponential smoothing techniques are used, the projection concerning the use of care during the planning period requires: (1) the forecast of use derived for the current period and (2) the extent to which the actual use of care during the current period has deviated from the forecast for this period. The basic forecasting formula for exponential smoothing can be expressed in the form

$$\begin{matrix} \text{New Forecast} \\ \text{of Use} \end{matrix} = \begin{matrix} \text{Current Forecast} \\ \text{of Use} \end{matrix} + \alpha \left( \begin{matrix} \text{Current} \\ \text{Use} \end{matrix} - \begin{matrix} \text{Current Forecast} \\ \text{of Use} \end{matrix} \right)$$

where $\alpha$ is a smoothing constant that lies between 0 and 1. Here, the term *new forecast of use* refers to the forecast developed for the planning period. The new forecast is simply the current forecast of use plus an adjustment based on some fraction, $\alpha$, of the error in the current projection.

To develop this technique more formally, we let $P$ represent the projection or forecast of use and $\mu$ the actual use of care. We also represent the current period by the subscript $t$; the preceding period by the subscript $t - 1$, and the period for which the forecast pertains by the subscript $t + 1$. Thus, $P_t$ corresponds to the forecast developed in period $t - 1$ and pertains to the current period, $P_{t+1}$ to the forecast in period $t$ for the period $t + 1$, $\mu_t$ to the use of service during the current period, and $\mu_{t+1}$ the use of care in period $t + 1$.

Using this notation, we may express the basic exponential smoothing formula as follows

$$P_{t+1} = P_t + \alpha(\mu_t - P_t) \tag{13.3}$$

After slight manipulation, Equation 13.3 may be expressed in the form

$$P_{t+1} = (1 - \alpha)P_t + \alpha\mu_t \tag{13.4}$$

The only information required to calculate $P_{t+1}$ is the current forecast, $P_t$, and the current use of care, which is symbolized by $\mu_t$. In turn, the calculation of the forecast for the period $t + 2$ requires the projection for the period $t + 1$ (i.e., $P_{t+1}$) and the use of service during the period $t + 1$ that is symbolized by the term $\mu_{t+1}$. Thus, we find that

$$P_{t+2} = (1 - \alpha)P_{t+1} + \alpha\mu_{t+1} \tag{13.5}$$

$$= (1 - \alpha)^2 P_t + (1 - \alpha)(\alpha)\mu_t + \alpha\mu_{t+1}$$

This forecast for the period $t + 2$ is a weighted average based on the actual use of service during previous periods. The data pertaining to the more distant past are assigned lower weights in exponential smoothing. This may be seen by observing that the term $(1 - \alpha)$ is a value between 0 and 1. As a result, the term $(1 - \alpha)^k$ becomes smaller and smaller as $k$ increases in value. The rate of decline in $(1 - \alpha)^k$ depends on the value assigned to $\alpha$. The higher the value of $\alpha$, the more rapid the decline in $(1 - \alpha)^k$, and vice versa. Stated another way, the higher the value of $\alpha$, the more the forecast depends on the utilization experience in the most recent periods.

One of the major problems in exponential smoothing is to determine the value that should be assigned to $\alpha$. If $\alpha$ is too low, the forecasting method does not respond quickly to changes in use; if $\alpha$ is too high, the resulting forecast may be overly sensitive to erratic movements in use during more recent periods. As a practical matter, $\alpha$ may be assigned a value between .10 and .15 initially. Thereafter, its value may be adjusted to obtain more accurate projections.

To illustrate this technique, let us refer to Table 13-2, where 22,035 days of care were provided in 1980. Suppose that $P_{1980} = 21,000$ days of care. If we now let $\alpha = .15$, an application of Equation 13.3 suggests that

$$P_{1981} = P_{1980} + \alpha(\mu_{1980} - P_{1980})$$

$$= 21,000 + .15(22,035 - 21,000)$$

$$\cong 21,155$$

days of care. Similarly, if 25,000 days of care were provided in 1981, we find that

$$P_{1982} = 21,155 + .15(25,000 - 21,155)$$

$$\cong 21,732$$

days of care. This procedure may then be used when developing projections for subsequent periods.

### 13.2.3 Regression Analysis

Although the details of regression are not considered here, an indication of the basic approach and its usefulness in estimating the work load of the hospital is described briefly. Those interested in a technical discussion of regression analysis should consult the references at the end of this chapter.

The basic concept of multiple regression analysis is to produce a linear combination of independent variables that will correlate as highly as possible with the dependent variable. The general form of the linear combination is

$$y = b_0 + b_1 x_1 + b_2 x_2 + \cdots + b_n x_n + e \qquad (13.6)$$

where $y$ is the dependent variable, the $b$s are the regression coefficients, the $x$s are the independent variables and the $e$ is an error term. This linear combination may be used to predict the dependent variable in terms of known or assumed values of the independent variables. The difference between the value of the dependent variable and the value predicted by the regression equation is referred to as a residual, which is measured by $e$ in Equation 13.6.

In estimating the work load of the hospital during the budget period, the number of patient days of care may be used as the dependent variable while factors that are expected, or have been found, to influence the number of days of care are incorporated as the independent variables of Equation 13.6. For example, it might be expected that the number of patient days would be influenced by

1. the incidence of disease or injury
2. changes in the size of the population served
3. changes in the demographic composition of the population served
4. changes in medical technology

Similar factors may then be made operational and incorporated as the independent variables of the equation. Once the relation between the dependent variable (patient days of care) and the independent variables (size of population served, etc.) has been estimated, values of the independent variables that are expected to prevail during the budget period may be substituted into the resulting regression equation. Management then may develop projections concerning the dependent variable, which is the work load for the hospital.

Although the advantages of regression analysis in estimating the hospital's work load are many, only a few are mentioned here. First, depending on the number of available observations, management may estimate the influence of a large number of factors on the work load, which permits evaluation of the activities of the institution in terms of the existing and expected operating environment. Second, regression analysis permits evaluation of the statistical significance of the relation between hospital activity and each of the independent variables while controlling the other factors in the analysis as well as the relative importance of each of the independent variables in determining hospital activity. Such an analysis identifies factors in which changes are likely to have considerable impact on the work load. Third, regression analysis permits the construction of confidence intervals for predicted values of the dependent variable. Management then can assert with a known and specified probability that the actual work load will lie in the range defined by the upper and lower limits of the confidence interval. Since the independent variables influence predictions concerning the dependent variable, management must ensure that the values of the set of independent variables have been estimated as accurately as possible.

## 13.3 EXPENSE BUDGET

Once the elements of the work load have been estimated, management must develop the details of the operating plan by which the expected output is to be produced. In the traditional approach to budgeting, the details of the operating plan are expressed in the expense budget, which consists of a salary and wage budget and a supply expense budget.

### 13.3.1 The Salary and Wage Budget

In the average hospital, salaries and wages represent more than 60 percent of the total expense budget. As a result, the salary and wage budget must be prepared with the utmost care and accuracy.

As was seen in Chapter 12, the development of the salary and wage budget consists of two steps. The first is to estimate the real resources required in producing the expected work load. In the case of the salary and wage budget, real resource requirements are expressed in terms of the number of staff hours of each type of labor that management estimates will be needed to produce the anticipated level of output. The second step is to translate the expected real resource requirements into monetary or financial terms. This is accomplished by the application of relevant factor prices to the estimated resource requirements.

The results of the first of these steps are presented in Table 13-4, where the estimated personnel requirements for only one unit of the hospital—the surgical nursing ward—are summarized. The process of estimating the number of staff hours of each type of labor required to produce the anticipated work load must be repeated in each of the other areas of activity. In developing the estimated resource requirements for the ward, it is assumed that the work load has been estimated using one of the techniques mentioned earlier. As a result, the objective of management is to estimate the number of hours of each type of labor required to produce that volume of service.

To assist management in estimating personnel requirements, each type of labor is given a code classification, which appears in the first column of the table. For example, code A might correspond to the floor supervisor of the unit, while code D may indicate a nurse's aide. Such a classification should pinpoint the skills and responsibilities of the individual occupying the position.

Suppose that the work load of this unit is expressed in terms of the total number of days of care it is expected to provide during each month and during the budget year. Management must estimate the staffing requirements for the year and for each month of the budget period to ensure that the requisite amount of labor is available to provide the corresponding amount of care. In terms of the example, the following assumptions can be made:

1. the normal work week of the hospital is 40 hours
2. each full-time employee is given a two-week paid vacation each year
3. each full-time employee is given six paid holidays each year

On the basis of these assumptions, a full-time employee is scheduled for 1,952 hours of work each year, calculated as follows:

| | | | |
|---|---|---|---|
| Total paid hours (including vacation time) | = | 40 hours/week × 52 | = 2,080 |
| Less  Holiday time: 6 days × 8 hours | = | | 48 |
| Vacation time: 2 weeks × 40 hours | = | | 80 |
| Total scheduled work time/employee/year | = | | 1,952 |

During this phase of the estimation process, it is necessary to consider changes in the complement of the unit as well as the number and type of hours required to compensate for the absence of personnel on holiday or vacation. As seen in the table, the work load of this unit is expected to require an additional 952 hours of type C labor for the year. It also is expected that the additional person will not be required until February, or month 2, of the budget year.

**Table 13-4** Estimated Personnel Requirements for Surgical Nursing Ward

| Code | Name | Total Scheduled Work Hours | Vacation Hours | Holiday Hours | Total Paid Hours | Scheduled Work Hours | | | | |
|---|---|---|---|---|---|---|---|---|---|---|
| | | | | | | *1* | *2* | *3* | *4* | *12* |
| A | J. Jones | 1,952 | 80 | 48 | 2,080 | 157 | 165 | 164 | 165 | 157 |
| B | K. Smith | 1,952 | 80 | 48 | 2,080 | 157 | 84 | 164 | 165 | 157 |
| B | S. Gable | 1,952 | 80 | 48 | 2,080 | 157 | 84 | 165 | 164 | 157 |
| C | T. Hagan | 1,952 | 80 | 48 | 2,080 | 157 | 164 | 165 | 164 | 91 |
| C | — | 952 | 40 | 48 | 1,040 | — | 97 | 98 | 97 | 157 |
| C | A. Hardy | 1,952 | 80 | 48 | 2,080 | 157 | 164 | 165 | 164 | 157 |
| D | J. Bane | 2,152 | 80 | 48 | 2,280 | 175 | 183 | 184 | 184 | 177 |
| | Totals | 12,864 | 520 | 336 | 13,720 | 960 | 941 | 1,105 | 1,103 | 1,053 |
| **Other:** | | | | | | | | | | |
| | Overtime hours | 200 | | | | 16 | 16 | 17 | 16 | 16 |
| | Vacation relief | 500 | | | | | 160 | | | |
| | Holiday relief | 150 | | | | 40 | | | | 48 |
| | On-call duty | 2,688 | | | | 224 | 224 | 224 | 224 | 224 |
| | Total other | 3,538 | | | | 280 | 400 | 241 | 240 | 288 |
| | Total Hours | 16,402 | | | | 1,240 | 1,341 | 1,346 | 1,343 | 1,341 |

The estimate of vacation and holiday relief also are incorporated into the unit's personnel requirements. Vacation and holiday relief should be estimated and recorded only for periods in which the expected level of activity cannot be maintained by rescheduling the present work force to compensate for absent staff members.

The final entries in the table that require elaboration are the premium pay hours and the on-call duty requirements. The premium pay hours are scheduled work time that exceeds the normal work week of the hospital and are therefore subject to extra remuneration—overtime. In many hospital units such as the operating room, the emergency room, and the surgical nursing ward, it is necessary to have one or more persons stand by and be available to return to duty in the event of an emergency. In terms of our example, it is assumed that stand-by personnel are required seven days each week for eight hours per day. Assuming a four-week month, the stand-by requirement per month is 224 hours or 2,688 hours of on-call duty services for the budget year.

The translation of the operating plan into financial or monetary terms is summarized in Table 13-5. Several aspects of this table deserve comment. One involves an estimate of the wage and salary expense for each employee during each month of the budget period as adjusted for increases in those payments expected during the budget period. The values in the "Current Rate" column represent the amount of the periodic payments made currently to each employee. The "Increase Effective Date" column indicates the first day of the month in which it is expected that wage or salary payments to the individual will change. For example, J. Jones is paid $1,850 per month but on 2/1/79, this is expected to increase by $100 per month. The total budgeted increase for the period is $1,100 ($100 per month × 11 months) and the total salary payment to Jones for the year is expected to be $23,300 ($1,850 for one month + $1,950 per month for 11 months).

The computation of expected wage payments to individuals paid on an hourly basis is somewhat more complicated. Consider, as an example, the expected wage payments to J. Bane, who is paid $10.00 per hour and has agreed to work an additional four hours per week for a total of 200 premium pay hours during the year. Moreover, Bane is entitled to six paid holidays and a two-week paid vacation per year.

In most hospitals, premium payments usually are made to individuals who are paid on an hourly basis and work a number of hours beyond the normal workweek. In such cases, the hospital usually pays time and a half for the extra hours. Thus, Bane's annual salary, including overtime, vacation, and holiday pay is computed as follows:

1. total number of hours paid at the normal rate for the year:
   Normal          40 hours × 52 weeks     = 2,080

**Table 13-5** Wage and Salary Budget for the Surgical Nursing Ward

| Code | Name | Number of Paid Hours | Current Rate | Increase Effective Date | Total | Month 1 | 2 | 3 | 4 | 12 | Total Budgeted Increase |
|---|---|---|---|---|---|---|---|---|---|---|---|
| A | J. Jones | 2,080 | $1,850/mo. | 2/19 | $23,300 | $1,850 | $1,950 | $1,950 | $1,950 | $1,950 | $1,100 |
| B | K. Smith | 2,080 | 1,200/mo. | 3/19 | 14,900 | 1,200 | 1,200 | 1,250 | 1,250 | 1,250 | 500 |
| B | S. Gable | 2,080 | 1,000/mo. | 7/19 | 12,300 | 1,000 | 1,000 | 1,000 | 1,000 | 1,050 | 300 |
| C | T. Hagan | 2,080 | 800/mo. | 6/19 | 9,950 | 800 | 800 | 800 | 800 | 850 | 350 |
| C | — | 1,040 | 700/mo. | 10/19 | 8,550 | — | 700 | 700 | 700 | 750 | 150 |
| C | A. Hardy | 2,080 | 600/mo. | 11/19 | 7,300 | 600 | 600 | 600 | 600 | 650 | 100 |
| D | J. Bane | 2,280 | 10.00/hr. | — | 22,800 | 1,894 | 1,894 | 1,904 | 1,904 | 1,894 | — |
| | Total | | | | 99,100 | 7,344 | 8,144 | 8,204 | 8,204 | 8,394 | 2,500 |
| **Other:** | | | | | | | | | | | |
| | Premium pay | | | | 1,000 | 80 | 80 | 85 | 80 | 80 | |
| | Vacation relief | | | | 3,100 | | 2,200 | | | | |
| | Holiday | | | | 425 | 120 | | | | 161 | |
| | On Call | | | | 18,816 | 1,568 | 1,568 | 1,568 | 1,568 | 1,568 | |
| | Total other | | | | 23,341 | 1,768 | 3,848 | 1,653 | 1,648 | 1,809 | |
| | Total nursing unit | | | | 122,441 | 9,112 | 11,992 | 9,857 | 9,852 | 10,203 | |

| Overtime | 4 hours × 50 weeks | = | 200 |
| --- | --- | --- | --- |
| Total hours paid at normal rate | | = | 2,280 |

2. wage payments calculated at normal rate:
   2,280 × $10.00 = $22,800/year
3. premium pay expected during year:
   200 hours × 1/2($10.00) = $1,000/year
4. total expected wage payments to Bane for year:
   $22,800 + $1,000 = $23,800

In estimating the labor expenses for the department for each month, it is necessary to calculate the wage payments to Bane for each month during the budget period. Consider as an example the $1,894 payment expected during January, or the first month of the budget period. The expected payment to Bane is composed of three components: (1) payment for the number of hours actually worked; (2) a paid holiday; and (3) the amount of vacation pay earned during the month.

As seen in Table 13-4, Bane is scheduled for 175 hours of work during the first month of the coming year. The payment corresponding to the number of hours actually worked is:

$$175 \text{ hours} \times \$10.00 = \$1,750.00$$

During the first month, it is assumed that the employee is entitled to one paid holiday, which results in a payment of

$$8 \text{ hours} \times \$10.00 = \$80$$

Finally, during the year the individual earns vacation pay equal to $800 ($10.00 × 40 hours/week × 2 weeks). Since the vacation pay is earned over a 50-week period, $16 of vacation pay is earned each week and, assuming a four-week month, the person earns vacation pay of $64 per month. The regular pay expense associated with Bane during the first month is the sum of the three components, or

$$\$1,750 + \$80 + \$64 = \$1,894.00$$

The other entries of the table are calculated in a similar fashion.

Bane also is scheduled to work 200 overtime hours, of which 16 are scheduled for January—the first month of the budget period. The premium payment for 16 hours of overtime is

$$16 \times \$5.00 = \$80.00$$

Thus, the total expected wage expense associated with Bane for the first month, including regular and premium pay, is $1,894 + $80, or $1,974. The premium payments for each of the other months in the budget period are calculated in similar fashion.

A second major aspect of Table 13-5 involves translating the number of hours of holiday and vacation relief into financial or monetary terms. For example, consider the expected wage and salary payments required to obtain the additional staff needed to provide vacation relief. K. Smith and S. Gable occupy a category B position and are scheduled to take their vacations in February, the second month of the budget period. As Table 13-5 indicates, it is expected that a salary expense of $2,200 will be required to obtain the 160 hours of vacation relief to replace these two individuals. Similar estimates must be made for the other months in which it is expected that vacation and holiday relief will be required to sustain the expected level of activity.

As noted earlier, it may be necessary for one or more individuals to stand by on call and be available for a return to duty in the event of an emergency. Hospitals generally are required to remunerate employees even though an emergency does not require their services. The cost of on-call personnel is calculated by multiplying the wage rate by the number of hours required each month. In Table 13-5, it is assumed that the wage rate is $7.00 per hour.

Summing over all rows of the table results in a value that reflects the expected wage and salary payments for the year and for each month during the budget period. Summing over all months results in anticipated expenditures for the budget year.

The detailed wage and salary budgets for all departments and all divisions are then summarized and totaled to provide the compensation budget for the hospital. The detailed worksheets, however, should be retained and presented with the tentative wage and salary budget to the administrator or the budget officer.

## 13.3.2 Supply Expense Budget

Costs of consumable supplies usually are more responsive to quantitative demands for service than are wages and salary. This is true to a large extent in departments or units that provide services directly to the patient and to a lesser extent in departments that offer general support services. In the laboratory, for example, consumable supplies should vary proportionally with the number of laboratory tests performed; these, in turn, should relate to the number of patient days of care. On the other hand, supplies used by the housekeeping department in maintaining a fixed number of square feet would not be expected to increase or decrease in response to a gain or decline in the number of patient days. Thus, for departments whose output is provided directly to patients, the changes in the cost of service may be estimated by assuming that the number of procedures per patient day, the real resource requirements per unit of service, and factor prices will remain constant. Under these assumptions, the change in cost attributable to changes in volume from one year to the next is given by

$$C_{t+1} = \frac{C_t}{S_t} \times \frac{S_t}{PD_t} \times PD_t \times (1 + \%\Delta PD) \tag{13.7}$$

where

$C_{t+1}$ = the expected costs of the unit during the budget period
$C_t$ = the current costs of the department
$S_t$ = the number of services provided during the current period and
$PD_t$ = the number of patient days provided during the current period

Observe that $C_t$ is nothing more than the sum of the products of the physical quantities of resources used in production and their respective factor prices, which is given by

$$C_t = \sum_{i=1}^{i=y} P_i Q_i \qquad (i = 1, 2, \cdots, y) \tag{13.8}$$

where

$P_i$ = the price of resource $i$
$Q_i$ = the quantity of resource $i$

If resource prices remain constant from one year to the next, the use of the ratio $C_t/S_t$ in calculating the expected supply cost for the budget period is tantamount to assuming that the relation between factor inputs and the corresponding output is invariant. A similar assumption is involved when the ratio $S_t/PD_t$ is used in estimating the supply cost for the budget period. If these assumptions are valid, the expected supply cost of the unit for the budget period reduces to:

$$C_{t+1} = C_t(1 + \%\Delta PD) \tag{13.9}$$

The last step in calculating the expected supply expenses is to adjust $C_{t+1}$ to reflect anticipated changes in resource or factor prices.

These assumptions are invoked in estimating the supply expense budget of the surgical nursing ward shown in Table 13-6. The first row of the table corresponds to the supply costs incurred by this center during the current year and during each month of the current period. Thus, the values in the first row correspond to the argument $C_t$ in Equation 13.9. Each of these values is adjusted to reflect the percent change in the number of patient days of care expected

**Table 13-6** Supply Expense Budget—Surgical Nursing Ward

| Component | Total | | | | Month | | |
|---|---|---|---|---|---|---|---|
| | | 1 | 2 | 3 | 4 | 11 | 12 |
| $C_t$ | 40,859 | 3,269 | 3,300 | 2,800 | 3,200 | 4,542 | 5,000 |
| % Δ in *PD* | 6% | 6% | 10% | 4% | 2% | 6% | 8% |
| $C_{t+1}$ | 43,310 | 3,465 | 3,630 | 2,912 | 3,264 | 4,815 | 5,400 |
| % Δ in $P_i$ | 10% | 10% | 10% | 10% | 10% | 10% | 10% |
| Adjusted $C_{t+1}$ | 47,641 | 3,812 | 3,993 | 3,203 | 3,590 | 5,296 | 5,940 |

during the budget period. For example, if the number of days of care is expected to increase by 6 percent during the first month of the budget period, the unadjusted supply expense expected in that month is found by

$$\$3,269(1 + .06) = \$3,465$$

Each of the values in the $C_{t+1}$ row was calculated in a similar fashion.

The second step in the table is to adjust $C_{t+1}$ for changes in factor prices expected during the budget year. It is assumed that, on the average, prices will increase by 10 percent during the year. As an example, the adjusted supply expense for the first month of the budget period is given by

$$\$3,465(1 + .10) \cong \$3,812$$

where .10 is the expected price increase. A similar adjustment is made for each of the other expense projections.

Under the traditional approach to budgeting, a similar technique may be used in estimating the supply budget for each of the other units providing direct patient services. Assuming no change in the level of activity associated with units providing indirect services, the current level of expenditure is simply adjusted to reflect price changes in the supplies used in each area of activity.

Summarizing and totaling the supply budgets of each unit and each division generates the supply expense budget of the hospital. Combining the wage and salary budget with the supply budget results in the overall expense budget for the hospital.

## 13.4 THE REVENUE BUDGET

As mentioned, the second major element of the operating budget depicts the revenue the hospital expects to earn during the period involved. If management is to ensure the financial viability of the hospital, the revenues earned must be equal to or greater than the costs incurred during the period. As a consequence, the revenue budget must be developed with extreme care to ensure that *all* of the costs expected during the budget period will be returned to the hospital in the form of revenue.

In the case of a commercial company that produces or sells a single commodity, total revenue is calculated by multiplying the price at which the product sells by the quantity sold. Thus, total revenue, $TR$, is defined by

$$TR = P \cdot Q$$

where $P$ is the product price and $Q$ is the quantity sold.

The hospital, however, produces a wide variety of products or services and the calculation of its total revenue should reflect the heterogeneous nature of its output. Thus, the hospital's total revenue is defined as the sum of the products between the quantities of each identifiable output or service produced and a corresponding charge or price. Thus, the total revenue of the hospital may be defined as

$$TR = \sum_{i=1}^{n} F_i V_i \qquad (i = 1, \cdots, n) \qquad \textbf{(13.10)}$$

where

$F_i$ = the price of service $i$
$V_i$ = the volume of service $i$

In terms of developing the revenue budget, the $F_i'$s are multiplied by the number of each service *expected* to be produced during the budget period. Thus, the expected total revenue, $E(TR)$, is given by

$$E(TR) = \sum_{i=1}^{n} F_i E(V_i) \qquad (i = 1, \cdots, n) \qquad \textbf{(13.11)}$$

where $E(V_i)$ corresponds to the volume of service expected during the budget period. Obviously, the argument $E(V_i)$ is the expected work load corresponding to service or output $i$. Since this already has been computed by one of the methods mentioned earlier, the primary task of management in deriving the revenue budget is to revise or establish the prices or charges that comprise the hospital's fee schedule.

In dealing with the rate structure, hospital management must ensure that all costs are reflected in the prices charged. The *full costs* of a given revenue-generating center might be defined as the sum of: (1) direct production costs, (2) internal indirect costs, (3) an equitable share of external indirect costs, and (4) an equitable share of the unassigned cost, which includes a provision for bad debts, courtesy discounts, and contractual adjustments.

The production costs refer to expenditure items incurred by the direct involvement of labor, consumable supplies, and capital equipment in providing the services for which the revenue-generating center is responsible. Conversely, the internal indirect costs are expenditure items that are assigned to the revenue center but are not traceable to direct patient care. Examples of internal indirect costs are the salaries of department heads and supervisors. The sum of the direct and internal indirect costs represents the costs assigned to the revenue-generating center.

External indirect costs refer to expenditures associated with general support services such as those provided by the laundry, housekeeping, and plant maintenance departments. The sum of the direct production costs and an equitable share of the indirect costs might be referred to as the basic production costs of the revenue-generating center. When determining these basic production costs, management might use one of the cost-finding techniques described earlier.

Fees charged for the services of the revenue-generating center also must reflect an equitable share of the hospital's unassigned cost. This cost component includes such items as heat, light, and power; plant and equipment needs; working capital needs; and expenses that are purely financial in nature.

The inclusion of working capital and plant needs in the full cost of operating the revenue-generating center is necessary to maintain the productive capability of the institution. In particular, the basic production costs usually are based, in part, on the historical expense of acquiring plant and equipment. Management also should include a return on investment when revising or prospectively developing the fee schedule. The return on investment should at least compensate the hospital for differences between the historical and the replacement costs of plant and equipment.

The full costs of operating the revenue-generating center, and hence the fee schedule, also must reflect a set of purely financial expenses. That the hospital is not likely to receive full payment on all charges is well known. For example, the presence of third party payers has not completely eliminated bad debts, free or charity care, and courtesy discounts. Of particular importance are the contractual allowances that are granted to third party payers in the United States and, to a lesser extent, in Canada. Since the provision of service to insured patients reduces a hospital's collection costs and bad debt expenses, third party payers demand and receive a contractual allowance that permits the purchase of care at a price that is less than the full cost of service. In this case, however, contractual allowances represent a real cost that must be recovered to preserve the hospital's financial viability.

Viewing the development of the rate structure in terms of the full costs of operation is of value from a theoretical perspective and can increase understanding of how to establish charges used in developing the revenue budget. The discussion turns next to how such charges should be estimated and used in estimating the revenues that management expects to earn during the budget period.

Services that earn revenue for the hospital may be divided into four categories: (1) standardized direct patient services, (2) stay-specific services, (3) services measurable in terms of hours of use, and (4) services related to the performance of a merchandising function. The methods of estimating the revenues resulting from each of the four types of services are described next.

## 13.4.1 Standardized Services

Several units of the hospital such as the laboratory and the radiology department produce more or less standardized services. The estimation of the revenue from such activities should involve the average cost per weighted procedure or service produced by the unit. When estimating this cost, it is necessary to assign a value to each service provided by the center that reflects the time, resources, and skills required in producing that service relative to some other one that is used as a basis of comparison.

The next step is to multiply the unit weight of each service by the number of services expected to be produced during the planning period. The multiplication results in the total number of weighted units. Next, the anticipated full costs of the revenue-generating center are divided by the total number of weighted units, resulting in an estimate of the charge per weighted unit. Based on these calculations, the charge per service is determined by multiplying the charge per weighted unit by the relative value of the service.

To illustrate the technique, assume that we wish to estimate the revenue generated by providing laboratory services next year. Suppose further that the laboratory services consist of urinalyses ($UA$), blood chemistry examinations ($BC$), pathological examinations ($P$), hematological examinations ($H$), and serological examinations ($S$). Also assume that the anticipated full costs of this unit for the next year are \$720,000 and that the corresponding projection concerning the volume of each of these services is as follows:

| Service | Expected Rate of Production |
|---------|-----------------------------|
| UA | 60,000 |
| BC | 20,000 |
| P | 40,000 |
| H | 10,000 |
| S | 20,000 |

Finally, assume that the hospital assigns the following relative weights to each of the services:

| Service | Relative Weight |
|---------|-----------------|
| UA | .5 |
| BC | 1.0 |
| P | 1.5 |
| H | 2.0 |
| S | 2.5 |

Blood chemistry examinations are assigned a unit weight of 1.0; this procedure therefore represents the service to which all others are compared. For example, urinalyses are assigned the relative weight of .5, which implies that providing this procedure requires half of the resources needed for one blood chemistry examination.

The total number of weighted units then is calculated by multiplying the expected annual rate of producing each service by its relative weight:

| Service | Relative Weight | × | Expected Rate of Production | = | Weighted Rate of Production |
|---------|-----------------|---|------------------------------|---|------------------------------|
| UA | .5 | | 60,000 | | 30,000 |
| BC | 1.0 | | 20,000 | | 20,000 |
| P | 1.5 | | 40,000 | | 60,000 |
| H | 2.0 | | 10,000 | | 20,000 |
| S | 2.5 | | 20,000 | | 50,000 |
| | | | Total number of weighted units | = | 180,000 |

Once the total number of weighted units has been computed, the cost or charge per weighted unit is derived by dividing the full costs of $720,000 by the number of weighted units. Thus, the charge per weighted unit, $CWU$, is given by

$$CWU = \frac{\$720,000}{180,000} = \$4/\text{Weighted unit} \qquad (13.12)$$

The charge per service is derived by multiplying the charge per weighted unit by the relative weight of each service:

| Service | Relative Weight | Charge/ Weighted Unit | Charge/ Service |
|---------|-----------------|------------------------|-----------------|
| UA | .5 | $4 | $2 |
| BC | 1.0 | 4 | 4 |
| P | 1.5 | 4 | 6 |
| H | 2.0 | 4 | 8 |
| S | 2.5 | 4 | 10 |

On the basis of these calculations, the total revenue expected next year by providing laboratory services may be estimated as follows:

| Service | Projected Volume of Service | × | Prospective Fee Schedule | = | Revenue Budget |
|---------|------------|---|----------|---|----------------|
| UA | 60,000 | | $2 | | $120,000 |
| BC | 20,000 | | 4 | | 80,000 |
| P | 40,000 | | 6 | | 240,000 |
| H | 10,000 | | 8 | | 80,000 |
| S | 20,000 | | 10 | | 200,000 |
| | | | | Total | 720,000 |

The expected revenues of the department are just equal to the anticipated full costs of $720,000. In such a situation, the laboratory department is said to break even since neither losses nor economic profits are anticipated. The prospective fee schedule also should be combined with projections of the monthly cost of providing laboratory service to develop a monthly revenue budget for this component of hospital activity.

It should be noted that several relative value scales have been developed for laboratory, pathological, and radiological services. Before using existing schedules as the basis for developing the rate structure, management must examine the extent to which the schedule reflects the hospital's cost structure. Failing to validate an existing relative value schedule could result in the development of an erroneous fee schedule and an inaccurate revenue budget.

### 13.4.2 Stay-Specific Services

Stay-specific services may be defined as those that depend only on the number of days of care provided during a given period. When estimating the income generated by providing stay-specific services, it is convenient to consider the revenue earned from a day of care in (1) a ward, (2) a semiprivate room, (3) a private room. In Canadian hospitals, it also is necessary to estimate the revenues associated with authorized charges.

For illustration, assume that management uses one of the techniques described earlier to develop the projections of the annual number of days of care by type of accommodation that are presented below. The relative values of 1.0, 1.5, and 2.0 are assigned to a day of care in a ward, semiprivate accommodation, and a private room, respectively.

| Factors | Type of Facility | | | Total |
|---|---|---|---|---|
| | Ward | Semiprivate | Private | |
| Expected days | 60,000 | 6,000 | 4,000 | 70,000 |
| Relative value | 1.0 | 1.5 | 2.0 | |
| Total weighted units | 60,000 | 9,000 | 8,000 | 77,000 |

Once the expected number of patient days of care has been estimated, the next step is to determine the charges assessed for occupancy in a ward (the standard ward rate) and for a private or semiprivate accommodation (differential charges). In turn, these rates are used to derive the revenue budget for this component of hospital activity. The technique by which these charges may be computed is similar to the method used in deriving the rate schedule for the set of standardized services.

To determine the cost per weighted unit, suppose the full costs of providing the number of days of care that have been estimated and classified are as follows:

1. The costs to be apportioned on the basis of the expected number of un-weighted days of care are $8,400,000. This estimate represents the cost elements that are applied more or less uniformly to all patients and includes expenditures associated with dietary services, nursing care, medical records, etc.
2. The costs to be apportioned on the basis of unit values are $770,000. This amount corresponds to cost elements that cannot or should not be allocated on the basis of unweighted patient days but that reflect intrinsic differences that exist among the three types of accommodations. Examples of cost elements that should be apportioned on the basis of unit values are house-keeping, plant operations, and estimates of bad debt expenses.

On the basis of these estimates, the component of charges based on the number of unweighted patient days is given by

$$PDC = \frac{\text{Costs to be allocated on the basis of patient days}}{\text{Expected number of days}} \qquad \textbf{(13.13)}$$

where *PDC* corresponds to the portion of the daily room charge that is based on the number of unweighted days of care. In terms of our example, this portion of the daily room charge is computed as follows:

$$PDC = \frac{8,400,000}{70,000} = \$120$$

Similar to the discussion in Section 13.4.1, we find that

$$UVC = \frac{\text{Costs to be allocated on basis of unit values}}{\text{Total weighted units}} \qquad \textbf{(13.14)}$$

where $UVC$ represents the unit value charge. In terms of our example, $UVC$ is found to be

$$UVC = \frac{770,000}{77,000} = \$10/\text{unit value}$$

The weighted charge per unit is derived by multiplying the relative value of each type facility by the unit value charge:

| Type of Facility | Relative Value | × | Unit Value Charge | = | Weighted Charge/Unit |
|---|---|---|---|---|---|
| Ward | 1.0 | | $10 | | $10 |
| Semiprivate | 1.5 | | 10 | | 15 |
| Private | 2.0 | | 10 | | 20 |

The daily charge for each of the facilities is found by simply adding the patient day charge and the weighted charge per unit:

| Type of Facility | Patient Day Charge | + | Weighted Charge per Unit | = | Charge/ Day |
|---|---|---|---|---|---|
| Ward | $120 | + | $10 | = | $130 |
| Semiprivate | 120 | + | 15 | = | 135 |
| Private | 120 | + | 20 | = | 140 |

The ward rate or the charge assessed for the occupancy of a standard ward accommodation thus is $130. The differential for occupying a semiprivate room is $5 per day ($135 − $130) while the differential for occupying a private room is $10 per day ($140 − $130).

| Type of Facility | Projected Volume of Service | Charge/ Day | Projected Revenue |
|---|---|---|---|
| Ward | 60,000 | 130 | $7,800,000 |
| Semiprivate | 6,000 | 135 | 810,000 |
| Private | 4,000 | 140 | 560,000 |
| Total | | | 9,170,000 |

On the basis of these calculations, we may develop projections concerning the revenue generated by providing stay-specific services during the budget period. The projected revenues of $9,170,000 are just equal to the expected full costs of providing stay-specific services (i.e., $8,400,000 + $770,000). Consequently, neither net losses nor economic profits are anticipated, which implies that the institution expects to break even when providing this component of care. As discussed earlier, management should combine the prospective charge per day and monthly estimates of the days of care by type of accommodation to develop a revenue budget for each month of the budget period.

### 13.4.3 Services Measured by Hours of Use

Several hospital units produce services that are measurable in terms of the annual or monthly number of hours of use—anesthesiology, physiotherapy, and the operating room. When developing the revenue budget for these and other departments with measurable output, the fee schedule should reflect either the cost per hour of use or per staff hour of use.

As an example, consider the operating room, for which the expected full costs amount to $420,000. Suppose also that the anticipated annual use of these facilities is 6,000 hours and that, on the average, five persons are required to perform each operative procedure. On the basis of these data, the prospective hourly rate for each procedure involving five staff persons is given by

$$\text{Rate/Hour} = \frac{\text{Economic Cost}}{\text{Hours of Use}} = \frac{\$420,000}{6,000} = \$70 \qquad \textbf{(13.15)}$$

Thus, for each procedure involving five staff persons, the hospital should charge a fee of $70 per hour of use.

Obviously, not all operative procedures will involve five staff people. As a result, it is necessary to calculate a rate or charge per staff hour of operating room use. The total number of such hours is given by multiplying the average number of staff persons per procedure by the projected number of hours of use (i.e., $5 \times 6,000 = 30,000$ staff hours). The prospective charge per hour is obtained by dividing anticipated full costs ($420,000) by the total number of staff hours (30,000). In the example, the charge per staff hour is found to be $14 and an operation that is expected to last two hours and involve four persons would generate $112 in revenue (8 staff hours $\times$ $14/staff hour). Once the hourly rates have been obtained, the revenue budget corresponding to the set of services measured by hours of use is obtained by multiplying the hourly charge by the expected hours of use during the year and each month of the budget period.

### 13.4.4 Merchandising Function

Several centers such as the pharmacy perform a merchandising function. The revenues generated by these units should be determined in terms of a surcharge on the goods they supply. Centers that handle or prepare goods for final sale or distribution should establish prospective charges and revenue budgets on the basis of the cost of the good plus a surcharge that reflects the costs of handling and processing.

As an example, consider the pharmacy for which the following information is available:

$$\frac{\text{Anticipated}}{\text{Full Costs}} = \$90,000$$

$$\text{Cost of Drugs} = \$60,000$$

In computing the markup on these drugs, the total surcharge is calculated by subtracting the cost of drugs from the expected full costs. Thus,

$$\text{Total Surcharge} = \text{Full Costs} - \text{Cost of Drugs}$$

$$= \$90,000 - \$60,000$$

$$= \$30,000$$

Once the total surcharge has been determined, the percent markup is calculated by

$$\text{\% Markup} = \frac{\text{Total Surcharge}}{\text{Cost of Drugs}} = \frac{\$30,000}{\$60,000} = .50 \qquad \textbf{(13.16)}$$

The surcharge for a given prescription is then given by

$$\text{Surcharge} = (\text{\% Markup})(\text{Cost of Drug})$$

As an example, consider a drug costing $12. In this case, the surcharge is

$$\text{Surcharge} = .5 \times \$12 = \$6.00$$

and the revenue generated by filling this prescription is the sum of the surcharge ($6) and the cost of the drug ($12). In general, the revenue from performing the merchandising function is the sum of the surcharge, as calculated above, and the cost of the goods or merchandise that are expected to be distributed during the planning period.

Once estimates of the revenue from standardized services, stay-specific services, those measured by hours of use, and those pertaining to the merchandising function have been calculated, they should be totaled and summarized in a single revenue budget. The total revenue for the period and the expected revenue for each month should be compared with corresponding expense estimates. The purpose of the comparison is to ensure that the total revenues of the period are at least equal to the full or economic costs of the period.

## 13.5 THE CAPITAL BUDGET

The primary purpose of the capital budget is to ensure that cash outlays for fixed assets are based on a carefully drawn program of development. As such, the capital budget is a detailed plan for replacements, betterments, and additions. Additions are represented by expenditures that will expand existing capacity, betterments are improvements to existing facilities, and replacements are substitutes for existing facilities that have become obsolete or worn out.

In developing the capital budget, replacements, betterments, and additions should be shown separately. If this procedure is followed, the analysis of which projects will be funded or which capital items will be acquired is facilitated. Since capital funding is limited in most hospitals, many requests for such expenditures cannot be approved. As a result, it is necessary to rank requests for these expenditures ordinally and thereby provide the basis for making decisions on allocating scarce capital funds.

All expenditures for plant expansion should be included in the capital budget. The number of items requested should be designated and an explanation or description of the proposed capital expenditure provided. Equipment, construction, and operating costs as well as the cash requirements for each month should be included for each group of priorities. Starting dates should be established for construction projects and purchasing dates for each budget item as well as completion dates for projects and receiving dates for equipment.

Since the usefulness of plant and equipment usually extends beyond the coming year, the capital budget for a given period should be integrated with a comprehensive long-range plan concerning the acquisition and disposal of capital equipment. Since such acquisitions can commit the community and the hospital to a specific course of action for many years, it also is desirable to develop a comprehensive three- to five-year capital budget that is integrated with the system by which health care is delivered to the population at risk. When developing such a budget it is necessary not only to coordinate the capital plans with the existing health care system but also to consider the impact of these plans on costs as well as on the fee schedule, revenues, and cash flows of the institution.

The integration of the hospital's capital plans with the health care delivery system can avoid duplication and reduce costs while ensuring that resources are available to meet the total health needs of the community. Increased attention has been devoted recently to the relationship between the rapid escalation in the costs of hospital care and capital expenditures in the industry. Most students of health care administration are aware of the increasing pressure to contain hospital costs by rationing capital acquisitions among institutions. These pressures have been reinforced by certificate-of-need legislation as well as the National Health Planning and Resources Development Act of 1974 (P.L. 93-641), which require more careful evaluation of capital acquisitions in the United States. Similarly, the rapid growth of District Health Councils in Canada is a reflection of governmental and public pressure to plan and provide integrated systems of health care delivery.

### 13.6 CASH BUDGET

As noted earlier, the cash budget is composed of a cash receipts budget, a cash disbursement budget, and a summary of the two. The availability of sufficient cash to meet current obligations is a requirement of sound fiscal practice and a budget program should be designed to ensure that funds will be available to meet obligations as they mature.

In addition, accurate estimates of cash requirements may reveal the availability of sizable sums of money that may be invested in short-term marketable securities and thereby earn investment income for the hospital. On the other hand, such an analysis also may reveal cash deficiencies that may necessitate negotiations for short-term loans to provide working capital or that may require the postponement of plant expansion plans.

### 13.6.1 Cash Receipts Budget

Essentially two methods of financing hospital care are used extensively in North America. The first is dominated by a series of nonrandom cash inflows intended to finance the use of care on a current basis. In the second, the hospital receives a retrospective reimbursement for services provided previously to patients. Under the second method, the cash inflows of a given period may be viewed as a random variable that, in large part, reflects payments on outstanding receivables. The cash receipts of the average hospital also are derived from returns on investments in marketable securities, donations, bequests, providing goods or service to a party other than the patient, and payments that occur more or less simultaneously with the provision of service.

For illustration, assume that a hypothetical hospital is guaranteed a nonrandom cash inflow of $500,000 per month that is intended to finance only a portion of its operations on a current basis. Assume also that the rest of the hospital's activities is financed on a retrospective basis through a series of random cash inflows from other third party payers and self-responsible patients. Obviously, if a hospital relies exclusively on the retrospective reimbursement method, the nonrandom cash is zero, and the lion's share of the cash it receives is from payments on outstanding receivables.

When the hospital receives a fixed or nonrandom cash payment each month and a series of more or less random cash receipts, some of the outstanding receivables will prove to be uncollectable. Thus, one of the first steps in preparing the cash receipts budget is to estimate the value of receivables that will prove to be uncollectable during the period. This may be accomplished by determining the percentage of the institution's receivables that have been written off previously as bad debts and applying this percentage to the projected value of receivables expected during the budget period. For obvious reasons, the cash receipts budget should be based on the value of expected receivables net of estimated bad debts.

A second important factor when developing the cash receipts budget involves the timing of the cash inflows that result from payments on outstanding receivables. It is reasonable to anticipate a lag between the recognition of income, as reflected in the revenue budget, and the resulting cash inflow. When estimating the timing of these cash receipts, management should examine the previous collection experience of the institution to ascertain the proportion of the time that payment is received within, say, 1–30, 31–60, 61–90, and 91–180 days after service has been provided. Other things held constant, these probabilities then may be used to estimate the timing of the cash receipts resulting from the expected net receivables of the budget period. For illustration, assume that, after an analysis of the collection experience of the hypothetical hospital, management determines that the probabilities of receiving cash 1–30, 31–60, and 61–90 days after revenue is earned are as follows:

| Time Lapse | Probability |
|---|---|
| 1–30 days | .60 |
| 31–60 days | .30 |
| 61–90 days | .10 |

Assume also that it is reasonable to apply these probabilities to the expected net receivables of the budgeting period.

The assumptions concerning the nonrandom cash receipt of $500,000 per month and the probabilities concerning the nonrandom component of the cash inflows of the hospital are incorporated in Table 13-7, where the cash receipts budget has been developed. The table shows that net receivables of $63,700 are expected to be generated during the first month of the year. Management expects

**Table 13-7** Cash Receipts Budget

| Source of Cash | Total | Month | | | | | |
| --- | --- | --- | --- | --- | --- | --- | --- |
| | | 1 | 2 | 3 | 4 | 5 | 12 |
| Nonrandom: | | | | | | | |
| Third party payer | $6,000,000 | $500,000 | $500,000 | $500,000 | $500,000 | $500,000 | $500,000 |
| Accounts Receivable beginning balance: | | | | | | | |
| 2 months old | 25,000 | 25,000 | | | | | |
| 1 month old | 24,000 | 18,000 | 6,000 | | | | |
| Current | 84,000 | 50,400 | 25,200 | 8,400 | | | |
| Budget period: | | | | | | | |
| 1st month | 63,700 | 38,220 | 19,110 | 6,370 | | | |
| 2nd month | 60,300 | | 36,180 | 18,090 | 6,030 | | |
| 3rd month | 65,000 | | | 39,000 | 19,500 | 6,500 | |
| ... | | | | | | | |
| 12th month | 62,300 | | | | | | |
| Subtotal | 6,774,000 | 631,620 | $586,490 | 571,860 | | | |
| Other | 31,000 | 3,000 | 7,000 | 1,000 | | | |
| Total cash | 6,805,000 | 634,620 | 593,490 | 572,860 | | | |

that 60 percent of this amount, or $38,220, will be collected during the first month of the budget period; 30 percent, or $19,110, in the second month; and 10 percent, or $6,370, in the third month. Similar estimates of the cash flows from net receivables in the remaining months of the budget period also are listed.

In addition to the nonrandom cash receipts from the private or public third party payer and the payments made in settlement of outstanding receivables, the hospital also receives cash inflows related to returns on investments, contributions, and so on. These cash receipts are grouped in the "other" category in the next to last line of the table. The bottom line is obtained by summing over all rows, which results in an estimate of the cash inflows expected during the year and during each month of the budget period.

## 13.6.2 Cash Disbursement Budget

The cash disbursement budget for the hypothetical hospital (Table 13-8) is based on three major cash outflows: (1) for wages and salaries, (2) for the acquisition of consumable supplies, and (3) for the acquisition of plant and equipment.

Since the first component—wage and salary expenses—has been prepared previously and pay periods are known with certainty, the amount of cash required for these items is determined easily. When deriving the cash outflows for the payment of wages and salaries, the accrued payroll at the beginning and at the end of each period as well as the amounts withheld from the payroll should be reflected in the cash disbursement budget.

The second major component of the cash disbursement budget involves the amount of cash required to acquire consumable supplies. Obviously, the magnitude of these cash disbursements are related closely to the supply expense budget and to the terms of trade credit offered by suppliers. Similar to the discussion of the cash outflows for the payment of wages and salaries, anticipated cash disbursements to acquire consumable supplies should reflect outstand-

**Table 13-8** Cash Disbursement Budget

| Item | Total | 1 | 2 | 3 | 4 | 12 |
|---|---|---|---|---|---|---|
| Wages and salaries | $3,391,000 | $296,350 | $261,750 | $261,750 | $300,950 | $290,000 |
| Supplies | 1,698,850 | 140,750 | 139,640 | 144,330 | 138,830 | 120,000 |
| Capital | 905,000 | 99,000 | 72,000 | 54,000 | 50,000 | 47,000 |
| Other | 570,000 | 19,790 | 47,500 | 47,500 | 47,500 | 47,500 |
| Total disbursements | 6,564,850 | 555,890 | 520,890 | 507,580 | 537,280 | 504,500 |

ing accounts payable at the beginning and end of the period as well as expected price discounts.

Finally, the cash disbursement budget must reflect outlays involving previous and planned capital acquisitions. The amount and maturity dates of long-term and short-term debt instruments for previous capital acquisitions are known with relative certainty. The magnitude and timing of cash disbursements to finance the planned acquisition of plant and equipment may be derived from the capital budget. In this case, the amount and timing of cash outlays are related to the outright purchases of equipment planned during the budget period. In addition, the planned acquisition of plant and equipment may require the issuance of several debt instruments that are expected to mature during the budget period. Obviously, the liquidation of such a liability also must be reflected in the hospital's cash disbursement budget.

### 13.6.3 Summary of Cash Receipts and Disbursements

The cash receipts and cash disbursements budgets provide the basis for projecting the cash position of the hospital during each month of the budget period. Table 13-9 is a summary of anticipated cash receipts, cash disbursements, and ending cash balances for the budget period and each month of the coming year. In this table, the sum of the beginning cash balance and the cash receipts of the period represents the amount of cash available. When the estimated cash disbursements are subtracted from the amount of cash available to the hospital, the end-of-period cash balance is obtained. The ending cash balance of one period is the beginning cash balance of the next.

**Table 13-9** Summary of Cash Receipts and Cash Disbursements

| Item | Total | 1 | 2 | 3 ... |
|------|-------|---|---|-------|
| Beginning balance | $279,000 | $279,000 | $357,730 | $430,330 |
| Cash receipts | 6,805,000 | 634,620 | 593,490 | 572,860 |
| Available cash | 7,084,000 | 913,620 | 951,220 | 1,003,190 |
| Less: Disbursements | 6,564,850 | 555,890 | 520,890 | 507,580 |
| Ending cash balance | 519,150 | 357,730 | 430,330 | 495,610 |

REFERENCES

American Hospital Association. *Budgeting Procedures for Hospitals.* Chicago: American Hospital Association, 1971.

Benston, G. J. "Multiple Regression Analysis of Cost Behavior." *The Accounting Review,* October 1966, pp. 657–672.

Bishop, W. "Patient Service Units, the First Step Towards Better Comparisons." *Hospital Financial Management,* vol. 26, no. 3, March 1972, pp. 15–16.

Chambers, J. C., et al. "How to Choose the Right Forecasting Technique." *Harvard Business Review,* vol. 49, no. 4, July–August 1971, pp. 45–74.

Clark, B. B., and Lamont, G. S. "Accurate Census Forecasting Leads to Cost Containment." *Hospitals,* JAHA, vol. 50, no. 12, June 1, 1976, pp. 38–47.

Draper, N., and Smith, H. *Applied Regression Analysis.* New York: John Wiley & Sons Inc., 1966.

Donlon, V. W. "Statistical Methods to Forecast Volume of Service for the Revenue Budget." *Hospital Financial Management,* vol. 29, no. 4, April 1975, pp. 38–47.

Eberhard, M., et al. "The HRU—Measuring Input to Find Productivity." *Hospital Financial Management,* vol. 00, no. 0, February, 1976, pp. 44–48.

Grapes, T. A., and Grown, T. "A Review of Prescription Pricing and A Call for Equitable Rates." *Hospitals,* JAHA, vol. 50, no. 13, July 1, 1976, pp. 91–98.

Hanning, V. "Advancing Averages Develop Trends for Budget Projection." *Hospital Financial Management,* vol. 30, no. 2, October 1976, pp. 44–50.

Herkimer, A. G. "Treatment Degree: A Standard Unit of Measure for All Components of the Health Care Industry." *Hospital Financial Management,* vol. 26, no. 3, March 1972, pp. 7–13.

Horwitz, R. M. "Flexible Budgeting: Tips for Switching." *Hospital Financial Management,* vol. 31, no. 3, March 1977, pp. 48–50, 52.

Houser, R. "How to Build and Use a Flexible Budget." *Hospital Financial Management,* vol. 28, no. 8, August 1974, pp. 12–20.

Jensen, R. "A Multiple Regression Model for Cost Control—Assumptions and Limitations." *The Accounting Review,* April 1967, pp. 265–272.

Kenneth, R. J., and Lampi, G. "When the Cash Comes In—How to Forecast." *Hospital Financial Management,* vol. 31, no. 7, July 1977, pp. 38–41.

Kretschmar, C. G. "How to Forecast Your Rates Without Guessing." *Hospital Financial Management,* vol. 30, no. 7, July 1976, pp. 44–50.

Koza, R. "Times Series Data Is Essential to Health Care Planning." *Hospital Financial Management,* vol. 23, no. 1, January 1974, pp. 32–39.

Lay, C. M., and Broyles, R. W. *Statistics in Health Administration,* Volume II. Germantown, Md.: Aspen Systems Corporation, 1980.

Rowley, C. S. "Which Is the Best (Method) to Find Cost Behavior." *Hospital Financial Management,* vol. 30, no. 4, April 1976, pp. 18–26.

Schinderle, D. A., and Joslen, R. A. "Does the Breakeven Point Still Mean Anything?" *Hospital Financial Management,* vol. 30, no. 11, November 1976, pp. 32–36.

Weston, J. F., and Brigham, E. F. *Managerial Finance,* 5th ed. Hinsdale, Ill.: The Dryden Press, 1975, Ch. 4.

Wheelwright, S. C. and Makyidakis, S. G. *Forecasting Methods for Management.* New York: John Wiley & Sons, Inc., 1973.

# Chapter 14

# Traditional Systems of Internal Control and Reporting

## Objectives

After completing this chapter, you should be able to:

1. Understand the basic principles of internal control.
2. Understand, prepare, and use work performance reports.
3. Understand, prepare, and use reports depicting cost variances.
4. Understand and use reports depicting revenues and expenses.

This chapter examines the usefulness of the budget and indexes of operating results in evaluating and controlling the performance of a hospital. The objective is twofold: (1) to describe the fundamental elements of the system by which the performance of the hospital is controlled, (2) to review the types of reports and reporting mechanisms that traditionally have been used in the hospital industry.

## 14.1 BASIC PRINCIPLES OF INTERNAL CONTROL

The importance of the budget in controlling hospital activity is seen in Figure 14-1. This assumes that a comparison of current and desired performance results in the identification of a problem that may be resolved by the discretionary action of management. Once the problem has been identified and its parameters have been specified clearly, management should develop a remedial plan or course of action. After implementing the plan, the effects of the discretionary action on operating results must be measured, recorded, and reported to appropriate administrative personnel.

Of critical importance in the paradigm of internal control is the function of recording and reporting the results of operational activity. Unless these results are reported in real as well as in financial terms on a timely and accurate basis,

**Figure 14-1** Internal Control Flow Chart

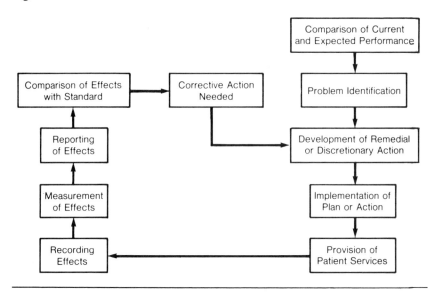

management's ability to control hospital activities will be impaired. Once the effects of the plan have been reported to management, the extent to which the discretionary actions resolve the problem or create additional problems must be evaluated. Obviously, if the plan is not completely successful in solving the problem or generates new problems, management must develop and implement alternate courses of action that must be evaluated in a similar manner.

It is useful to summarize the types of reports received by the various levels of managerial responsibility. Assume that the hospital is composed of two divisions, I and II, each of which consists of two responsibility centers (Figure 14-2). In turn, each of the responsibility centers consists of two cost centers. In such a situation, information concerning the number of staff hours used, work units performed, and number of patients treated are forwarded from the cost centers, responsibility centers, and divisional units to the fiscal services division. That division collects information from the organizational units and prepares summary reports in which actual operations are compared with budgetary projections.

To discharge the responsibility of controlling operational performance, managers of the responsibility centers should receive reports from the fiscal services division that identify differences between: (1) the actual and expected use of resources, (2) the actual and expected work load, and (3) the actual and expected costs of their centers. Similarly, divisional managers should receive a summary report on the performance of the units comprising the divisions for which they

**Figure 14-2** Hospital Division Into Responsibility and Cost Centers

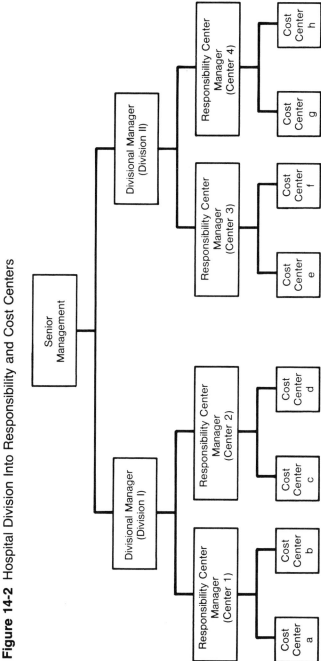

are responsible. Finally, senior management should receive summary reports on the divisions comprising the hospital enterprise. It also is desirable to ensure that divisional and senior managers receive the reports prepared for their subordinates.

## 14.2 BASIC STATISTICAL REPORTS

The statistical reports described in this section are grouped into two categories. The first measures the work performance of an organizational unit by providing an overview of the relation between the use of resources and the provision of service. The second group provides an overview of the difference between the expected costs and actual costs incurred by a responsibility center or divisional unit of the hospital.

### 14.2.1 Work Performance Reports

When describing the group of management reports that seek to relate the use of resources to service demands, it is convenient to distinguish between units that provide stay-specific services and those that offer ancillary services. The nursing department is used here as an example of a responsibility center that provides stay-specific services while the laboratory department serves as an example of a responsibility center that provides ancillary services.

Consider first reports on providing stay-specific services. At least two types of information are required for the unit: (1) the quantity and composition of patients currently receiving care, (2) the staffing and use of consumable supplies in providing nursing care.

The information on the unit's patient population can be reported in the daily census that is collected routinely by most hospitals. The objective of the daily census is to determine which bed is occupied and by what type of patient. The information that should be collected includes the room number and bed number (if appropriate) as well as the name, age, sex, and diagnostic condition of the patient. It also is of value to include the level of care required by the patient. These data may be used to construct a profile of the patients currently receiving care in the nursing unit as well as to determine the percentage of the total bed complement occupied.

The patient profile of a nursing unit may be of considerable value when determining day-to-day staffing patterns. The quantity and composition of resources required to care for a set of aged patients with serious conditions probably differ significantly from the resources needed for a group of younger patients presenting less serious or less complicated conditions. Thus, staffing decisions concerning a nursing ward or department should reflect not only the occupancy rate of the unit but also the diagnostic mix and the severity of the cases.

The frequency and the intensity of nursing contacts depends on both the time of day and the phase of the patient's hospital stay. For example, nurse-patient contacts in a case of acute appendicitis are more frequent and more intensive immediately following admission and during the preoperative and postoperative phases of treatment than just before discharge. Systems that coordinate staffing levels or patterns with the level of care provided are available and used by nursing departments in many hospitals.

The daily census of each nursing unit can include data that provide the basis for developing a profile for each patient; this, in turn, influences the staffing pattern during the next 24-hour period. As an example, Table 14-1 is a census report for a surgical nursing unit on the third floor of the north wing. The information on the number of occupied beds provides the basis for calculating the occupancy rate. Similarly, information pertaining to characteristics of the individual patients coupled with the presenting diagnosis provides the basis for estimating the number of nursing hours by type of nurse that will be required in managing each of the patients.

Assume that the nursing services division is composed of the various nursing units of the hospital. The data in the census reports of the nursing units can be summarized for the divisional manager in a form such as Table 14-2. The daily census reports provides management with information on the occupancy rate in each unit, the occupancy rate for the hospital, the distribution of patients by severity of condition, and the estimated number of nursing hours by type of nurse that will be required during the next 24-hour period.

The second set of data for evaluating the performance of a unit is, as noted, a measure of the resources actually used in providing service. One of the most common such measures is the number of labor hours per unit of service. If the nursing unit is used as an example, the number of nursing hours per patient day by type of nurse is employed as a measure of the use of labor in providing care. Table 14-3 is an example of a report that depicts the number of hours worked in a given nursing unit by type of nurse during each of three shifts. These data permit the calculation of

1. the total number of hours worked during each of the three shifts by type of nurse
2. the total number of hours worked during the day by type of nurse
3. the total number of nursing hours worked during each of the three shifts
4. the total number of nursing hours worked during the day.

The total number of nursing hours worked during the day divided by the number of patients yields the average number of hours per patient. Similarly, the number

**Table 14-1** Census Report for a Nursing Unit

Unit 3N                                                      Date _____

| Room & Bed # | Name | Age | Sex | Dx[1] | Level of Required Care | Estimated # of Nursing Hours R.N. | L.P.N. | Aide |
|---|---|---|---|---|---|---|---|---|
| 301-1 | | | | | | | | |
| 2 | | | | | | | | |
| 302-1 | | | | | | | | |
| 2 | | | | | | | | |
| 303-1 | | | | | | | | |
| 2 | | | | | | | | |
| 304-1 | | | | | | | | |
| 2 | | | | | | | | |
| 305-1 | | | | | | | | |
| 2 | | | | | | | | |
| 306-1 | | | | | | | | |
| 2 | | | | | | | | |
| | | | | | Total | | | |

Bed complement _____
Number of patients _____
Occupancy rate _____

[1] Dx refers to diagnostic condition.

**Table 14-2** Daily Census Report for Divisional Manager

Date _____

| Unit | Bed Complement | Occupied Beds | Occupancy Rate | Head Nurse | Estimated # Nursing Hours R.N. | L.P.N. | Aide |
|---|---|---|---|---|---|---|---|
| 2N | | | | | | | |
| 2S | | | | | | | |
| 2W | | | | | | | |
| 2E | | | | | | | |
| 3N | | | | | | | |
| 3S | | | | | | | |
| 3W | | | | | | | |
| 3E | | | | | | | |
| CCU | | | | | | | |
| ICU | | | | | | | |
| Nursery | | | | | | | |
| Total | | | | | | | |

Average occupancy _____

% Very Seriously Ill _____
% Seriously Ill _____
% Ill _____

**Table 14-3** Nursing Roster

| Unit 3N | | | Date | |
|---|---|---|---|---|
| Nursing Category & Employee | 12–8 a.m. | Shift 8 a.m.–4 p.m. | 4–12 p.m. | Total |
| **R.N.:** | | | | |
| Jane Smith | 4 | 4 | | 8 |
| Joan Block | | 8 | | 8 |
| Barbara Schultz | 8 | | | 8 |
| Mary Jones | | 4 | | 4 |
| Helen Jackson | | | 8 | 8 |
| Subtotal | 12 | 16 | 8 | 36 |
| **L.P.N.:** | | | | |
| Barbara Dole | 4 | 4 | | 8 |
| Karen Black | | 4 | 4 | 8 |
| Virginia Myer | 4 | 4 | | 8 |
| Donna Blue | | | 8 | 8 |
| Subtotal | 8 | 12 | 12 | 32 |
| **Aide:** | | | | |
| Cheryl Kara | | 8 | | 8 |
| Joanne Carson | | | 8 | 8 |
| Subtotal | | 8 | 8 | 16 |
| Total | 20 | 36 | 28 | 84 |

| | | | | | | |
|---|---|---|---|---|---|---|
| Total hours | 84 | Total hours: morning shift | 20 | Average hours/pt: | 4.2 |
| Total hours: R.N. | 36 | Total hours: afternoon shift | 36 | Average hours: R.N. | 1.8 |
| Total hours: L.P.N. | 32 | Total hours: evening shift | 28 | Average hours: L.P.N. | 1.6 |
| Total hours: Aide | 16 | Total patients: | 20 | Average hours: Aide | .8 |

of hours of each nursing category in the unit divided by the number of patients provides an estimate of the average number of hours of nursing care per patient by type of nurse. When this estimate is compared with the planned number of nursing hours per patient, the manager of the responsibility center may evaluate the extent to which adequate care is being provided in the unit. No mention is made of the time worked by the nursing supervisor or other staff members who might have provided care. The hospital might want to allocate a portion of the number of hours these persons worked to the unit or charge their time to nursing administration.

The data on the census and number of hours worked in each nursing unit might then be summarized weekly or monthly for divisional managers as in Table 14-4. The first column lists the total number of available bed days, which is given by the product of the bed complement of the unit and the number of days in the month. The second column contains the number of days of care provided in each of the units during the month. Dividing entries in the second column by the corresponding value in the first yields the average occupancy rate

**Table 14-4** Summary of Departmental Census and Hours Worked for the Month of _____

| Unit | Number of Available Bed Days for Month (1) | Patient Days for Month (2) | Occupancy Rate for Month (2) ÷ (1) | Nursing Hours Total | R.N. | L.P.N. | Aide | Average Nursing Hours per Patient Day All nurses | R.N. | L.P.N. | Aide |
|------|------|------|------|------|------|------|------|------|------|------|------|
| 2N | | | | | | | | | | | |
| 2S | | | | | | | | | | | |
| 2W | | | | | | | | | | | |
| 2E | | | | | | | | | | | |
| 3N | | | | | | | | | | | |
| 3S | | | | | | | | | | | |
| 3W | | | | | | | | | | | |
| 3E | | | | | | | | | | | |
| CCU | | | | | | | | | | | |
| ICU | | | | | | | | | | | |
| Nursery | | | | | | | | | | | |
| Total | | | | | | | | | | | |

for the unit during the month. Similarly, dividing the hospital's total number of days of care by the total available bed days of care yields the institution's average occupancy rate. The other columns are self-explanatory.

Consider next a department that provides ancillary services. The work load of such a unit might be measured by the frequency with which each service in the set of departmental services is provided. For example, the work load of the laboratory department might be defined in terms of either the total volume of all services provided during a given period or the volume of each type of laboratory examination during the period. In turn, resource use might be measured in terms of (1) the total number of staff hours worked, (2) the total number of hours worked by type of labor, or (3) the total number of hours worked by type of labor by type of service. Accordingly, the performance of the unit might be evaluated in terms of (1) the average amount of labor used per laboratory test, (2) the average number of staff hours by type of labor used per laboratory test, and (3) the average number of staff hours by type of labor used per service by type of test. When these statistics are compared with budget estimates, management may evaluate whether these resources are being used as efficiently as planned.

A similar set of reports can be constructed for units that provide indirect patient care. For example, in the laundry or dietary departments, the work load might be measured in terms of the number of pounds of laundry processed and the number of meals served, respectively. The resources used in providing these services then might be measured in terms of the total number of hours worked and the number of hours worked by type of labor. Similar to the management reports for the nursing department, the ratio of staff hours worked per unit of service (pounds of laundry processed or meals served) may be used in evaluating the unit.

## 14.2.2 Cost Variances: A Summary View

The primary purpose of reporting cost variances in a departmental unit or responsibility center is to provide line management with information on differences between current expenditures and work load as compared to the corresponding budget projection. For example, in Table 14-5 variances in the personnel and supply costs for the month and year to date are reported for the laboratory department. Differences between actual and expected labor costs, supply costs, staff hours/unit of service, and work load of the department are summarized for the manager. As should be verified, the data indicate that the operational activity of the unit has deviated from the standard set in the budget and that remedial action may be required to achieve assigned goals.

**Table 14-5** Budget Report for the Month of _____

Unit: Laboratory

| Component* | Month | | | Year to Date | | |
|---|---|---|---|---|---|---|
| | Budget | Actual | Variance | Budget | Actual | Variance |
| Personnel cost | $10,500 | $11,750 | $1,250 | $80,000 | $97,500 | $17,500 |
| Supply cost | 4,500 | 8,000 | 3,500 | 60,500 | 82,760 | 22,260 |
| Total | 15,000 | 19,750 | 4,750 | 140,500 | 180,260 | 39,760 |
| Staff hours/ service | 1.5 | 1.8 | .3 | 1.5 | 1.7 | .2 |
| Volume of service | 10,000 | 9,500 | (500) | 45,000 | 36,500 | (8,500) |

* In sufficient detail to satisfy the needs of various levels of managerial responsibility.

In addition to the monthly expense report prepared for line managers, the directors of the divisional units of the hospital should receive a monthly summary of the cost variances of the units or departments for which they are responsible. Suppose that one of the divisions of the hospital is composed of the radiology. laboratory, pharmacy, and anesthesiology departments. An example of the monthly summary report for this division is presented in Table 14-6.

Finally, a monthly summary report depicting the cost variances in each of the departmental units of the hospital should be prepared for senior management. The primary objective of such a report is to indicate the cost variances in each department by type of expenditure (e.g., wages and salaries, supply costs, etc.). This report also should identify cost variances that are significant or excessive as defined in statistical terms or in terms of a specified percentage deviation from the expectation that was negotiated previously. A detailed listing of cost variances as well as an identification of significant differences between actual costs and budget projections provide a valuable data base on which management can develop appropriate policies and plans of action to reduce or eliminate exceptions to the budget.

## 14.3 REPORTING REVENUES AND EXPENSES

As noted earlier, one of management's basic objectives is to ensure the financial viability of the hospital and one of its primary responsibilities is to evaluate the extent to which revenues are at least equal to total economic costs.

In this evaluation, the income earned by the various revenue-generating centers should be compared with the total costs of these units on a monthly or quarterly basis. Such a comparison is of greatest value to management when the

**Table 14-6** Summary Report on Cost Variances

| Department/ Unit | Month Budget | Actual | Variance | Year to Date Budget | Actual | Variance |
|---|---|---|---|---|---|---|
| Laboratory | $15,000 | $19,750 | $4,750 | $140,500 | $180,260 | $39,760 |
| Pharmacy | | | | | | |
| Anesthesiology | | | | | | |
| Radiology | | | | | | |
| Total | | | | | | |

**Table 14-7** Summary of Revenues and Expenditures by Department for the Period Ending _____

| Department | Month Revenues | Costs | Net Revenue or Loss | Year to Date Revenues | Costs | Net Revenue or Loss |
|---|---|---|---|---|---|---|
| Nursing department | | | | | | |
| Radiology | | | | | | |
| Laboratory | | | | | | |
| Emergency room | | | | | | |
| Anesthesiology | | | | | | |
| Physical/occupational therapy | | | | | | |
| Surgery | | | | | | |
| Total | | | | | | |

cost-finding techniques described earlier are used to derive the total expenditures of each of the centers.

Table 14-7 is an example of a report for senior management that summarizes the revenues and expenses of the departments that earn income for the hospital on a monthly or quarterly basis. This information is of obvious value in determining which units are earning revenues that at least equal total economic costs and in identifying departments that are incurring net losses. This identifies areas in which management might consider possible ways of either (1) reducing the costs of the revenue-generating center or (2) altering the hospital fee schedule to reduce the imbalance between revenues and expenditures. Many hospitals operate revenue-generating centers that are expected to incur a net loss. For those units, the summary of revenues and expenditures provides information that is germane to the determination of the extent to which current net losses are within tolerable limits.

A more detailed analysis of the net income or the net loss for each service provided by the revenue-generating centers serves to identify specific areas in

**Table 14-8** Revenue Cost Report for the Period Ending _____

*Unit: Laboratory Department*

| | Month | | | Year to Date | | |
|---|---|---|---|---|---|---|
| *Service Component* | *Revenue* | *Cost* | *Net Income or Loss* | *Revenue* | *Cost* | *Net Revenue or Loss* |
| Blood chemistry | | | | | | |
| Serology examination | | | | | | |
| Pathology examination | | | | | | |
| Hematological examination | | | | | | |
| Total | | | | | | |

which adjustments are appropriate and desirable. Table 14-8 is an example of a revenue/cost report for a department that produces a set of more or less standardized services. The primary purpose of this report is to compare the revenue earned and costs incurred in a given revenue-generating center by major category of service. The development of such a report requires the apportionment of total departmental costs among the services produced by the unit as well as an estimate of the revenue earned by providing each of the services. The departmental cost may be allocated to each of the services by using the weighted value technique described earlier, while the revenues earned by providing each of the services may be obtained by

$$TR_k = F_k Q_k$$

where $TR_k$ corresponds to the total revenue earned by providing service $k$, $F_k$ is the full established rate charged for the use of service $k$, and $Q_k$ represents the quantity of the service provided during the current period. Comparing the income earned by providing each service with the total costs generated in earning that revenue will identify areas in which management might alter the hospital's fee schedule or introduce policies and actions designed to improve the efficiency of operations. Moreover, for services regarded as "loss leaders," the information in the detailed analysis of revenues and costs provides the basis for evaluating the extent to which the current net loss is within normal or acceptable limits.

In addition to these interim reports, most hospitals provide a set of annual reports that depict performance as expressed in actual expenditures and revenues as well as the end-of-period assets, liabilities, and fund balances. These data also provide a basis for formulating both financial and operational decisions and policies.

**REFERENCES**

American Hospital Association. *Internal Control and Internal Auditing for Hospitals.* Chicago: American Hospital Association, 1969.

Anthony, R. N., and Reece, J. S. *Management Accounting: Texts and Cases.* Homewood: Richard D. Irwin, Inc., 1975, Ch. 14.

Chazen, C., Herkimer, A. G., and Landis, I. M. "What You (and Your Board) Should Know About Audit Committees." *Hospital Financial Management,* vol. 31, no. 9, September 1977, pp. 24–31.

Garrett, R. D. *Hospitals—A Systems Approach.* Philadelphia: Auerbach Publishers, Inc., 1973, Ch. 4.

Hay, L. *Budgeting and Cost Analysis for Hospital Management,* 2nd ed. Bloomington, Ind.: Pressler Publications, 1963.

Seawell, L. V. *Hospital Financial Accounting: Theory and Practice.* Chicago: Hospital Financial Management Association, 1975.

Schwartz, M. D. "Status of Hospital Information Systems." *Hospital Progress,* vol. 51, no. 6, June 1970, pp. 53–60.

# Chapter 15

# Program Budgeting

## Objectives

After completing this chapter, you should be able to:

1. Define the program area in terms of diagnostic nomenclature.
2. Describe the basic components of care required by the program area.
3. Understand and prepare the operational budget of the program area, including:
   a. the diagnostic mix.
   b. service mix.
   c. resource mix.
4. Estimate the labor and supply costs of the program area.
5. Determine the full costs of operating the program area.

## 15.1 INTRODUCTION*

As described in Chapter 11, program budgeting is a managerial tool for reaching macrolevel decisions on the allocation of resources while responsibility budgeting represents one of the major tools for controlling the day-to-day activities of the hospital. When developing the program budget, it is necessary to use a technique that permits an evaluation of the activities of the various responsibility centers in relation to the goals and objectives of the program areas as well as in terms of the common objective of the hospital enterprise. Since the rates of

---

* In this and in the next three chapters the notation and operations of matrix algebra are used extensively. Readers unfamiliar with this area of mathematics should review Chapter 4 before proceeding.

activity in centers providing direct patient care are determined by the demands exerted by the various program areas, the discussion of alternate approaches to the preparation of the budget begins with this level of analysis.

## 15.2 THE PROGRAM AREA

The various program areas comprising hospital activity can be described in terms of well-defined sets of diseases or injuries. Such a procedure recognizes that medical knowledge and technology frequently serve as guidelines to indicate the quantity and composition of service that should be used in diagnosing, monitoring, therapeutically managing, and otherwise supporting patients. Thus, it might be argued that the objective of a given program is to provide diagnostic, therapeutic, and support services to patients who are hospitalized with the set of conditions that define the program area. When program areas are described in terms of sets of well-defined diagnoses, the patient and the related condition may be used as the unit of analysis which, in turn, permits a specification of the relationship of the goals of the responsibility center, the program area, and the hospital enterprise.

For illustration, assume that the hospital uses diagnostic nomenclature to define $v$ programs represented by the subscripts $(1, \cdots, g, \cdots, v)$. The interrelationship of the goals of the hospital, the program areas, and the responsibility centers is presented in Figure 15-1. Defining program areas in terms of diagnostic nomenclature ensures that the goals of the three levels of analysis are consistent and mutually supportive.

In slightly more operational terms, it might be argued that the common goal of the hospital is to improve, restore, or maintain (or prevent a further deterioration in) the health status of a patient population presenting the set of conditions

$$M^* = \{M_1, \cdots, M_t\} \tag{15.1}$$

by providing the set of services

$$S^* = \{S; N; AGS\} \tag{15.2}$$

at an acceptable level of quality and at minimum costs. With respect to Equation 15.2, let: (1) $S$ represent the set of ancillary services $(S_1, \cdots, S_k, \cdots, S_x)$; (2) $N$ represent the set of stay-specific services $(N_1, \cdots, N_r, \cdots, N_n)$, where $N_r$ is the number of days of care provided in nursing department $r$; and (3) $AGS$ represent the set of general support and administrative services offered on behalf of the patient. The elements of $S$, $N$, and $AGS$ are departmentally specific and providing these services requires the use of labor, consumable supplies, and

**Figure 15-1** Interrelationship of Hospital Goals, Program Areas, and Responsibility Centers

Goals of the Hospital

To provide required services at an acceptable level of quality and at minimum cost while preserving the long-run and short-run viability of the institution.

Goals of Program Areas $P_1, \ldots, P_g, \ldots, P_v$

To provide services required by patients presenting conditions that define the program area at an acceptable level of quality and at minimum costs.

Goals of the Responsibility Centers

To provide services required by all program areas at an acceptable level of quality and at minimum costs.

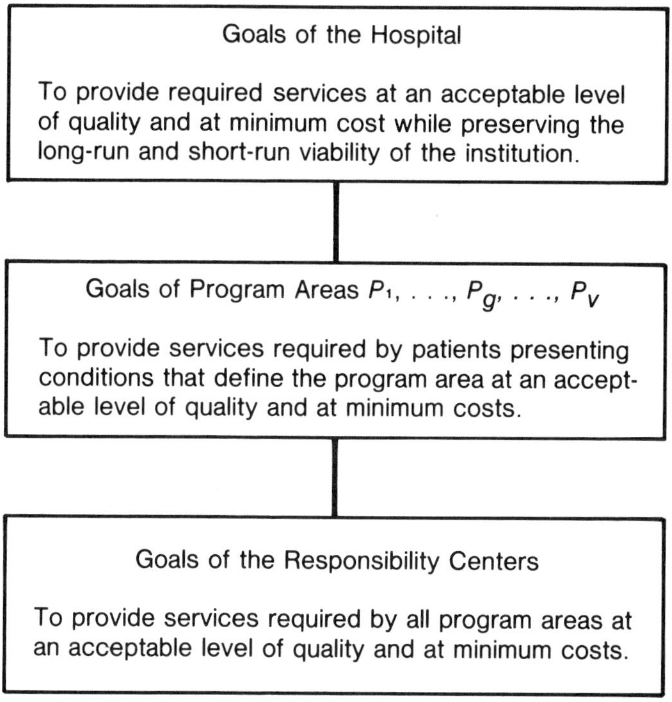

capital equipment. Since the objective is to develop an operating budget for the program area of activity, this chapter focuses on the labor and supply requirements associated with varying rates of production.

For purposes of discussion, assume that program $P_g$ is defined by the set of diagnoses

$$M_g = \{M_1, \cdots, M_i, \cdots, M_z\}$$

In this case, the elements of $M_g$ are a subset of $M^*$ that is represented symbolically by $M_g \subseteq M^*$.

## 15.3 THE COMPONENTS OF HOSPITAL CARE

Before discussing the budgeting procedure, it is necessary to consider the various components of hospital care. Presented in Table 15-1 is a group of

**Table 15-1** Identification, Measurement, and Symbolic Representation of Departmentally Specific Services

| Department of Care, Department and Subcategory of Service | Measure of Output by Number of: | Symbolic Representation |
|---|---|---|
| *Ancillary Services:* | Units | $S_k$ |
| Operating room | procedures by type of procedure | |
| Laboratory | procedures by type of procedure | |
| Radiology | exposures by type of exposure | |
| Inhalation therapy | procedures by type of procedure | |
| Physical therapy | procedures by type of procedure | |
| Other ancillary services | procedures by type of procedure | |
| *Stay-Specific Service:* | | $N_r$ |
| Nursing care by specialty department | days of care | |
| Nonprofessioral stay-specific services | | |
| Dietary | 3 meals/day × number of days of care | |
| Hotel services | days of care | |
| *Administrative and General Support Services:* | | |
| Plant maintenance | square feet | |
| Plant operation | square feet | |
| Medical records | records | |
| General administration | employees | |
| Laundry | pounds | |

representative departments that are assumed to comprise the hospital. With the exception of stay-specific services, the components of care provided directly to the patient are measured in terms of the number of services or procedures offered by the various departments during the period. For example, the production of the laboratory department may be defined as the number of (1) urinalyses, (2) hematology examinations, (3) blood chemistry examinations, (4) bacteriological examinations, (5) serology examinations, (6) pathologies, and (7) clinical microscopic examinations provided in managing a set of specified morbidities.

On the other hand, the quantity of hotel services (i.e., maid and janitorial) may be measured by the number of unweighted days of care during a given period. In this case, assume that bedding is changed daily and that the other housekeeping functions are performed on a more or less daily basis. Similarly, the number of meals provided by the dietary department depends on the number of days of care in a given period.

Nursing and other nonsurgical professional care also may be measured in terms of the number of days of care. However, without further specification or weighting, the number of days of care fails to reflect the various dimensions of this category. Specifically, the unweighted number of days of care does not reflect the frequency or intensity of patient-nurse contacts, which probably varies during a 24-hour period. With the possible exception of the intensive care unit and the coronary care unit, the number of patient-nurse contacts probably is greater during the day and early evening hours than when patients normally sleep. In addition, for most diagnoses, nursing care is more or less intensive depending on the stage of the hospital episode. For example, the frequency and intensity of care for a patient undergoing surgery (cholecystectomy) for gall bladder disease is greater before and immediately after the operation than during the later stages of recovery or just before discharge.

In an effort to overcome the difficulties of using the unweighted number of days of care as a proxy variable for this component of hospital output, nursing service and the other components of nonsurgical professional care are measured by the length of stay as classified by diagnosis and by department. Thus, the dimensions of nursing care in a given department are similar for cases of a specific diagnosis.

For example, a penetrating chest wound frequently requires dressing changes, initiating and monitoring intravenous solutions, administering medications, and monitoring vital signs. To the extent that a patient who presents a specific diagnosis and receives service in a given department requires a similar set or series of nursing activities, the classification of days of care by morbidity and department recognizes differences in the care required by different medical conditions and may be viewed as a reasonable surrogate for the services supplied by nursing personnel and the nonsurgical professional staff.

## 15.4 AN OVERVIEW

The process of developing an operational budget for the program area is outlined in Figure 15-2. The first step in developing the operational budget is to estimate the total number of patients expected to receive hospital care during the budget period. In the second step, once the size of the patient population has been forecast, the anticipated number of patients is distributed in terms of presenting condition and service requirements. The third step, which represents the bridge between the diagnostic and resource mixes of the program area, requires that management estimate the standard bundle of services as well as the total associated service requirements. The fourth step involves estimation of the standard staff hours and standard supply requirements by type of input per unit of service, which provides the basis for estimating the resource needs of the program area.

**Figure 15-2** Developing Operational and Financial Budget for Program Area

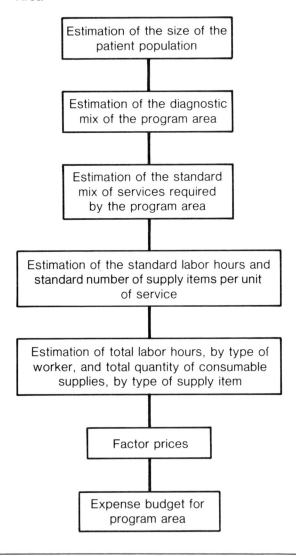

Once the real resources required by the program area have been estimated, management may transform the operational budget into financial terms. As indicated in Figure 15-2 the translation is accomplished by applying appropriate factor prices to the corresponding forecast of resource use.

## 15.5 THE OPERATIONAL BUDGET OF THE PROGRAM AREA

The development of the operational budget for the program (Figure 15-2) requires projections concerning: (1) the size of the patient population, (2) the distribution of the patient population in terms of diagnoses and service requirements, (3) the standard mix of services, and (4) the standard resource requirements. The purpose of this section is to consider the techniques by which these projections might be developed.

### 15.5.1 The Size of the Patient Population

The size of the patient population anticipated during the budget period may be estimated using one of the techniques described earlier. That is, management may use the geometric mean as applied to a moving average, exponential smoothing, or regression analysis for this estimate. For the purposes of future discussion, we use the symbol $\rho$ (the Greek letter rho) to represent the size of the patient population expected during the budget period.

### 15.5.2 The Expected Diagnostic Mix

The patient population may be distributed in terms of diagnosis and service requirements by applying the principles of mathematical expectation. Consider first the number of patients who are expected to present diagnosis $i$ and require ancillary service $k$. The statement of mathematical expectation that provides such a distribution might be expressed in words as follows:

$$\begin{bmatrix} \text{Expected Number of} \\ \text{Patients Presenting} \\ \text{Diagnosis } i \text{ and Requiring} \\ \text{Ancillary Service } k \end{bmatrix}$$

$$= \begin{bmatrix} \text{Size of} \\ \text{Expected Patient} \\ \text{Population} \end{bmatrix} \times \begin{bmatrix} \text{Probability of a} \\ \text{Patient's Presenting} \\ \text{Diagnosis } i \text{ and Requiring} \\ \text{Ancillary Service } k \end{bmatrix}$$

Similarly, we may distribute the expected population in terms of diagnosis and nursing department by

$$\begin{bmatrix} \text{Expected Number of} \\ \text{Patients Presenting} \\ \text{Diagnosis } i \text{ and Requiring} \\ \text{Service in Nursing Department } r \end{bmatrix}$$

$$= \begin{bmatrix} \text{Size of} \\ \text{Expected} \\ \text{Patient} \\ \text{Population} \end{bmatrix} \times \begin{bmatrix} \text{Probability of a} \\ \text{Patient's Presenting} \\ \text{Diagnosis } M_i \text{ and Requiring} \\ \text{Care in Nursing Department } r \end{bmatrix}$$

which, of course, pertains to the use of stay-specific services. As an example of the first distribution mentioned, suppose that the probability of a patient presenting diagnosis $M_i$ and requiring ancillary service $S_1$ is .02. If the hospital expects to treat 1,500 patients during the budget period, we find that

$$.02(1,500) = 30$$

patients are expected to present diagnostic condition $M_i$ and require ancillary service $S_1$. In the following discussion we let

$P(S_k \cap M_i)$ represent the probability of a patient presenting diagnosis $M_i$ and requiring ancillary $S_k$; and

$P(D_r \cap M_i)$ represent the probability of a patient presenting diagnosis $i$ and requiring care in nursing department $D_r$.

Suppose that the operational activity of the institution is limited to ancillary services $S_1$, $S_2$, and $S_3$ as well as stay-specific services $N_1$ and $N_2$ in nursing departments $D_1$ and $D_2$ to patients presenting conditions $M_1$, $M_2$, $M_3$, and $M_4$. Assume further that program $P_1$ is defined by conditions $M_1$ and $M_2$ while program $P_2$ is defined by diagnoses $M_3$ and $M_4$. Suppose that an examination of the medical records of 1,000 individuals who were discharged in the previous year yielded the distribution of patients presented in Table 15-2. On the basis of these data, we may calculate $P(S_1 \cap M_i)$ as follows

$$P(S_1 \cap M_1) = .020$$

$$P(S_1 \cap M_2) = .180$$

$$P(S_1 \cap M_3) = .150$$

$$P(S_1 \cap M_4) = .030$$

**Table 15-2** Historical Distribution of Patients by Diagnosis and Service Requirements

| Program and Diagnosis | Number of Patients Who Required Service $S_1$ | Number of Patients Who Did Not Require Service $S_1$ | Total |
|---|---|---|---|
| $P_1$: | | | |
| $M_1$ | 20 | 260 | 280 |
| $M_2$ | 180 | 120 | 300 |
| $P_2$: | | | |
| $M_3$ | 150 | 170 | 320 |
| $M_4$ | 30 | 70 | 100 |
| Total | 380 | 620 | 1,000 |

Now, suppose we replicated this analysis for the other components of care and obtained the results presented in Table 15-3.

The data in that table provide the basis for distributing the patient population in terms of diagnosis and service requirements. Considering first the patient population of program $P_1$, we may extract the data in the first three rows and the first two columns of the table, and form the matrix

$$\mathbf{A}_1 = \begin{bmatrix} .020 & .180 \\ .100 & .072 \\ .030 & .020 \end{bmatrix}$$

where the attached subscript specifies the program area. If we now multiply each element of matrix $\mathbf{A}_1$ by the size of the expected patient population (i.e., $\rho = 1,500$), we obtain

**Table 15-3** Probability Distribution of Patients by Diagnosis and Service Requirements

| Service | Diagnosis | | | |
|---|---|---|---|---|
| | $M_1$ | $M_2$ | $M_3$ | $M_4$ |
| Ancillary services | | | | |
| $S_1$ | .020 | .180 | .150 | .030 |
| $S_2$ | .100 | .072 | .090 | .020 |
| $S_3$ | .030 | .020 | .060 | .012 |
| Stay-specific services | | | | |
| $D_1$ | .280 | .150 | .000 | .030 |
| $D_2$ | .000 | .150 | .320 | .070 |

$$\mathbf{C}_1 = 1{,}500 \begin{bmatrix} .020 & .180 \\ .100 & .072 \\ .030 & .020 \end{bmatrix} = \begin{bmatrix} 30 & 270 \\ 150 & 108 \\ 45 & 30 \end{bmatrix}$$

where the first column of the resulting matrix represents the number of patients presenting diagnosis $M_1$ who are expected to require each of the ancillary services and the second column represents the number presenting condition $M_2$ who are expected to require ancillary services $S_1$, $S_2$, and $S_3$.

Employing a similar approach, we may distribute the expected patient population associated with program $P_1$ in terms of diagnosis and nursing department by forming the matrix

$$\mathbf{B}_1 = \begin{bmatrix} .28 & .15 \\ .00 & .15 \end{bmatrix}$$

As before, we multiply each element of $\mathbf{B}_1$ by the size of expected patient population and obtain

$$\mathbf{E}_1 = 1{,}500 \begin{bmatrix} .28 & .15 \\ .00 & .15 \end{bmatrix} = \begin{bmatrix} 420 & 225 \\ 0 & 225 \end{bmatrix}$$

These findings suggest that management expects 420 patients to present condition $M_1$ and require nursing care in department $D_1$. The other entries in the matrix are interpreted in a similar fashion.

Referring to program $P_2$, we may use the techniques outlined above to obtain

$$\mathbf{C}_2 = \begin{bmatrix} 225 & 45 \\ 135 & 30 \\ 90 & 18 \end{bmatrix}$$

and

$$\mathbf{E}_2 = \begin{bmatrix} 0 & 45 \\ 480 & 105 \end{bmatrix}$$

where $\mathbf{C}_2$ represents the distribution of patients associated with this program area in terms of diagnosis and service requirements while $\mathbf{E}_2$ corresponds to the distribution of patients in terms of diagnosis and nursing department. At this point in the analysis, it is convenient to summarize the results of the calculations as seen in Table 15-4, the four sections of which correspond to the matrices $\mathbf{C}_1$, $\mathbf{C}_2$, $\mathbf{E}_1$, and $\mathbf{E}_2$.

## 15.5.3 Service Requirements of the Program Area

Once the patient population has been distributed in terms of diagnosis and service requirements, management's next task is to estimate the volume of care required by the program area. As before, we consider ancillary and stay-specific services separately. Considering ancillary services first, the general approach in this text may be expressed as follows

$$
\begin{bmatrix} \text{Expected Demand for} \\ \text{Service } k \text{ by Patients} \\ \text{Presenting Diagnosis } i \end{bmatrix}
$$

$$
= \begin{bmatrix} \text{Expected Number of} \\ \text{Patients Presenting} \\ \text{Diagnosis } i \text{ and} \\ \text{Requiring Service } k \end{bmatrix} \times \begin{bmatrix} \text{Standard Number of} \\ \text{Units of Service } k \\ \text{Provided to a Patient} \\ \text{Presenting Diagnosis } i \\ \text{and Requiring the Service} \end{bmatrix}
$$

If we sum this result with respect to diagnoses $(1, \cdots, i, \cdots, z)$, the volume of ancillary service $k$ required by the program area is obtained. Similarly, when considering program demands for stay-specific services we find that

$$
\begin{bmatrix} \text{Expected Number of} \\ \text{Days of Care Associated} \\ \text{with Patients Presenting} \\ \text{Diagnosis } i \text{ and} \\ \text{Receiving Care in} \\ \text{Nursing Department } r \end{bmatrix}
$$

$$
= \begin{bmatrix} \text{Expected Number of} \\ \text{Patients Presenting} \\ \text{Diagnosis } i \text{ and} \\ \text{Requiring Care in} \\ \text{Nursing Department } r \end{bmatrix} \times \begin{bmatrix} \text{Standard Length of} \\ \text{Stay Associated with} \\ \text{Patients Presenting} \\ \text{Diagnosis } i \text{ and} \\ \text{Requiring Care in} \\ \text{Nursing Department } r \end{bmatrix}
$$

As in the case of ancillary services, summing over all diagnostic groups yields the volume of stay-specific services required by the program area.

**Table 15-4** Distribution of Expected Patient Population of Program $P_1$ and $P_2$ in Terms of Diagnostic Condition and Service Requirements

| Service | Diagnosis | | | |
|---|---|---|---|---|
| | $M_1$ | $M_2$ | $M_3$ | $M_4$ |
| Ancillary services | $(C_1)$ | | $(C_2)$ | |
| $S_1$ | 30 | 270 | 225 | 45 |
| $S_2$ | 150 | 108 | 135 | 30 |
| $S_3$ | 45 | 30 | 90 | 18 |
| Stay-specific services | $(E_1)$ | | $(E_2)$ | |
| $D_1$ | 420 | 225 | 0 | 45 |
| $D_2$ | 0 | 225 | 480 | 105 |

As implied, projections concerning the volume of service demanded by the program area require an estimation of the standard service mix. We may define the standard volume of a given service as the number of units which should be provided to the average patient who is hospitalized with a given condition and requires that component of care. Suppose that the care provided by the institution has been the subject of continuous scrutiny by an internal review committee composed of physicians who have determined that the care offered previously was of acceptable quality. In such a situation, historical data, as modified to reflect recent or anticipated changes in medical practice, might be used to construct the mix of services required by a patient presenting a given diagnosis.

Referring to the example, suppose that the volume of care rendered to those patients who required service $S_1$ is as follows:

| Diagnosis | Volume of Service $S_1$ Provided to Previous Patients Hospitalized with Diagnostic Condition $M_i$ (1) | ÷ | Number of Previous Patients Who Required Service $S_1$ (2) | = | Standard Volume of Service $S_1$ (3) |
|---|---|---|---|---|---|
| $M_1$ | 40 units | | 20 | | 2.0 |
| $M_2$ | 180 units | | 180 | | 1.0 |
| $M_3$ | 600 units | | 150 | | 4.0 |
| $M_4$ | 90 units | | 30 | | 3.0 |

In this case, the standard volume of service $S_1$ is obtained by dividing the entries in column (1) by the corresponding value in column (2). Replicating this process for each component of care results in the standard mix of services associated with each diagnositc category.

Combining the standard volume of ancillary service $S_1$ with the data in the first row of Table 15-4, we find that

1. 2.0(30) or 60 units of service $S_1$ will be required by patients presenting diagnosis $M_1$;
2. 1.0(270) or 270 units of service $S_1$ will be required by patients presenting diagnosis $M_2$;
3. 4.0(225) or 900 units of service $S_1$ will be required by patients presenting diagnosis $M_3$; and
4. 3.0(45) or 135 units of service $S_1$ will be required by patients presenting diagnosis $M_4$.

As can be verified, the demand for ancillary service $S_1$ generated by program $P_1$ is found to be 2.0(30) + 1.0(270) or 330 units. Similarly, the demand for ancillary service $S_1$ generated by program $P_2$ is given by 4.0(225) + 3.0(45) or 1,035 units.

To complete the data requirements for this section, suppose that the coefficients in Table 15-5 represent the standard mix of services, as expressed in per capita terms, for each of the diagnostic groups $M_1$, $M_2$, $M_3$, and $M_4$. Focusing on the projected volume of ancillary services required by program $P_1$, we form the matrix

$$S_1 = \begin{bmatrix} 2.0 & 2.0 & 2.0 \\ 1.0 & 5.0 & 7.0 \end{bmatrix}$$

which has been partitioned into three columns as indicated by the dotted lines. In a similar fashion, we partition the matrix

$$C_1 = \begin{bmatrix} 30 & 270 \\ 150 & 108 \\ 45 & 30 \end{bmatrix}$$

into three rows. In this case, the product on the first row of $C_1$ and the first column of $S_1$ yields

$$\begin{bmatrix} 30 & 270 \end{bmatrix} \begin{bmatrix} 2.0 \\ 1.0 \end{bmatrix} = 30(2.0) + 270(1.0) = 330 \text{ units}$$

**Table 15-5** Standard Per Capita Use of Ancillary and Stay-Specific Services During the Hospital Episode

| Diagnosis and Program | Per Capita Use of Ancillary Service (in Units of Service) | | | Per Capita Use of Stay-Specific Services (in Days of Care) | |
|---|---|---|---|---|---|
| | $S_1$ (1) | $S_2$ (2) | $S_3$ (3) | $N_1$ (4) | $N_2$ (5) |
| Program $P_1$: | | | | | |
| $M_1$ (1) | 2.0 | 2.0 | 2.0 | 5.00 | 0 |
| $M_2$ (2) | 1.0 | 5.0 | 7.0 | 4.36 | 12.00 |
| Program $P_2$: | | | | | |
| $M_3$ (3) | 4.0 | 5.0 | 5.0 | 0 | 3.75 |
| $M_4$ (4) | 3.0 | 3.0 | 2.5 | 9.0 | 5.20 |

which agrees with the projections developed earlier. In a similar fashion, we find that

$$[150 \quad 108] \begin{bmatrix} 2.0 \\ 5.0 \end{bmatrix} = 840 \text{ units}$$

and

$$[45 \quad 30] \begin{bmatrix} 2.0 \\ 7.0 \end{bmatrix} = 300 \text{ units}$$

yield projections concerning the volume of ancillary services $S_2$ and $S_3$ required by program $P_1$. For purposes of future references, it is convenient to let

$$\mathbf{s}_1 = \begin{bmatrix} 330 \\ 840 \\ 300 \end{bmatrix}$$

where the subscript attached to the column vector $\mathbf{s}$ refers to the program area.

A similar approach may be used when projecting the volume of stay-specific services required by each of the program areas. Referring again to program $P_1$, Table 15-5 reveals that we may form the matrix

$$\mathbf{N}_1 = \begin{bmatrix} 5.00 & 0.00 \\ 4.36 & 12.00 \end{bmatrix}$$

that has been partitioned into two columns. Recall that the distribution of the program population by diagnosis and nursing department is given by

$$E_1 = \left[ \begin{array}{cc} 420 & 225 \\ \hline 0 & 225 \end{array} \right]$$

that has been partitioned into two rows.

In this case, the product of the first row of $E_1$ and the first column of $N_1$ is given by

$$[420 \quad 225] \begin{bmatrix} 5.00 \\ 4.36 \end{bmatrix} = 3,081$$

days of care, which represents the projection concerning the requirements of the program area for stay-specific services provided in nursing department $D_1$. In a similar fashion,

$$[0 \quad 225] \begin{bmatrix} 0.00 \\ 12.00 \end{bmatrix} = 2,700$$

days of care will be required by program $P_1$ in nursing department $D_2$. As in the discussion of ancillary services, it is convenient to let

$$\mathbf{n}_1 = \begin{bmatrix} 3,081 \\ 2,700 \end{bmatrix}$$

Consider next the service requirements generated by program $P_2$ (Table 15-6). The techniques described above should be used to verify that

$$\mathbf{s}_2 = \begin{bmatrix} 1,035 \\ 765 \\ 495 \end{bmatrix}$$

while

$$\mathbf{n}_2 = \begin{bmatrix} 405 \\ 2,346 \end{bmatrix}$$

**Table 15-6** Projected Volume of Ancillary and Stay-Specific Services by Program Area

| Program and Diagnosis | Volume of Ancillary Services (in Units) | | | Volume of Stay-Specific Services (in Days) | |
|---|---|---|---|---|---|
| | $S_1$ | $S_2$ | $S_3$ | $N_1$ | $N_2$ |
| Program $P_1$: | | | | | |
| $M_1$ | 60 | 300 | 90 | 2,100 | 0 |
| $M_2$ | 270 | 540 | 210 | 981 | 2,700 |
| Subtotal $(P_1)$ | 330 | 840 | 300 | 3,081 | 2,700 |
| Program $P_2$: | | | | | |
| $M_3$ | 900 | 675 | 450 | 0 | 1,800 |
| $M_4$ | 135 | 90 | 45 | 405 | 546 |
| Subtotal $(P_2)$ | 1,035 | 765 | 495 | 405 | 2,346 |

As seen earlier, the standard volume of care symbolized by $S_{ik}$ and $N_{ir}$ represent the normative amount of service $k$ and the normative number of days of care in nursing department $r$ that should be provided to a patient presenting diagnosis $i$ and requiring the component of care. We may use the average amount of each ancillary service and the average length of stay in department $r$ to estimate $S_{ik}$ and $N_{ir}$ respectively. It is important to note, however, that the mean rates of providing ancillary and stay-specific services provide the basis for estimating only a single volume of service. Since the mean rate of use is only one measure of the distributional properties associated with each component of care demanded by the program area, it is quite possible for the actual rate of production to differ from the expected or mean rate of production. As a result, the derivation of the operational budget for the program area requires the estimation of various levels of activity and the incorporation of a methodology by which each level of activity may be evaluated.

In the development of a flexible budget, the variation or dispersion surrounding the mean constitutes a reasonable vehicle by which various levels of activity may be predicted and evaluated statistically. As implied above, if there are differences in case severity, physician characteristics, and patient characteristics such as age, sex, etc., variation might be expected in providing each component of hospital output while controlling for diagnosis.

Assuming that $S_{ik}$ and $N_{ir}$ are distributed normally and that the estimates of $\rho$ as well as the distribution of patients by diagnosis and service requirements are accurate, the low and high rates of providing each ancillary service may be projected. Using general notation, let

$$
\mathbf{S}_g = \begin{bmatrix} S_{11} & \cdots & S_{1k} & \cdots & S_{1x} \\ \vdots & & \vdots & & \vdots \\ S_{i1} & \cdots & S_{ik} & \cdots & S_{ix} \\ \vdots & & \vdots & & \vdots \\ S_{z1} & \cdots & S_{zk} & \cdots & S_{zx} \end{bmatrix}
$$

and

$$
\sigma_g = 1.96 \begin{bmatrix} \sigma_{11} & \cdots & \sigma_{1k} & \cdots & \sigma_{1x} \\ \vdots & & \vdots & & \vdots \\ \sigma_{i1} & \cdots & \sigma_{ik} & \cdots & \sigma_{ix} \\ \vdots & & \vdots & & \vdots \\ \sigma_{z1} & \cdots & \sigma_{zk} & \cdots & \sigma_{zx} \end{bmatrix}
$$

where $\sigma_{ik}$ represents the standard deviation of the distribution of the variable $S_{ik}$. In turn, the matrices formed by

$$
\mathbf{G}_g = \mathbf{S}_g - \sigma_g \tag{15.3.1}
$$

and

$$
\mathbf{H}_g = \mathbf{S}_g + \sigma_g \tag{15.3.2}
$$

may be used in estimating the high and low rates of providing services $S_1, \cdots,$ $S_i, \cdots, S_k$ to patients associated with program $g$. A similar operation yields the high and low number of expected patient days of care by diagnosis and by department. The resulting matrices are then employed as demonstrated to obtain the high and low predictions of producing these components of hospital output.

### 15.5.4 Estimation of Resource Requirements

As seen earlier, the production of each service in the sets $S$ and $N$ require the use of capital, labor, and consumable supplies. When developing the operating budget for the program, the focus of the analysis is on estimating personnel requirements by type of labor and supply requirements by type of supply item. As a result, if it is assumed that the stock of equipment is constant, the major objective is to estimate the standard amount of labor and consumable supplies that should be used in providing a unit of each element of the sets $S$, $N$, and, to a lesser extent, *AGS*.

One of the primary functions of the coefficients that reflect the resource requirements per unit of service is to translate the expected service mix into a forecast of the total amount of labor and consumable supplies that will be required to provide care to patients associated with the program area. The unit resource coefficients should reflect standards attainable through efficient operations. When resource coefficients are expressed in terms of attainable standards, employees are motivated to achieve stated productivity goals since the standard represents a reasonable future performance rather than an ideal goal or an objective based solely on past performance.

In general, the approach in estimating resource requirements may be expressed in the form

$$\begin{bmatrix} \text{Estimated} \\ \text{Resource} \\ \text{Requirements} \end{bmatrix} = \begin{bmatrix} \text{Projected} \\ \text{Volume of} \\ \text{Service} \end{bmatrix} \times \begin{bmatrix} \text{Standard Resource} \\ \text{Requirements Per} \\ \text{Unit of Service} \end{bmatrix}$$

In the following, assume that the labor employed by the hospital is grouped into the categories represented by the set $L = \{L_1, \cdots, L_j, \cdots, L_y\}$. The labor category $L_j$ may consist of laboratory technicians or registered nurses. Similarly, assume that the consumable supplies are grouped into several categories represented by the set $R = \{R_1, \cdots, R_q, \cdots, R_w\}$. For example, the supply category $R_q$ may consist of bandages, oxygen, or blood. The objective, then, is to estimate the amount of labor and consumable supplies, by type of resource, required to provide the anticipated volume of service.

For illustration, suppose that the hospital employs labor of type $L_1$, $L_2$, and $L_3$ as well as consumable supplies of type $R_1$ and $R_2$ in providing ancillary and stay-specific services. Suppose also that the coefficients in Table 15-7 represent the amount of resources required on each occasion that each of the services is provided. In this table, let

$SMH_j$ represent the standard staff hours of type $j$ labor required to produce a *unit* of service or a day of care and

$SSR_q$ represent the standard quantity of supply item $q$ needed to produce a *unit* of service or a day of care.

This table shows that 2.0 standard hours of type $L_1$ labor are required for each unit of service $S_3$ provided by the hospital. Similarly, a standard supply requirement of 7.0 units of supply item 1 is needed on each occasion that ancillary service $S_3$ is provided. The other entries are interpreted in similar fashion.

To illustrate this general approach, recall that program $P_1$ is expected to require 330, 840, and 300 units of ancillary services $S_1$, $S_2$, and $S_3$, respectively. As seen in Table 15-7, 1.0, 0.0, and 2.0 hours of type $L_1$ labor are needed on each occasion that the hospital provides ancillary services $S_1$, $S_2$, and $S_3$, respectively. As a result, the number of hours of type $L_1$ labor to provide ancillary services in support of program $P_1$ is given by

**Table 15-7** Standard Hours and Supply Requirements per Unit of Service

| Service Component | Standard Resource Requirement | | | | |
| --- | --- | --- | --- | --- | --- |
| | Standard Staff Hours | | | Standard Supply Requirements | |
| | $SMH_1$ | $SMH_2$ | $SMH_3$ | $SSR_1$ | $SSR_2$ |
| Ancillary Service | | | | | |
| $S_1$ | 1.0 | 0.0 | 2.0 | 0.0 | 3.5 |
| $S_2$ | 0.0 | 1.5 | 0.0 | 1.0 | 8.2 |
| $S_3$ | 2.0 | 2.5 | 2.6 | 7.0 | 3.6 |
| Stay-Specific Service | | | | | |
| $N_1$ | 1.8 | 2.9 | 4.0 | 0.0 | 2.1 |
| $N_2$ | 2.5 | 3.6 | 3.1 | 2.0 | 0.0 |

$$330(1.0) + 840(0) + 300(2.0) = 930$$

staff hours.

Referring to Table 15-7, we find that the coefficients in the first three columns may be used to form the matrix

$$\mathbf{L} = \begin{bmatrix} 1.0 & 0.0 & 2.0 \\ 0.0 & 1.5 & 0.0 \\ 2.0 & 2.5 & 2.6 \\ \hline 1.8 & 2.9 & 4.0 \\ 2.5 & 3.6 & 3.1 \end{bmatrix} = \begin{bmatrix} \mathbf{L}_a \\ \text{---} \\ \mathbf{L}_s \end{bmatrix}$$

where the submatrix $\mathbf{L}_a$ contains the standard staff hours, by type of labor, involved in providing the set of ancillary services while the submatrix $\mathbf{L}_s$ contains the standard hours required to provide stay-specific services in the two nursing departments. We may employ the vectors $\mathbf{s}_1$ and $\mathbf{s}_2$ to form the matrix

$$\mathbf{S} = \begin{bmatrix} 330 & 840 & 300 \\ \hline 1{,}035 & 765 & 495 \end{bmatrix} = \begin{bmatrix} \mathbf{s}_1' \\ \text{---} \\ \mathbf{s}_2' \end{bmatrix}$$

Consequently, the hours, by type of labor, that management expects to employ in providing ancillary services to patients comprising the two program areas are given by

$$\hat{\mathbf{L}}_a = \mathbf{S}\mathbf{L}_a \qquad (15.4)$$

$$= \begin{bmatrix} 330 & 840 & 800 \\ 1{,}035 & 765 & 495 \end{bmatrix} \begin{bmatrix} 1.0 & 0.0 & 2.0 \\ 0.0 & 1.5 & 0.0 \\ 2.0 & 2.5 & 2.6 \end{bmatrix}$$

$$= \begin{bmatrix} 930 & 2{,}010 & 1{,}440 \\ 2{,}025 & 2{,}385 & 3{,}357 \end{bmatrix}$$

These calculations indicate that 930, 2,010, and 1,440 hours of labor of type $L_1$, $L_2$, and $L_3$, respectively, will be required by program $P_1$. Similarly, the elements in the second row of $\hat{\mathbf{L}}_a$ indicate that 2,025, 2,385, and 3,357 hours of labor of type $L_1$, $L_2$, $L_3$, respectively, will be needed to provide ancillary services to patients in program $P_2$.

A similar approach may be used when estimating the staff hours required to provide stay-specific services to patients associated with the two program areas. In this case, we let,

$$\mathbf{N} = \begin{bmatrix} 3{,}081 & 2{,}700 \\ \hline 405 & 2{,}346 \end{bmatrix} = \begin{bmatrix} \mathbf{n}_1' \\ \hline \mathbf{n}_2' \end{bmatrix}$$

and, as a result

$$\hat{\mathbf{L}}_s = \mathbf{N}\mathbf{L}_s \qquad (15.5)$$

$$= \begin{bmatrix} 12{,}295.8 & 18{,}654.9 & 20{,}694.0 \\ 6{,}594.0 & 9{,}620.1 & 8{,}892.6 \end{bmatrix}$$

As before, the elements in the first row of $\hat{\mathbf{L}}_s$ represent the personnel requirements, by type of labor, of program $P_1$ and the elements in the second row correspond to the staffing estimates, by type of labor, of program $P_2$.

At this point in the analysis, we may determine the quantity and composition of staff hours, by type of labor, required to provide ancillary *and* stay-specific services to patients associated with the two programs by

$$\hat{\mathbf{L}} = \hat{\mathbf{L}}_a + \hat{\mathbf{L}}_s \qquad (15.6)$$

In terms of our example, we find that

$$
\hat{\mathbf{L}} = \begin{bmatrix} 930 & 2,010 & 1,440 \\ 2,025 & 2,385 & 3,357 \end{bmatrix} + \begin{bmatrix} 12,295.8 & 18,654.9 & 20,694.0 \\ 6,594.0 & 9,620.1 & 8,892.6 \end{bmatrix}
$$

$$
= \begin{bmatrix} 13,225.8 & 20,664.9 & 22,134.0 \\ 8,619.0 & 12,005.1 & 12,249.6 \end{bmatrix}
$$

The elements in the first row of $\hat{\mathbf{L}}$ indicate that 13,225.8, 20,664.9, and 22,134.0 hours of labor of type $L_1$, $L_2$, and $L_3$, respectively, will be required to provide ancillary and stay-specific services to patients in program $P_1$. Similarly, the elements in the second row of the matrix refer to the personnel required to provide ancillary and stay-specific services in program $P_2$.

Consider next the projection concerning the quantity and composition of supplies required to provide service to the two program areas. In this case, we simply extract the coefficients in the last two columns of Table 15-7 and form the matrix

$$
\mathbf{R} = \begin{bmatrix} 0.0 & 3.5 \\ 1.0 & 8.2 \\ 7.0 & 3.6 \\ \hline 0.0 & 2.1 \\ 2.0 & 0.0 \end{bmatrix} = \begin{bmatrix} \mathbf{R}_a \\ \hline \mathbf{R}_s \end{bmatrix}
$$

Consequently, we find that

$$
\hat{\mathbf{R}}_a = \mathbf{S}\mathbf{R}_a \tag{15.7}
$$

$$
= \begin{bmatrix} 2,940 & 9,123.0 \\ 4,230 & 11,677.5 \end{bmatrix}
$$

which implies that 2,940 and 9,123 units of consumable supply $R_1$ and $R_2$, respectively, will be needed to provide ancillary services $S_1$, $S_2$, and $S_3$, to patients associated with program $P_1$. Similarly, the elements in the second row of $\hat{\mathbf{R}}_a$ indicate the quantity and composition of supplies required to provide ancillary services $S_1$, $S_2$, and $S_3$ for program $P_2$.

Also notice that the expression

$$\hat{\mathbf{R}}_s = \mathbf{N}\mathbf{R}_s \qquad (15.8.1)$$

yields the quantity and composition of consumable supplies necessary to provide stay-specific services for the two program areas. Returning to our numeric example, it can be verified that

$$\hat{\mathbf{R}}_s = \begin{bmatrix} 5{,}400.0 & 6{,}470.1 \\ 4{,}692.0 & 850.5 \end{bmatrix}$$

As before, the elements in the first row of $\hat{\mathbf{R}}_s$ pertain to program $P_1$, while those in the second row represent the supply requirements associated with stay-specific services for the program $P_2$.

Finally, the quantity and composition of consumable supplies for ancillary and stay-specific services in the two program areas are given by

$$\hat{\mathbf{R}} = \hat{\mathbf{R}}_a + \hat{\mathbf{R}}_s \qquad (15.8.2)$$

In terms of our example, we find that

$$\hat{\mathbf{R}} = \begin{bmatrix} 8{,}340.0 & 15{,}593.1 \\ 8{,}922.0 & 12{,}528.0 \end{bmatrix}$$

For purposes of future reference, the projections developed in this section are summarized in Table 15-8.

## 15.6 LABOR AND SUPPLY COSTS OF THE PROGRAM AREA

The expense budget for the program area is derived by simply multiplying the estimated resource requirements by standard factor prices that, for purposes here, may be defined as the hourly wage that management expects to pay each group of hospital employees and the prices of consumable supplies expected to prevail during the budget period. In this case, the standard labor costs may be found by

$$\begin{bmatrix} \text{Standard} \\ \text{Labor Cost} \end{bmatrix} = \begin{bmatrix} \text{Projected} \\ \text{Number of} \\ \text{Hours} \end{bmatrix} \times \begin{bmatrix} \text{Standard} \\ \text{Wage Rate} \end{bmatrix}$$

**Table 15-8** Estimated Resource Requirements for Programs $P_1$ and $P_2$

| Program and Dimension of Service | Total Standard Labor Hours | | | Standard Supply Requirements | |
|---|---|---|---|---|---|
| | $L_1$ (1) | $L_2$ (2) | $L_3$ (3) | $R$ (4) | $R_2$ (5) |
| *Program 1:* | | | | | |
| Ancillary services (1) | 930.0[1] | 2,010.0[1] | 1,440.0[1] | 2,940.0[4] | 9,123.0[4] |
| Stay-specific services (2) | 12,295.8[2] | 18,654.9[2] | 20,694.0[2] | 5,400.0[5] | 6,470.1[5] |
| (Subtotal) (3) | 13,225.8[3] | 20,664.9[3] | 22,134.0[3] | 8,340.0[6] | 15,593.1[6] |
| *Program 2:* | | | | | |
| Ancillary services (4) | 2,025.0[1] | 2,385.0[1] | 3,357.0[1] | 4,230.0[4] | 11,677.5[4] |
| Stay-specific services (5) | 6,594.0[2] | 9,620.1[2] | 8,892.6[2] | 4,692.0[5] | 850.5[5] |
| (Subtotal) (6) | 8,619.0[3] | 12,005.1[3] | 12,249.6[3] | 8,922.0[6] | 12,528.0[6] |
| Total | 21,844.8 | 32,670.0 | 34,383.6 | 17,262.0 | 28,121.1 |

[1] Value given by $\hat{L}_a = SL_a$
[2] Value given by $\hat{L}_s = NL_s$
[3] Value given by $\hat{L} = \hat{L}_a + \hat{L}_s$
[4] Value given by $\hat{R}_a = SR_a$
[5] Value given by $\hat{R}_s = NR_s$
[6] Value given by $\hat{R} = \hat{R}_a + \hat{R}_s$

while the process of projecting standard supply costs may be expressed in the form

$$\begin{bmatrix} \text{Standard} \\ \text{Supply Cost} \end{bmatrix} = \begin{bmatrix} \text{Projected} \\ \text{Use of} \\ \text{Supplies} \end{bmatrix} \times \begin{bmatrix} \text{Standard} \\ \text{Supply} \\ \text{Price} \end{bmatrix}$$

We consider next the set of factor prices expected to prevail during the budget period.

### 15.6.1 Standard Factor Prices

With respect to the standard hourly wage rate, it is assumed that the current money wage paid to employees in labor category $j$ will be adjusted during the budget period to reflect: (1) the general increase in consumer prices and (2) an increase in the *real* income of the labor group. The first component of the adjustment in the money wage serves only to maintain the real income of the labor group. Suppose we let $W$ represent the money wage paid and $CPI$ represent an appropriate consumer price index. In this case, the real wage, $W/CPI$, is held constant only if the rates of change in $W$ and the $CPI$ are equal. In this discussion, the symbol $\alpha$ represents the factor required to maintain a constant real wage. It also may be necessary to increase the real wage paid to employees in labor category $j$. The percentage increase in the real wage paid to these employees is represented by the symbol $\theta_j$. Using this notation, the standard wage paid to labor of type $L_j$ is given by

$$SWR_j = W_{jt}(1 + \alpha + \theta_j)$$

where

$W_{jt}$ = the current money wage of labor category $j$;
$SWR_j$ = the expected money wage of labor category $j$ that is expected to prevail during the budget period.

In a similar fashion, let $SSP_q$ represent the price the institution expects to pay for supply item $q$ during the budget period. In this case we find that

$$SSP_q = P_{qt}(1 + \beta_q)$$

where $P_{qt}$ represents the current price of supply item $q$ and $\beta_q$ correspond to the expected percentage change in the price of supply $R_q$.

Returning to the example, suppose that the standard hourly wage rates for labor of type $L_1, L_2$, and $L_3$ are \$7.70, \$11.50, and \$8.80, respectively and that the standard costs per unit of supply item $R_1$ and $R_2$ are \$7.20 and \$3.90, respectively. On the basis of these projections, management may translate the operational budgets of programs $P_1$ and $P_2$ into monetary terms as follows.

## 15.6.2 Labor Costs

Returning first to the labor costs of the two program areas, recall that

$$\hat{L}_a' = \begin{bmatrix} 930 & 2{,}025 \\ 2{,}010 & 2{,}385 \\ 1{,}440 & 3{,}357 \end{bmatrix} \quad \text{and} \quad \hat{L}_s' = \begin{bmatrix} 12{,}295.8 & 6{,}594.0 \\ 18{,}654.9 & 9{,}620.1 \\ 20{,}694.0 & 8{,}892.6 \end{bmatrix}$$

represent the personnel management expects to employ in providing ancillary and stay-specific services to patients in the two program areas. We now let

$$\mathbf{w}' = [\$7.70 \quad \$11.50 \quad \$8.80]$$

Observe that the elements of $\mathbf{w}'$ correspond to the wage rates expected to prevail during the budget period. As a result, we find that

$$\mathbf{c}'_l = \mathbf{w}' \,\hat{\mathbf{L}}'_a + \mathbf{w}' \,\hat{\mathbf{L}}'_s \tag{15.9}$$

yields the labor costs of providing ancillary and stay-specific services to the patient populations of the two programs. As can be verified, an application of Equation 15.9 to our numeric example yields

$$\mathbf{c}'_l = [\$7.70 \quad \$11.50 \quad \$8.80] \begin{bmatrix} 930.0 & 2{,}025.0 \\ 2{,}010.0 & 2{,}385.0 \\ 1{,}440.0 & 3{,}357.0 \end{bmatrix}$$

$$+ [\$7.70 \quad \$11.50 \quad \$8.80] \begin{bmatrix} 12{,}295.8 & 6{,}594.0 \\ 18{,}654.9 & 9{,}620.1 \\ 20{,}694.0 & 8{,}892.6 \end{bmatrix}$$

$$= [\$42{,}948.00 \quad \$72{,}561.60] + [\$491{,}316.21 \quad \$239{,}659.83]$$

$$= [\$534{,}264.21 \quad \$312{,}221.43]$$

These findings indicate that the expected costs of providing these services to the two program areas amount to \$534,264.21 and \$312,221.43, respectively. The elements of the vector-matrix product $\mathbf{w}'\hat{\mathbf{L}}'_a$ indicate that the expected labor costs for ancillary services in programs $P_1$ and $P_2$ are \$42,948.00 and \$72,561.60, respectively. Similarly, the elements of the vector-matrix product $\mathbf{w}'\hat{\mathbf{L}}'_s$ indicate that the expected labor costs of stay-specific services for patients in programs $P_1$ and $P_2$ are \$491,316.21 and \$239,659.83, respectively.

For purposes of internal control, it is desirable to estimate standard labor costs, by type of labor, of providing ancillary and stay-specific services to the patient population of a given program area. In this case, we employ the elements of the row vector $\mathbf{w}'$ to form the matrix

$$\mathbf{W} = \begin{bmatrix} \$7.70 & 0 & 0 \\ 0 & \$11.50 & 0 \\ 0 & 0 & \$8.80 \end{bmatrix}$$

The labor costs, by type of labor, may then be estimated by

$$\mathbf{C}_j^l = \mathbf{W}\hat{\mathbf{L}}_a' + \mathbf{W}\hat{\mathbf{L}}_s' \qquad (15.10)$$

Applying Equation 15.10 to our numeric example, we find that

$$\mathbf{C}_j^l = \begin{bmatrix} \$7.70 & 0 & 0 \\ 0 & \$11.50 & 0 \\ 0 & 0 & \$8.80 \end{bmatrix} \begin{bmatrix} 930 & 2,025 \\ 2,010 & 2,385 \\ 1,440 & 3,357 \end{bmatrix}$$

$$+ \begin{bmatrix} \$7.70 & 0 & 0 \\ 0 & \$11.50 & 0 \\ 0 & 0 & \$8.80 \end{bmatrix} \begin{bmatrix} 12,295.8 & 6,594.0 \\ 18,654.9 & 9,620.1 \\ 20,694.0 & 8,892.6 \end{bmatrix}$$

$$= \begin{bmatrix} \$7,161.00 & \$15,592.50 \\ 23,115.00 & 27,427.50 \\ 12,672.00 & 29,541.60 \end{bmatrix} + \begin{bmatrix} \$94,677.66 & \$50,773.80 \\ 214,531.35 & 110,631.15 \\ 182,107.20 & 78,254.88 \end{bmatrix}$$

$$= \begin{bmatrix} \$101,838.66 & \$66,366.30 \\ 237,646.35 & 138,058.65 \\ 194,779.20 & 107,796.48 \end{bmatrix}$$

These findings indicate that the costs of employing labor of type $L_1$, $L_2$, and $L_3$ to provide these services to program $P_1$ are expected to amount to \$101,838.66, \$237,646.35, and \$194,779.20, respectively. Similarly, the elements in the second column of $\mathbf{C}_j^l$ represent the expected costs of employing labor of type $L_1$, $L_2$, and $L_3$ for program $P_2$.

Consider next the product matrices $\mathbf{W}\hat{\mathbf{L}}'_a$ and $\mathbf{W}\hat{\mathbf{L}}'_s$. In this case, the elements in the first column represent the expected costs of employing labor, by type of worker, in providing ancillary and stay-specific services to patients associated with program $P_1$ respectively; similarly, the second column refers to the labor costs, by type of labor, for program $P_2$. These and the other cost estimates derived thus far in the analysis are summarized in Table 15-9.

## 15.6.3 Supply Costs

Consider next the costs of consumable supplies in providing patient care. Returning to our earlier work, we may summarize the assumptions concerning the standard supply prices as follows:

| Supply Item | Standard Price |
|---|---|
| $R_1$ | $7.20 |
| $R_2$ | $3.90 |

**Table 15-9** Summary of Labor Costs for Programs $P_1$ and $P_2$ by Type of Labor and Type of Service

| Component of Care and Program | Labor Costs | | | Total |
|---|---|---|---|---|
| | $L_1$ | $L_2$ | $L_3$ | Total |
| **Program $P_1$:** Ancillary services | $7,161.00[1] | $23,115.00[1] | $12,672.00[1] | $42,948.00[4] |
| Stay-specific services | 94,677.66[2] | 214,531.35[2] | 182,107.20[2] | 491,316.21[5] |
| Subtotal ($P_1$) | 101,838.66[3] | 237,646.35[3] | 194,779.20[3] | 534,264.21[6] |
| **Program $P_2$:** Ancillary services | 15,592.50[1] | 27,427.50[1] | 29,541.60[1] | $72,561.60[4] |
| Stay-specific services | 50,773.80[2] | 110,631.15[2] | 78,254.88[2] | 239,659.83[5] |
| Subtotal ($P_2$) | 66,366.30[3] | 138,058.65[3] | 107,796.48[3] | 312,221.43[6] |
| Total | 168,204.96 | 375,705.00 | 302,575.68 | 846,485.64 |

[1] Value appears in the product matrix $\mathbf{W}\hat{\mathbf{L}}'_a$
[2] Value appears in the product matrix $\mathbf{W}\hat{\mathbf{L}}'_s$
[3] Value appears in the matrix given by $\mathbf{W}\hat{\mathbf{L}}'_a + \mathbf{W}\hat{\mathbf{L}}'_s$
[4] Value appears in the vector-matrix product $\mathbf{w}'\hat{\mathbf{L}}'_a$
[5] Value appears in the vector-matrix product $\mathbf{w}'\hat{\mathbf{L}}'_s$
[6] Value given by $\mathbf{w}'\hat{\mathbf{L}}'_a + \mathbf{w}'\hat{\mathbf{L}}'_s$

In the following discussion, we let

$$\mathbf{p}' = [\$7.20 \quad \$3.90]$$

while

$$\mathbf{P} = \begin{bmatrix} \$7.20 & 0 \\ 0 & \$3.90 \end{bmatrix}$$

At this point, the similarities between the row vectors $\mathbf{w}'$ and $\mathbf{p}'$ as well as the matrices $\mathbf{W}$ and $\mathbf{P}$ should be obvious.

Similar to the earlier discussion, management may estimate the costs of consumable supplies by

$$\mathbf{c}_s' = \mathbf{p}'\hat{\mathbf{R}}_a' + \mathbf{p}'\hat{\mathbf{R}}_s' \tag{15.11}$$

The vector-matrix product $\mathbf{p}'\hat{\mathbf{R}}_a'$ yields the expected costs of using consumable supplies for ancillary services in each program area while the elements of $\mathbf{p}'\hat{\mathbf{R}}_s'$ represent the costs of consumable supplies for stay-specific services.

As in the discussion of labor costs, it is useful to estimate supply costs by type of consumable supply. In this case, we find that

$$\mathbf{C}_q^s = \mathbf{P}\hat{\mathbf{R}}_a' + \mathbf{P}\hat{\mathbf{R}}_s' \tag{15.12}$$

The coefficients of $\mathbf{P}\hat{\mathbf{R}}_a'$ and $\mathbf{P}\hat{\mathbf{R}}_s'$ represent the supply costs, by type of supply, for ancillary and stay-specific services to each program area, respectively. At this point, Equations 15.11 and 15.12 should be used to verify the results summarized in Table 15-10.

## 15.7 OVERHEAD AND DIRECT EQUIPMENT COSTS OF PROGRAM AREAS

Thus far this analysis has considered only the direct labor and supply costs of the program area. To determine the full program costs, however, it also is necessary to consider direct equipment and overhead expenses.

Consider first, the direct equipment costs of a program area. Suppose that capital equipment of type $E_1$, $E_2$, and $E_3$ is used exclusively in providing ancillary services $S_1$, $S_2$, and $S_3$, respectively, while equipment of type $E_4$ is used

**Table 15-10** Supply Expenses by Type of Supply Item for Programs $P_1$ and $P_2$

| Program and Component of Care | Consumable Supply Item | | Total |
|---|---|---|---|
| | $R_1$ | $R_2$ | |
| **Program $P_1$:** | | | |
| Ancillary services | $21,168.00[1] | $35,579.70[1] | $56,747.70[4] |
| Stay-specific services | 38,880.00[2] | 25,233.39[2] | 64,113.39[5] |
| Subtotal ($P_1$) | 60,048.00[3] | 60,813.09[3] | 120,861.09[6] |
| **Program $P_2$:** | | | |
| Ancillary services | 30,456.00[1] | 45,542.25[1] | 75,998.25[4] |
| Stay-specific services | 33,782.40[2] | 3,316.95[2] | 37,099.35[5] |
| Subtotal ($P_2$) | 64,238.40[3] | 48,859.20[3] | 113,097.60[6] |
| Total | 124,286.40 | 109,672.29 | 233,958.69 |

[1] Value appears in the product matrix $\mathbf{P\hat{R}_a'}$
[2] Value appears in the product matrix $\mathbf{P\hat{R}_s'}$
[3] Value appears in the matrix given by $\mathbf{P\hat{R}_a'} + \mathbf{P\hat{R}_s'}$
[4] Value appears in the vector-matrix product $\mathbf{p'\hat{R}_a'}$
[5] Value appears in the vector-matrix product $\mathbf{p'\hat{R}_s'}$
[6] Value given by $\mathbf{p'\hat{R}_a'} + \mathbf{p'\hat{R}_s'}$

in providing nursing service. Suppose further that the depreciation charges per unit of service are as follows:

| Equipment | Depreciation Charge* |
|---|---|
| $E_1$ | $4.50/unit $S_1$ |
| $E_2$ | $7.60/unit $S_2$ |
| $E_3$ | $2.75/unit $S_3$ |
| $E_4$ | $10.40/day of care |

In this case, the equipment cost of program $P_1$ is given by

$$\$4.50(330) + \$7.60(840) + \$2.75(300) + \$10.40(3{,}081 + 2{,}700) = \$68{,}816.40$$

while

$$\$4.50(1{,}035) + \$7.60(765) + \$2.75(495) + \$10.40(405 + 2{,}346) = \$40{,}443.15$$

* This assumes that the productivity method is used to calculate depreciation charges.

represents the direct equipment cost of program $P_2$. In these calculations, the values in parentheses were obtained from Table 15-6 and represent the program area's demand for each component of service.

Consider next the overhead component of the full cost of each program area. As in the earlier discussion, overhead costs may be viewed as the sum of the internal direct costs of the units that provide direct patient care and an equitable share of the external overhead that consists in large part of the cost of providing the general or support services required by the hospital.

As described previously, cost finding or cost analysis is a technique for allocating the cost of providing general or support services. Alternate methods of determining the amount of overhead assigned to a given program area also are considered. As before, the resources represented by overhead costs may be viewed as factor inputs that are used in providing services that earn revenue for the hospital. In this case, to determine the program's overhead cost, we might use

1. the overhead cost per hour of direct labor;
2. the overhead cost per unit of consumable supplies;
3. the overhead cost per dollar of direct labor, direct supply, or direct equipment cost; or
4. the overhead cost per dollar of direct cost.

After reviewing the budgets prepared for the general support centers, suppose that expected overhead costs are $888,984.00. Using the hours of direct labor as the basis of allocating the total overhead, we find that:

| | |
|---|---|
| Total overhead | $888,984.00 |
| ÷ Total direct labor | 88,898.40 |
| Overhead/hour of direct labor | $10/hour |

On the basis of these calculations, Table 15-8 demonstrates that

$$13,225.8 + 20,664.9 + 22,134$$

or 56,024.7 hours of direct labor are expected to be used in support of program $P_1$ while

$$8,619 + 12,005.1 + 12,249.6$$

or 32,873.7 hours are likely for program $P_2$. As a result, the overhead cost of $888,984.00 is allocated to programs $P_1$ and $P_2$ as follows

| Program | Program Overhead |
|---------|------------------|
| $P_1$ | $560,247.00 |
| $P_2$ | 328,737.00 |
| Total | 888,984.00 |

When the equipment and overhead cost projections are combined with the estimates of labor and supply expenses developed earlier, management may determine the anticipated full costs of each program area.

## 15.8 FULL PROGRAM COSTS

The financial budgets of programs $P_1$ and $P_2$ are summarized in Table 15-11. This table depicts the full costs of each of the programs as composed of direct labor, supply, and equipment expenses as well as an equitable share of the overhead associated with providing general support services. If the programs

**Table 15-11** Summary of Budget Projections for Programs $P_1$ and $P_2$

| Cost Component | Program Costs | | Total |
|----------------|---------------|----|-------|
| | $P_1$ | $P_2$ | |
| Labor: | | | |
| $L_1$ | $101,838.66 | $66,366.30 | $168,204.96 |
| $L_2$ | 237,646.35 | 138,058.65 | 375,705.00 |
| $L_3$ | 194,779.20 | 107,796.48 | 302,575.68 |
| Total Labor Cost | 534,264.21 | 312,221.43 | 846,485.64 |
| | | | |
| Consumable Supplies: | | | |
| $R_1$ | 60,048.00 | 64,238.40 | 124,286.40 |
| $R_2$ | 60,813.09 | 48,859.20 | 109,672.29 |
| Total Supply Cost | 120,861.09 | 113,097.60 | 233,958.69 |
| Total Labor and Supply Cost | 655,125.30 | 425,319.03 | 1,080,444.33 |
| | | | |
| Direct Equipment: | | | |
| $E_1$ | 1,485.00 | 4,657.50 | |
| $E_2$ | 6,384.00 | 5,814.00 | |
| $E_3$ | 825.00 | 1,361.25 | |
| $E_4$ | 60,122.40 | 28,610.40 | |
| Total Equipment cost | 68,816.40 | 40,443.15 | 109,259.55 |
| Overhead | 560,247.00 | 328,737.00 | 888,984.00 |
| Total | 1,284,188.70 | 794,499.18 | 2,078,687.88 |

are mutually exclusive and collectively exhaustive, the projected cost of hospital operations is given by the sum $1,284,188.70 + $794,499.18 or $2,078,687.88.

## 15.9 OBTAINING THE DATA

The data required for implementing the approach presented in this chapter are considerable but not prohibitive. Much of the information is available already in most hospitals. As an example, the wage and price information should be obtained readily from the fiscal services division and from the purchasing department. Similarly, information pertaining to the service mix required in the management of a particular morbidity may be obtained from the medical records of previous patients. However, a few comments regarding the retrieval of information from patients' medical records are in order.

If the medical record of each patient is not stored electronically (i.e., in a computerized medical record system), management may obtain the information from a sample of medical records that has been stratified so that the proportion of patients hospitalized with a given condition is the same as the corresponding proportion in the population from which the sample is drawn.

The problem of retrieving medical information is reduced greatly when the records are stored electronically. As an example of the many possible formats that might be designed for the typical record, we might devote the various fields as follows:

1. the first series to information identifying the patient;
2. the second series to patient-specific information such as age, sex, address, insurance status, etc.;
3. the third series to admission and discharge information such as date and hour of admission and discharge as well as the service into which the patient was admitted;
4. the fourth series to the primary and secondary admitting diagnoses as well as the primary discharge diagnosis;
5. the fifth series to information concerning the use of each service that may be classified by the department providing the service; and
6. the sixth series to information concerning the discharge status of the patient.

Organizing the medical record in this fashion permits examination of the medical records of an individual patient or of groups of patients who have been chosen by morbidity or nursing department. Such a system also is valuable in evaluating the use of a specific service (e.g., x-ray) by all patients irrespective of their presenting condition.

In estimating the relation between the provision of a given service and the resources required to produce that service, management frequently is forced to measure the amount of work and supplies involved in the production process. Among the various techniques of work measurement are: estimates based on expert opinion, averaging of historical data, logging, batching, time-motion analyses, and work sampling techniques. Each of these methods is described briefly.

Estimates of the resources required to produce a particular service may be obtained by seeking *expert opinion*. Under this approach, an expert, such as the department head or appropriate supervisor, is asked to list, in detail, the number of hours of each type of labor and the number of units of each type of supply required to produce a unit of each identifiable service. The major advantage of this approach is its simplicity and the ease with which estimates may be obtained; the major disadvantage is that it does not provide a basis on which estimates may be verified or subjected to statistical analysis.

By *averaging historical data*, the number of staff hours by type of labor and the amount of supplies used in providing each service are depicted. The major advantages of this approach are that the calculations do not require an understanding of sophisticated mathematical techniques and the results are easily understood; the major disadvantage is that it may foster a perpetuation of past inefficiencies or errors. If the historical information reflects inefficient production processes, the resulting averages also will reflect existing inefficiencies. Since this approach does not force management to evaluate the process by which resources are combined and used in the production process, simple averaging is not amenable to improving the efficiency of hospital operations.

A responsible employee or the individual providing the service may be required to *log* the amount of time by type of labor and the number of units of consumable resource by type of supply that were expended in producing a given procedure during a specified period. The obvious advantage of such an approach is that the resulting data are subject to verification and statistical analysis. However, the estimates will reflect current operational activity as well as any inefficiencies that might have existed previously. As a result, this approach is subject to the same criticisms as apply to the averaging method. Moreover, it is important to note that the validity of the resulting data depend, to a significant extent, on the accuracy with which information is recorded—a consideration that also may be a disadvantage.

When the *batching* process is used, a known number of work units are assigned to an individual and the time required to perform the assigned work is recorded. On the basis of the time required to complete the batch, an average time per unit of work may be obtained. Unfortunately, the approach is not particularly appropriate for the measurement of consumable supplies.

As an example of *time-and-motion* studies and *work sampling*, nursing activities such as counting narcotics, dispensing medication, initiating intravenous solutions, and monitoring vital signs on a given ward are identified and the amount of time to perform each is recorded. Frequently, the time required to perform each activity is recorded by an external observer, which may be the major disadvantage. The observer may record information incorrectly, fail to observe all activities, or influence the rate at which each activity is performed. Thus, the possibility of observer bias may cast doubt on the results obtained from the time-and-motion or work sampling techniques of calculating information concerning the resources required to perform a series or a set of related tasks.

---

**ADDITIONAL READINGS***

Bently, J. and P. Butler. "Case Measures/Diagnosis Related Groups," paper presented at the AHA/CHA Conference, Montreal, July 31, 1980.

Goodisman, L. D. and T. Trompeter. "Hospital Case Mix and Average Charge per Case: an Initial Study." *Health Services Research,* vol. 14, no. 1, Spring, 1979, pp. 44–55.

MacDonald, L. and L. Reuter. "A Patient Specific Approach to Cost Accounting." *Health Services Research,* 102, Summer 1973.

Fetter, R. B., R. Mills, D. C. Riedel and J. D. Thompson. "The Application of Diagnostic Specific Cost Profiles to Cost and Reimbursement Control in Hospitals." *Journal of Medical Systems* 1(2): 137, Nov., 1977.

Fetter, R. B., J. D. Thompson and R. Mills. "A System For Cost and Reimbursement Control in Hospitals." *The Yale Journal of Biology and Medicine* 49(2): 123, May 1976.

Thompson, J., R. Averill and R. Fetter. "Planning, Budgeting, and Controlling—One Look at the Future: Case-mix Cost Accounting." *Health Services Research* 14(2): 111, Summer 1979.

Thompson, J. D., R. B. Fetter and C. D. Mross. "Case Mix and Resource Use." *Inquiry* 12 (4): 300, Dec. 1975.

Mills, R., R. B. Fetter, D. C. Riedel and R. F. Averill. "AUTOGRP: An Interactive Computer System for the Analysis of Health Care Data." *Medical Care* 14(7): 603, July 1976.

---

* These readings would also be helpful as additional resources for Chapters 16 and 18.

# Chapter 16
# Responsibility Budgeting

## Objectives

After completing this chapter you should be able to:

1. Understand the relationship between the work load of the department and the demands for service from the program areas.
2. Translate the anticipated work load into the operational budget of the responsibility center.
3. Prepare the financial budget for the responsibility center.

## 16.1 INTRODUCTION

As suggested in Chapter 15, using the patient and related condition permits management to ensure that the goals of the responsibility center, the program area, and the hospital enterprise are consistent and mutually supportive. To understand the relationship between the program area and the responsibility center, assume that department $D_3$ provides ancillary services $S_1$, $S_2$, and $S_3$ while, as before, stay-specific services are provided in nursing departments $D_1$ and $D_2$. Table 16-1 summarizes Table 15-6. As seen in the bottom row of Table 16-1, the patient population is expected to require 1,365, 1,605, and 795 units of ancillary service $S_1$, $S_2$, and $S_3$, respectively. Assuming that programs $P_1$ and $P_2$ not only are mutually exclusive but also are collectively exhaustive, the sum of the program demands for ancillary services represents the anticipated work load of department $D_3$. Similarly, the data suggest that to support the anticipated activity in the various program areas, nursing department $D_1$ is expected to provide 3,486 days of care and nursing department $D_2$ 5,046 days. The anticipated work load of each departmental unit thus is dependent on the rate of

**Table 16-1**  Summary of Expected Quantity and Composition of Services Required by Anticipated Patient Population

| Program Area | Volume of Ancillary Services (in units) | | | Volume of Stay-Specific Services (in days of care) | |
|---|---|---|---|---|---|
| | $S_1$ | $S_2$ | $S_3$ | $N_1$ | $N_2$ |
| $P_1$ | 330 | 840 | 300 | 3,081 | 2,700 |
| $P_2$ | 1,035 | 765 | 495 | 405 | 2,346 |
| Departmental work load | 1,365 | 1,605 | 795 | 3,486 | 5,046 |

activity in the hospital's program areas. As a result, the departmental goal of satisfying projected work load requirements is consistent with the goals of the various program areas as well as the corporate objectives of the hospital.

Assume that the departmental unit and the responsibility center are synonymous. The objective is to develop budgets for those departments that provide ancillary and stay-specific services as well as an alternate frame of reference within which management might estimate the full costs of operating the organizational units that provide direct patient care.

## 16.2 OPERATIONAL BUDGET OF THE RESPONSIBILITY CENTER

The operational budgets of departments $D_1$, $D_2$, and $D_3$ are developed before estimating the financial resources required to sustain desired rates of activity. The operational budget of department $D_3$ is based on the resource coefficients in Table 16-2. The standard staff hours and standard supply requirements are identical to those in Table 15-7.

Similar to the approach used earlier, projections as to the resources needed to provide ancillary services $S_1$, $S_2$, and $S_3$ are developed by

$$\begin{bmatrix} \text{Estimated} \\ \text{Resource} \\ \text{Requirements} \end{bmatrix} = \begin{bmatrix} \text{Volume} \\ \text{of} \\ \text{Service} \end{bmatrix} \times \begin{bmatrix} \text{Standard Resource} \\ \text{Requirements Per} \\ \text{Unit of Service} \end{bmatrix}$$

In this case, we may represent the work load of department $D_3$ by the row vector

$$s'_3 = [1,365 \quad 1,605 \quad 795]$$

where the subscript now refers to the departmental unit. Concerning the standard resource requirements per unit of service, Table 16-2 suggests that we may form the matrix

$$\mathbf{I}_a = \begin{bmatrix} 1.0 & 0.0 & 2.0 & \vdots & 0.0 & 3.5 \\ 0.0 & 1.5 & 0.0 & \vdots & 1.0 & 8.2 \\ 2.0 & 2.5 & 2.6 & \vdots & 7.0 & 3.6 \end{bmatrix}$$

which has been partitioned to reflect the standard hours and standard supply requirements per unit of service. Employing $\mathbf{s}_3'$ and the matrix $\mathbf{I}_a$, we find that the resource requirements, by type of factor input, are given by

$$\mathbf{r}_3' = \mathbf{s}_3' \mathbf{I}_a \tag{16.1}$$

$$= [1{,}365 \quad 1{,}605 \quad 795] \begin{bmatrix} 1.0 & 0.0 & 2.0 & \vdots & 0.0 & 3.5 \\ 0.0 & 1.5 & 0.0 & \vdots & 1.0 & 8.2 \\ 2.0 & 2.5 & 2.6 & \vdots & 7.0 & 3.6 \end{bmatrix}$$

$$= [2{,}955 \quad 4{,}395 \quad 4{,}797 \quad \vdots \quad 7{,}170 \quad 20{,}800.5]$$

These calculations imply that 2,955, 4,395, and 4,797 hours of type $L_1$, $L_2$, and $L_3$ labor will be needed to produce the projected volume of ancillary services. Similarly, the last two elements of the row rector $\mathbf{r}_3'$ indicate that management expects to use 7,170 units of consumable supply $R_1$ and 20,800.5 units of consumable supply $R_2$.

We also might use a matrix of the form

$$\mathbf{S} = \begin{bmatrix} 1{,}365 & 0 & 0 \\ 0 & 1{,}605 & 0 \\ 0 & 0 & 795 \end{bmatrix}$$

to estimate the quantity of each resource required to sustain the expected rate of activity in the department. The diagonal elements of matrix $\mathbf{S}$ correspond to the volume of service $S_1$, $S_2$, and $S_3$ that is expected to be provided during the period. The resource requirements, by type of factor input and type of service, are given by

$$\mathbf{R}_3 = \mathbf{S} \mathbf{I}_a \tag{16.2}$$

**Table 16-2**  Standard Staff Hours and Standard Supply Requirements Per Unit of Service

| Service Component | Standard Staff Hours | | | Standard Supply Requirements | |
|---|---|---|---|---|---|
| | $SMH_1$ (1) | $SMH_2$ (2) | $SMH_3$ (3) | $SSR_1$ (4) | $SSR_2$ (5) |
| Ancillary service | | | | | |
| $S_1$ | 1.0 | 0.0 | 2.0 | 0.0 | 3.5 |
| $S_2$ | 0.0 | 1.5 | 0.0 | 1.0 | 8.2 |
| $S_3$ | 2.0 | 2.5 | 2.6 | 7.0 | 3.6 |
| Stay-specific service | | | | | |
| $N_1$ | 1.8 | 2.9 | 4.0 | 0.0 | 2.1 |
| $N_2$ | 2.5 | 3.6 | 3.1 | 2.0 | 0.0 |
| Standard factor price | $7.70 | $11.50 | $8.80 | $7.20 | $3.90 |

$$
= \begin{bmatrix} 1,365 & 0 & 0 \\ 0 & 1,605 & 0 \\ 0 & 0 & 795 \end{bmatrix} \begin{bmatrix} 1.0 & 0.0 & 2.0 & 0.0 & 3.5 \\ 0.0 & 1.5 & 0.0 & 1.0 & 8.2 \\ 2.0 & 2.5 & 2.6 & 7.0 & 3.6 \end{bmatrix}
$$

$$
= \begin{bmatrix} 1,365.0 & 0 & 2,370.0 & 0 & 4,777.5 \\ 0 & 2,407.5 & 0 & 1,605.0 & 13,161.0 \\ 1,590.0 & 1,987.5 & 2,067.0 & 5,565.0 & 2,862.0 \end{bmatrix}
$$

The rows of the matrix $R_3$ represent the resource requirements, by type of resource, for each service. For example, in providing 1,365 units of service $S_1$, we expect to use 1,365.0, 0, and 2,370.0 hours of labor of type $L_1, L_2,$ and $L_3,$ respectively, as well as 0 and 4,777.5 units of consumable supplies $R_1$ and $R_2,$ respectively.

Projections concerning the resource requirements of department $D_3$ are summarized in Table 16-3. The bottom row of the table is given by the vector-matrix product $s_3' I_a$ while the other entries correspond to the elements of the matrix $R_3$.

By analogy, the operational budget of nursing departments $D_1$ and $D_2$ may be developed as follows. The total number of hours of type $L_1, L_2,$ and $L_3$ labor as well as the quantity and composition of consumable supplies that management will need in these two units are given by

$$\mathbf{r}'_{1,2} = \mathbf{n}' \mathbf{I}_n \tag{16.3}$$

$$= [3{,}486 \quad 5{,}046] \begin{bmatrix} 1.8 & 2.9 & 4.0 & 0.0 & 2.1 \\ 2.5 & 3.6 & 3.1 & 2.0 & 0.0 \end{bmatrix}$$

$$= [18{,}889.8 \quad 28{,}275.0 \quad 29{,}586.6 \mid 10{,}092 \quad 7{,}320.6]$$

The elements of the row vector $\mathbf{n}'$ correspond to the anticipated work load of the two departments while the elements of the matrix $\mathbf{I}_n$ represent the standard amount of resources required to provide a day of care in nursing departments $D_1$ and $D_2$.

As to the amount of each type of resource that management expects to use in the departments providing stay-specific services, we may employ a matrix of the form

$$\mathbf{N} = \begin{bmatrix} 3{,}486 & 0 \\ 0 & 5{,}046 \end{bmatrix}$$

where the elements 3,486 and 5,046 represent the work load of departments $D_1$ and $D_2$, respectively. Accordingly, the product matrix

$$\boxed{\mathbf{R}_{1,2} = \mathbf{NI}_n \qquad\qquad (16.4)}$$

$$= \begin{bmatrix} 3{,}486 & 0 \\ 0 & 5{,}046 \end{bmatrix} \begin{bmatrix} 1.8 & 2.9 & 4.0 & 0.0 & 2.1 \\ 2.5 & 3.6 & 3.1 & 2.0 & 0.0 \end{bmatrix}$$

$$= \begin{bmatrix} 6{,}274.8 & 10{,}109.4 & 13{,}944.0 & 0 & 7{,}320.6 \\ 12{,}615.0 & 18{,}165.6 & 15{,}642.6 & 10{,}092 & 0 \end{bmatrix}$$

**Table 16-3** Projected Resource Requirements of Department $D_3$

| Resources | $S_1$ | $S_2$ | $S_3$ | Total |
|---|---|---|---|---|
| Hours of labor | | | | |
| $L_1$ | 1,365.0 | 0.0 | 1,590.0 | 2,955.0 |
| $L_2$ | 0.0 | 2,407.5 | 1,987.5 | 4,395.0 |
| $L_3$ | 2,730.0 | 0.0 | 2,067.0 | 4,797.0 |
| Units of supply | | | | |
| $R_1$ | 0.0 | 1,605.0 | 5,565.0 | 7,170.0 |
| $R_2$ | 4,777.5 | 13,161.0 | 2,862.0 | 20,800.5 |

represents the resources, by department and type of factor input, needed to provide the anticipated volume of stay-specific services. For example, to provide 3,486 days of care in department $D_1$, management expects to employ 6,274.8, 10,109.4, and 13,944.0 hours of labor of types $L_1$, $L_2$, and $L_3$, respectively, as well as 0 and 7,320.6 units of consumable supply $R_1$ and $R_2$, respectively.

The results of these calculations are summarized in Table 16-4. The entries in the bottom row were obtained by the vector-matrix product $\mathbf{n}'\mathbf{I}_n$, while the other entries correspond to the elements of the matrix $\mathbf{R}_n$ that were obtained by the product $\mathbf{NI}_n$.

At this point in the analysis, the operational budgets for departments $D_1$, $D_2$, and $D_3$ are complete. Of particular importance is the finding that the resource requirements derived using the department as the unit of analysis are identical to those derived when the program area was used as the unit of analysis. Regarding the estimates derived in this chapter, the total departmental demand for type $L_1$ labor is 21,844.8 hours (i.e., 2,955 + 18,889.8); type $L_2$ labor, 32,670 hours (4,395 + 28,275); type $L_3$ labor, 34,383.6 hours (4,797 + 29,586.6); supply item $R_1$ is 17,262 units (7,170 + 10,092), and supply item $R_2$ 28,121.1 units (20,800.5 + 7,320.6). These estimates are identical to those in the bottom row of Table 15-8. In this case, the observed equality is a mathematical necessity of the estimation procedures used in developing the forecasts of required resources. The equality also is a reflection of the presumption that the activities of the various departmental units must be consistent with and contribute to the attainment of the goals of the various program areas as well as the corporate objectives of the hospital enterprise.

## 16.3 FINANCIAL BUDGET OF THE RESPONSIBILITY CENTER

Once management has developed the projections for resource requirements, the supply expense budget and the wage and salary expense budget may be developed for each responsibility center. Similar to the discussion in the previous chapter, the operational budget is transformed into a financial budget simply by multiplying estimated resource requirements by corresponding factor prices.

In developing the financial budgets for departments $D_1$, $D_2$, and $D_3$, assume that, as before,

$$SWR_1 = \$7.70$$

$$SWR_2 = \$11.50$$

$$SWR_3 = \$8.80$$

represent the expected wage structure of the hospital while

$$SSP_1 = \$7.20$$

$$SSP_2 = \$3.90$$

correspond to the prices of consumable supply $R_1$ and $R_2$ that are expected to prevail during the coming period. The general approach in deriving the wage and salary expense budget of each responsibility center may be expressed in words as follows:

$$\begin{bmatrix} \text{Labor} \\ \text{Costs} \end{bmatrix} = \begin{bmatrix} \text{Estimated Labor} \\ \text{Requirements} \end{bmatrix} \times \begin{bmatrix} \text{Standard} \\ \text{Wage Rate} \end{bmatrix}$$

Similarly, the expression

$$\begin{bmatrix} \text{Supply} \\ \text{Expense} \end{bmatrix} = \begin{bmatrix} \text{Estimated Supply} \\ \text{Requirements} \end{bmatrix} \times \begin{bmatrix} \text{Standard} \\ \text{Resource} \\ \text{Price} \end{bmatrix}$$

represents the general approach for developing the supply expense budget of each responsibility center.

### 16.3.1 Financial Budget for Department $D_3$

Consider first the wage and salary expense budget for department $D_3$. In this case, we may employ the row vector

$$\mathbf{w}' = [\$7.70 \quad \$11.50 \quad \$8.80]$$

where each element corresponds to one of the expected wage rates. Similarly, we may extract data from Table 16-3 and form the matrix

$$T = \left[ \begin{array}{ccc} 1,365.0 & 0 & 1,590.0 \\ 0 & 2,407.5 & 1,987.5 \\ 2.730.0 & 0 & 2,067.0 \\ \hline 0 & 1,605.0 & 5,565.0 \\ 4,777.5 & 13,161.0 & 2,862.0 \end{array} \right] = \left[ \begin{array}{c} T_1 \\ \hline T_2 \end{array} \right]$$

**Table 16-4** Projected Resource Requirements of Nursing Departments $D_1$ and $D_2$

| Nursing Department | Number of Staff Hours | | | Number of Units | |
|---|---|---|---|---|---|
| | $L_1$ | $L_2$ | $L_3$ | $R_1$ | $R_2$ |
| $D_1$ | 6,274.8 | 10,109.4 | 13,944.0 | 0.0 | 7,320.6 |
| $D_2$ | 12,615.0 | 18,165.6 | 15,642.6 | 10.092.0 | 0.0 |
| Total | 18,889.8 | 28,275.0 | 29,586.6 | 10,092.0 | 7,320.6 |

where the submatrix $T_1$ contains the personnel requirements, by type of labor and ancillary service, while the elements of submatrix $T_2$ represent the quantity and composition of consumable supplies by type of service. We find that

$$c_{l3}' = w'T_1 \qquad (16.5)$$

$$= [\$7.70 \quad \$11.50 \quad \$8.80] \begin{bmatrix} 1,365.0 & 0 & 1,590.0 \\ 0 & 2,407.5 & 1,987.5 \\ 2,730.0 & 0 & 2,067.0 \end{bmatrix}$$

$$= [\$34,534.50 \quad \$27,686.25 \quad \$53,288.85]$$

represents the expected wage costs, by type of labor, for department $D_3$. These calculations suggest that the total costs of employing labor of type $L_1$ are expected to amount to $34,534.50. The other elements of $c_{l3}'$ are interpreted in a similar fashion.

It also is desirable to derive projections concerning departmental wage costs by type of labor and by type of service. In this case, we employ the elements of the row vector $w'$ to form the matrix

$$W = \begin{bmatrix} \$7.70 & 0 & 0 \\ 0 & \$11.50 & 0 \\ 0 & 0 & \$8.80 \end{bmatrix}$$

Referring to the wage and salary budget of department $D_3$, we find that

$$C_3^l = WT_1 \qquad (16.6)$$

$$= \begin{bmatrix} \$7.70 & 0 & 0 \\ 0 & \$11.50 & 0 \\ 0 & 0 & \$8.80 \end{bmatrix} \begin{bmatrix} 1,365.0 & 0 & 1,590.0 \\ 0 & 2,407.5 & 1,987.5 \\ 2,730.0 & 0 & 2,067.0 \end{bmatrix}$$

$$= \begin{bmatrix} \$10,510.50 & 0.00 & \$12,243.00 \\ 0.00 & \$27,686.25 & \$22,856.25 \\ \$24,024.00 & 0.00 & \$18,189.60 \end{bmatrix}$$

yields the labor costs by type of labor and service. For example, the elements of the first row indicate that costs of employing labor of type $L_1$ in providing service $S_1$, $S_2$, and $S_3$ are \$10,510.50, \$0.00, and \$12,243.00, respectively.

These findings are summarized in the first half of Table 16-5. The labor costs by type of service (i.e., \$34,534.50, \$27,686.25, and \$53,288.85) were obtained by the vector-matrix product $\mathbf{w}'\mathbf{T}_1$. The labor costs, by type of labor and type of service, correspond to the elements of the matrix $\mathbf{c}'_3$.

Consider next the supply expense budget for department $D_3$ and, as before, let

$$\mathbf{p}' = [\$7.20 \quad \$3.90]$$

---

**Table 16-5** Financial Budget for Department $D_3$

| Cost Component | Ancillary Service | | | Total |
|---|---|---|---|---|
| | $S_1$ | $S_2$ | $S_3$ | |
| Labor | | | | |
| $L_1$ | \$10,510.50 | \$0.00 | \$12,243.00 | \$22,753.50 |
| $L_2$ | 0.00 | 27,686.25 | 22,856.25 | 50,542.50 |
| $L_3$ | 24,024.00 | 0.00 | 18,189.60 | 42,213.60 |
| Labor cost | 34,534.50 | 27,686.25 | 53,288.85 | 115,509.60 |
| Supplies | | | | |
| $R_1$ | 0.00 | 11,556.00 | 40,068.00 | 51,624.00 |
| $R_2$ | 18,632.25 | 51,327.90 | 11,161.80 | 81,121.95 |
| Supply cost | 18,632.25 | 62,883.90 | 51,229.80 | 132,745.95 |
| Total cost | 53,166.75 | 90,570.15 | 104,518.65 | 248,255.55 |

Employing the submatrix $T_2$, which was defined earlier, we find that

$$c'_{s3} = p'T_2 \tag{16.7}$$

$$= [\$7.20 \quad \$3.90] \begin{bmatrix} 0 & 1,605.0 & 5,565.0 \\ 4,777.5 & 13,161.0 & 2,862.0 \end{bmatrix}$$

$$= [\$18,632.25 \quad \$62,883.90 \quad \$51,229.80]$$

yields a forecast of the supply cost, by type of consumable supply, for the department. In this example, the total supply costs of providing ancillary services $S_1$, $S_2$, and $S_3$ are expected to amount to $18,632.25, $62,883.90, and $51,229.80, respectively.

We now may use the elements of the row vector $p'$ and form the matrix

$$P = \begin{bmatrix} \$7.20 & 0 \\ 0 & \$3.90 \end{bmatrix}$$

Consequently, we find that

$$C_3^s = PT_1 \tag{16.8}$$

$$= \begin{bmatrix} \$7.20 & 0 \\ 0 & \$3.90 \end{bmatrix} \begin{bmatrix} 0 & 1,605.0 & 5,565.0 \\ 4,777.5 & 13,161.0 & 2,862.0 \end{bmatrix}$$

$$= \begin{bmatrix} \$0.00 & \$11,556.00 & \$40,068.00 \\ 18,632.25 & 51,327.90 & 11,161.80 \end{bmatrix}$$

represents the direct costs of using consumable supplies $R_1$ and $R_2$ in providing services $S_1$, $S_2$, and $S_3$. For example, the elements of the first row of matrix $C_3^s$ indicate that the costs of employing supplies of type $R_1$ in providing services $S_1$, $S_2$, and $S_3$ are $0.00, $11,556.00, and $40,068, respectively.

The supply expense budget for department $D_3$ is summarized in the bottom half of Table 16-5. As seen above, the total supply costs by type of service are given by the elements of the row vector $c'_{s3}$ while the direct costs by type of supply item and by type of service correspond to the elements of the matrix $C_3^s$.

## 16.3.2 Financial Budget for Departments $D_1$ and $D_2$

A similar approach may be used to develop the financial budget for departments responsible for stay-specific services. For example, data may be extracted from Table 16-4 to form the matrix

$$
\mathbf{H} = \begin{bmatrix} 6,274.8 & 12,615.0 \\ 10,109.4 & 18,165.6 \\ 13,944.0 & 15,642.6 \\ \hline 0 & 10.092.0 \\ 7,320.6 & 0 \end{bmatrix} = \begin{bmatrix} \mathbf{H}_1 \\ \hline \mathbf{H}_2 \end{bmatrix}
$$

where the submatrix $\mathbf{H}_1$ contains the personnel requirements of departments $D_1$ and $D_2$ and the submatrix $\mathbf{H}_2$ the quantity and composition of consumable supplies required by the two units.

Using the approach developed above, we find that

$$
\mathbf{c}_{l(2,3)} = \mathbf{w}'\mathbf{H}_1 \tag{16.9}
$$

yields the labor cost of the two nursing departments while the expression

$$
\mathbf{C}^l_{1,2} = \mathbf{W}\mathbf{H}_1 \tag{16.10}
$$

results in an estimate of the labor costs, by type of personnel, associated with departments $D_1$ and $D_2$. Similarly, the direct supply costs of the two departments may be estimated by

$$
\mathbf{C}^s_{1,2} = \mathbf{P}\mathbf{H}_2 \tag{16.11}
$$

while

$$
\mathbf{c}^s_{1,2} = \mathbf{P}\mathbf{H}_2 \tag{16.12}
$$

yields the supply expense budget, by type of supply item, for departments $D_1$ and $D_2$. At this point in the analysis, the approach outlined above should be used to verify the results in Table 16-6.

**Table 16-6** Financial Budget for Nursing Units $D_1$ and $D_2$

| Cost Component | Nursing Unit | | Total |
| | $D_1$ | $D_2$ | |
|---|---|---|---|
| Labor: | | | |
| $L_1$ | $48,315.96 | $97,135.50 | $145,451.46 |
| $L_2$ | 116,258.10 | 208,904.40 | 325,162.50 |
| $L_3$ | 122,707.20 | 137,654.88 | 260,362.08 |
| Labor cost | 287,281.26 | 443,694.78 | 730,976.04 |
| Supplies: | | | |
| $R_1$ | 0.00 | 72,662.40 | 72,662.40 |
| $R_2$ | 28,550.34 | 0.00 | 28,550.34 |
| Supply cost | 28,550.34 | 72,662.40 | 101,212.74 |
| Total cost | 315,831.60 | 516,357.18 | 832,188.78 |

## 16.4 EQUIPMENT AND OVERHEAD COSTS OF THE RESPONSIBILITY CENTER

In Chapter 15, it was assumed that the institution uses the productivity method of determining depreciation charges. Recall that equipment of type $E_1$, $E_2$, and $E_3$ is used exclusively in providing ancillary services $S_1$, $S_2$, and $S_3$, respectively, and equipment of type $E_4$ is used exclusively in the provision of stay-specific services. In addition, it was assumed that the depreciation charges per unit of service were as follows:

| Equipment | Depreciation Charge |
|---|---|
| $E_1$ | $4.50/unit of $S_1$ |
| $E_2$ | $7.60/unit of $S_2$ |
| $E_3$ | $2.75/unit of $S_3$ |
| $E_4$ | $10.40/days of care |

When viewed from the perspective of the responsibility center, the equipment costs of nursing departments $D_1$ and $D_2$ are found as follows:

| Nursing Department | Volume of Service | × | Depreciation Charge Per Unit | = | Equipment Cost |
|---|---|---|---|---|---|
| $D_1$ | 3,486 | | $10.40 | | $36,254.40 |
| $D_2$ | 5,046 | | 10.40 | | 52,478.40 |
| Total | | | | | 88,732.80 |

Similarly, the equipment costs of department $D_3$ may be obtained by

| Service | Volume of Service | × | Depreciation Charge Per Unit | = | Equipment Cost |
|---------|-------------------|---|------------------------------|---|----------------|
| $S_1$ | 1,365 | | $4.50 | | $6,142.50 |
| $S_2$ | 1,605 | | 7.60 | | 12,198.00 |
| $S_3$ | 795 | | 2.75 | | 2,186.25 |
| Total | | | | | 20,526.75 |

The data pertaining to the work load of each responsibility center were obtained from the bottom row of Table 16-1. The sum of the direct equipment costs of the responsibility centers ($88,732.80 + $20,526.75) is equal to the sum of the direct equipment cost ($109,259.55) assigned to the two program areas (see Table 15-11).

Concerning anticipated costs of providing general support services, management may use the techniques described in Chapter 7 to develop the financial budgets for the laundry, dietary, administrative services, housekeeping, medical records, and plant maintenance departments. As in the previous chapter, it is assumed that management expects the costs of providing general support services and the internal indirect costs will amount to $888,984.00. The objective in the following discussion is to allocate this sum among departments $D_1$, $D_2$, and $D_3$ as follows

$$\frac{\text{Allocated}}{\text{Overhead}} = \frac{\text{Overhead Cost}}{\text{per Direct Hour}} \times \frac{\text{Number of}}{\text{Direct Hours}}$$
$$\text{of Labor} \qquad \text{of Labor}$$

Tables 16-3 and 16-4 demonstrate that projections concerning the use of labor in each of the departments may be summarized as follows:

| Department | Expected Number of Staff Hours |
|------------|-------------------------------|
| $D_1$ | 30,328.2 |
| $D_2$ | 46,423.2 |
| $D_3$ | 12,147.0 |
| Total | 88,898.4 |

As a consequence, the overhead charges per hour of direct labor are, as before, $10 (see Section 15.7). Using this rate, the amount of overhead allocated to each department may be obtained as follows:

| Department | Expected Number of Staff Hours | × | Overhead Rate | = | Allocated Overhead |
|---|---|---|---|---|---|
| $D_3$ | 12,147.0 | | $10 | | $121,470.00 |
| $D_1$ | 30,328.2 | | 10 | | 303,282.00 |
| $D_2$ | 46,423.2 | | 10 | | 464,232.00 |
| Total | | | | | 888,984.00 |

When the costs calculated in this section are combined with the wage and salary expense budget and the supply expense budget developed earlier, management may determine the anticipated full costs of each departmental unit and the full costs of hospital operations.

## 16.5 FULL COSTS OF OPERATION

Table 16-7 summarizes the full costs of operating each of the departmental units and the full costs of the hospital enterprise. Several aspects of these summary data are worthy of note. Referring to Table 15-11, notice that for providing ancillary and stay-specific services to the patient population of programs $P_1$ and $P_2$, (1) projected labor and supply costs amounted to $1,080,444.33; (2) projected equipment costs were $109,259.55; (3) projected overhead totaled $888,984.00; and (4) the total expected cost was $2,078,687.88. In terms of Table 16-7, we find that (1) the projected labor and supply costs of operating departments $D_1$, $D_2$, and $D_3$ also amount to $1,080,444.33; (2) the sum of the projected equipment costs is $109,259.55; (3) projected overhead costs total $888,984.00; and (4) anticipated full costs are $2,078,687.88.

As a result, the financial requirements derived using the department as the unit of analysis are identical to those developed using the program area as the

**Table 16-7** Summary of Projected Full Costs of Departments $D_1$, $D_2$, and $D_3$

| Cost Component | Department | | | Total |
|---|---|---|---|---|
| | $D_1$ | $D_2$ | $D_3$ | |
| Labor | $287,281.26 | $443,694.78 | $115,509.60 | $846,485.64 |
| Supplies | 28,550.34 | 72,662.40 | 132,745.95 | 233,958.69 |
| Labor & supply cost | 315,831.60 | 516,357.18 | 248,255.55 | 1,080,444.33 |
| Equipment cost | 36,254.40 | 52,478.40 | 20,526.75 | 109,259.55 |
| Overhead cost | 303,282.00 | 464,232.00 | 121,470.00 | 888,984.00 |
| Total | 655,368.00 | 1,033,067.60 | 390,252.30 | 2,078,687.88 |

unit of analysis. As before, the equality is a mathematical necessity of the techniques used in deriving projections as to the financial resources required to sustain desired rates of operation. The equality also reflects the presumption that the allocation of financial resources among the various departmental units must be consistent with the goals of the program area as well as the corporate objective of the hospital enterprise.

## 16.6 RATE SETTING

The analysis now focuses on developing the prospective fee schedule for the institution. As seen earlier, the fee charged on each occasion that service is provided should reflect the full economic costs of operation, which are defined as the sum of

1. the direct labor costs
2. the direct supply costs
3. the direct equipment costs
4. an equitable share of the indirect or overhead costs

The objective of the following discussion is to develop the fee schedule for the set of ancillary services represented by $S_1$, $S_2$, and $S_3$. It should be noted, however, that this general approach also can be used to develop fees for stay-specific services.

### 16.6.1 Direct Costs

The fees charged by the institution must reflect the direct costs of using labor, consumable supplies, and capital equipment in providing service. Referring first to the direct labor and supply cost of providing units of service $S_1$, $S_2$, and $S_3$, the transpose of the matrix $\mathbf{I}_a$ is given by

$$\mathbf{I}'_a = \begin{bmatrix} 1.0 & 0.0 & 2.0 \\ 0.0 & 1.5 & 2.5 \\ 2.0 & 0.0 & 2.6 \\ 0.0 & 1.0 & 7.0 \\ 3.5 & 8.2 & 3.6 \end{bmatrix}$$

where each column represents the standard quantity of resources required to provide a unit of one service. We now let

$$\mathbf{f}' = [\$7.70 \quad \$11.50 \quad \$8.80 \quad \$7.20 \quad \$3.90]$$

where each element corresponds to one of the standard factor prices. Consequently, the direct labor and supply cost per unit of service is given by

$$\mathbf{c}'_p = \mathbf{f}'\mathbf{I}'_a$$

$$= [\$38.95 \quad \$56.43 \quad \$131.47]$$

These findings show that the direct labor and supply costs for each unit of $S_1$, $S_2$, and $S_3$ amount to $38.95, $56.43, and $131.47, respectively.

These results, when coupled with the direct equipment costs calculated earlier, allow us to summarize the direct costs per unit of service. In this example,

| Service | Direct Labor & Supply Costs | + | Direct Equipment Costs | = | Direct Cost Per Unit |
|---------|-----------------------------|---|------------------------|---|----------------------|
| $S_1$ | $38.95 | | $4.50 | | $43.45 |
| $S_2$ | 56.43 | | 7.60 | | 64.03 |
| $S_3$ | 131.47 | | 2.75 | | 134.22 |

the direct cost per unit of service $S_1$, $S_2$, and $S_3$ is given by the sum of the corresponding direct supply, labor, and equipment expenses.

## 16.6.2 Indirect or Overhead Costs

Section 16.4 noted that overhead charges amounted to $10 per hour of direct labor. As can be verified, the number of hours of direct labor per unit of service $S_1$, $S_2$, and $S_3$ may be calculated as follows:

| Type of Labor | Hours/Unit of Service | | |
|---------------|-------|-------|-------|
| | $S_1$ | $S_2$ | $S_3$ |
| $L_1$ | 1.0 | 0.0 | 2.0 |
| $L_2$ | 0.0 | 1.5 | 2.5 |
| $L_3$ | 2.0 | 0.0 | 2.6 |
| Total | 3.0 | 1.5 | 7.1 |

Consequently, the indirect costs of providing a unit of service $S_1$, $S_2$, and $S_3$ may be obtained as follows:

| Service | Direct Hours Per Unit | × | Overhead Cost Per Hour of Direct Labor | = | Indirect Cost Per Unit |
|---------|-----------------------|---|-----------------------------------------|---|------------------------|
| $S_1$ | 3.0 | | $10 | | $30 |
| $S_2$ | 1.5 | | 10 | | 15 |
| $S_3$ | 7.1 | | 10 | | 71 |

## 16.6.3 Full Cost Pricing

On the basis of the findings developed in Sections 16.6.1 and 16.6.2, the charge per unit of service may be derived as follows:

| Service | Direct Cost Per Unit | + | Indirect Cost Per Unit | = | Fee |
|---------|----------------------|---|------------------------|---|------|
| $S_1$ | $43.45 | | $30.00 | | $73.45 |
| $S_2$ | 64.03 | | 15.00 | | 79.03 |
| $S_3$ | 134.22 | | 71.00 | | 205.22 |

Using the notation developed earlier, recall that

$$s_3' = [1,365 \quad 1,605 \quad 795]$$

represents the work load of department $D_3$. Using the projected fee schedule developed above to form the column vector

$$\mathbf{r} = \begin{bmatrix} \$73.45 \\ 79.03 \\ 205.22 \end{bmatrix}$$

we find that revenue amounting to

$$y = s_3'\mathbf{r} \qquad\qquad \textbf{(16.13)}$$

$$= \$390,252.30$$

is generated by providing the set of services represented by the projected work load of department $D_3$. This department's revenue of $390,252.30 thus is just equal to the projected economic costs of operating the unit (Table 16-7). Consequently, when the fee schedule represented by column vector **r** is used, the operational activity of the department is expected to result in neither an economic profit nor an operating loss.

# Chapter 17

# Controlling the Program Area

## Objectives

After completing this chapter, you should be able to:

1. Define a cost variance.
2. Distinguish between a controllable and an uncontrollable cost.
3. Determine the total cost variance of the program area.
4. Partition the total variance in program costs into portions attributable to differences between the actual and expected
   a. diagnostic mix.
   b. service mix.
   c. resource mix.
   d. factor prices.
5. Prepare a summary report that depicts the performance of program areas of activity.

## 17.1 INTRODUCTION

The budget of the program area and the responsibility center may be viewed as the standard against which the current performance of those units can be compared. A comparison of actual performance with the expectations of management as expressed by the budget frequently will identify areas of activity where managerial attention and the implementation of remedial policies or plans of action are required. Thus, to discharge the responsibilities of monitoring, controlling, and evaluating operational activity effectively, the administrator must be provided with a set of timely and accurate management reports that depict differences between the current performance of the various aspects of hospital operations and the standard of performance as expressed by the budget.

When monitoring, evaluating, and controlling operational activity in a program area or responsibility center, it is necessary first to distinguish between controllable and uncontrollable costs. A component of cost may be regarded as controllable if the manager of a given *area of responsibility* is able to exert a *significant* influence over the expense.

That the concept of controllable cost always must refer to a specific center or area of responsibility is related to the notion that, when the organization is viewed as an entity, all costs may be viewed as controllable and influenced by some individual in the hospital. For example, senior management may reduce the costs of a nursing ward to zero simply by closing the unit. On the other hand, if the nursing unit is to continue operations, the labor costs may be modified by the discretionary actions of the director of nursing services or by the manager of the ward. Thus, the basic issue does not involve the identification of which cost items are controllable, since all costs may be influenced by the actions of some individual. Rather, management must identify cost components that are controllable in specific areas of responsibility since the internal control system must focus on these factors.

The second dimension of the definition of controllable costs emphasizes the extent to which they may be constrained by the director of a given area of responsibility. The extent to which costs are controlled by the discretionary actions of management always is a matter of degree. This is because only in rare cases does a single individual exert complete control over all factors which influence an item of cost. For example, direct labor expenses are cited frequently as an item of controllable cost. It is important to note that direct labor costs are the product not only of the quantity and mix of personnel in a given responsibility area, but also of the rates at which hospital employees are paid. Since departmental managers exert little or no control over the hospital's wage structure, they usually can influence only the quantity and mix of labor and the functions of individual employees. However, technological considerations frequently impose limitations on the extent to which management can influence even those elements.

Cost variance is defined as the difference between actual and budgeted costs. When evaluating unfavorable cost variances (i.e., actual costs in excess of budgeted costs), it is useful to identify portions of the difference that are attributable to: (1) the size and diagnostic mix of the patient population, (2) the quantity and composition of services provided to patients, (3) the use of real resources, and (4) the prices of factor inputs used by the hospital. It might be argued that the departmental manager can control factors that contribute to the third component. Conversely, the size and mix of the patient population depend more on the admitting policies of physicians than on the discretionary actions of line management. Similarly, it might be argued that the quantity and composition of services depends in large part on the prescribing pattern of the physicians, while the factor prices paid by the hospital are determined by the personnel department in accordance with market forces or the results of the collective bargaining process. Thus, line managers are able to redress only the portions of the cost variance that are attributable to the use of real resources. The purchasing department or a centralized purchasing agent usually is responsible for ensuring that resources are purchased at the most favorable prices and that the institution takes advantage of discounts offered by suppliers. Similarly, the remuneration paid to employees must conform with the wage and salary structure of the hospital. Obviously, deviations between actual and established wages or salaries may indicate a need to review and improve the functioning of the personnel department. Thus, when exceptions to the budget are partitioned to reflect the factors cited earlier, it is possible to identify the areas in which specific managers are responsible for developing and implementing remedial policies or actions designed to redress imbalances.

The development of the budget requires assumptions concerning such variables as the factor prices, diagnostic distribution, demand for service, medical technology, and other related elements that are likely to influence hospital activity during the budget period. Ultimately, the assumptions concerning these factors will prove to be correct or erroneous, and the expectations of management as expressed by the budget should be adjusted accordingly. If the budget projections are not adjusted to compensate for erroneous assumptions on variables over which management exerts little or no control, a comparison of actual performance with budget projections is likely to result in a distorted evaluation of the use of available resources. Conversely, comparing actual performance with a standard that has been adjusted to reflect the actual values of uncontrollable variables can identify deviations between current and expected performance that may be redressed by discretionary action of management.

## 17.2 AN OVERVIEW OF THE REPORTING SYSTEM

What types of reports should be provided to the various levels of management? Of obvious value to line managers is an analysis of the variance in the total costs of their responsibility centers. These managers should receive reports that indicate the portion of the cost variance attributable to controllable factors. The reports should be supplemented with an analysis of the extent to which real resources have been used as efficiently as originally planned after compensating for changes in patient load and other uncontrollable factors. Productivity reports, when coupled with a list of cost variances, provide the basis for identifying problem areas and specifying corrective actions.

Once the variance in the costs of all hospital departments has been analyzed, divisional unit directors should receive a monthly summary statement of the total variance in each of the departments for which they are responsible as well as the portions of the total variance attributable to factors over which line managers exert direct control and those over which they have little or no direct control. Summary information on efficiency of resource use also should be made available to the divisional directors on a monthly or quarterly basis.

Finally, senior management should be provided with a set of reports that depicts the performance of the departmental and divisional units as well as reports that portray the operational activities of the various program areas. Concerning the divisional and departmental units of the hospital, senior management receives summary information that quantifies:

1. the cost variances associated with each of the departmental and divisional units;
2. the portion of the cost variances which is the responsibility of an identifiable individual or group associated with the institution;
3. the extent to which departmental and divisional units are using resources as efficiently as planned after compensating for uncontrollable factors.

In addition, senior management should receive periodic reports on current operations of the program areas of activity as compared with budget projections. These reports should provide summary information regarding:

1. the extent to which the program costs differ from budget projections;
2. the portion of the total variance in program costs that is attributable to an identifiable individual or group associated with the institution;
3. the extent to which required services are being provided by the departmental units in support of the various program areas;
4. the extent to which resources allocated to the program areas are being used as efficiently as originally planned after compensating for uncontrollable factors.

The remaining sections of this chapter discuss the elements of the reporting system that pertain to monitoring, evaluating, and controlling program activity.

The primary objectives of this section are to: (1) develop techniques by which the total variance in program costs might be determined; (2) develop methods of partitioning the total variance in program costs into components that are attributable to the size and diagnostic mix of the patient population, the mix of services, the mix of real resources, and factor prices; (3) develop a set of control indexes; and (4) describe a set of reports that summarize operational activity in the program area.

## 17.3 THE TOTAL COST VARIANCE

A cost variance is the difference between actual and budgeted expenses. The total cost variance of a program area may be found by

$$
\begin{array}{c}\text{Total}\\\text{Cost Variance}\end{array} = \begin{array}{c}\text{Actual}\\\text{Program Costs}\end{array} - \begin{array}{c}\text{Budgeted}\\\text{Program Costs}\end{array}
$$

In turn, the actual costs of the program area may be determined by

$$
\begin{array}{c}\text{Actual}\\\text{Program}\\\text{Costs}\end{array} = \begin{bmatrix}\text{Volume of Service}\\\text{Provided to the}\\\text{Program Population}\end{bmatrix} \times \begin{bmatrix}\text{Actual Costs}\\\text{Per Unit}\\\text{of Service}\end{bmatrix}
$$

while

$$
\begin{array}{c}\text{Budgeted}\\\text{Program}\\\text{Costs}\end{array} = \begin{bmatrix}\text{Anticipated Volume}\\\text{of Service Required}\\\text{by the Program Population}\end{bmatrix} \times \begin{bmatrix}\text{Standard}\\\text{Costs Per}\\\text{Unit of Service}\end{bmatrix}
$$

represents a technique for estimating the program costs for the budget period.

For illustration, we again view the organizational structure of the hospital as consisting of a series of programs represented by $P_1, \cdots, P_g, \cdots, P_v$. Similar to the earlier discussion, each of the programs is defined as consisting of several subprograms and program elements that provide services to a set of well-defined conditions requiring hospital care. For purposes of future illustration, we consider a program, $P_g$, that is limited to providing care to patients presenting conditions $M_1$ and $M_2$. To simplify the example, assume that the patient population of the program area is hospitalized exclusively in nursing departments $D_1$ and $D_2$. We also assume that the ancillary services required by the program area are limited to laboratory service and surgical care, which we represent by $S_1$ and $S_2$, respectively.

To calculate the expected costs of the program area, we distribute the anticipated patient population of the program area in terms of diagnosis and service requirements. Table 17-1 presents the probabilities $P(S_k \cap M_i)$ and $P(D_r \cap M_i)$. Assuming that 10,000 patients were expected to receive treatment in the hospital, we find that

$$
\mathbf{P} = 10,000 \begin{bmatrix} .10 & .08 \\ .00 & .04 \\ \hline .30 & .20 \\ .07 & .12 \end{bmatrix} = \begin{bmatrix} 1{,}000 & 800 \\ 0 & 400 \\ \hline 3{,}000 & 2{,}000 \\ 700 & 1{,}200 \end{bmatrix}
$$

**Table 17-1** Probability Distribution of Patients, by Diagnosis and Service
Requirement

| | Diagnostic Condition | |
| --- | --- | --- |
| Component of Service | $M_1$ | $M_2$ |
| Ancillary services | | |
| $S_1$ | .10 | .08 |
| $S_2$ | .00 | .04 |
| Stay-specific services | | |
| $D_1$ | .30 | .20 |
| $D_2$ | .07 | .12 |

represents the distribution of the patient population in terms of diagnosis and
service requirements. The entries above the dotted lines correspond to the distribution of the patient population in terms of diagnosis and use of ancillary
services while those below the line involve the distribution in terms of diagnosis
and use of stay-specific services.

The results of these calculations are combined with the standard mix of services per patient in Table 17-2 to derive estimates concerning the anticipated
volume of services $S_1$, $S_2$, $N_1$, and $N_2$.

Using the approach introduced earlier, we find that

$$[1000 \quad 800] \begin{bmatrix} 2.5 \\ 4.0 \end{bmatrix} = 5{,}700 \text{ units}$$

$$[0 \quad 400] \begin{bmatrix} 0.0 \\ 1.0 \end{bmatrix} = 400 \text{ units}$$

represents the anticipated volume of ancillary services $S_1$ and $S_2$, respectively.
As a result, we may let

$$\mathbf{e}(\mathbf{s}_g) = \begin{bmatrix} 5{,}700 \\ 400 \end{bmatrix}$$

As can be verified, the anticipated number of days of care required in nursing
departments $D_1$ and $D_2$ may be summarized by letting

$$\mathbf{e}(\mathbf{n}_g) = \begin{bmatrix} 36{,}500 \\ 11{,}200 \end{bmatrix}$$

**Table 17-2** Standard Mix of Services per Patient

| | Component of Care | | | |
| --- | --- | --- | --- | --- |
| Condition | Laboratory Tests ($S_1$) | Operative Procedures ($S_2$) | Days of Care ($N_1$) | Days of Care ($N_2$) |
| $M_1$ | 2.5 | 0 | 6.5 | 5.2 |
| $M_2$ | 4.0 | 1.0 | 8.5 | 6.3 |

The next step in deriving expected program area expenditures is to estimate the standard unit costs of each component of care. These may be defined by

$$\begin{bmatrix} \text{Standard} \\ \text{Unit} \\ \text{Cost} \end{bmatrix} = \begin{bmatrix} \text{Standard} \\ \text{Factor} \\ \text{Price} \end{bmatrix} \times \begin{bmatrix} \text{Standard Resource} \\ \text{Requirements} \\ \text{Per Unit of Service} \end{bmatrix}$$

Using the notation developed earlier, we assume that the standard resource requirements per unit of service are represented by the coefficients in Table 17-3. The standard factor prices are given in the last column.

Referring to the approach outlined above, we form the vector

$$\mathbf{f}'_s = [\$10.00 \quad \$3.00 \quad \$6.00 \quad \$4.00 \mid \$4.00 \quad \$1.00 \quad \$2.00 \quad \$1.50]$$

where the first four elements correspond to the expected wage structure of the hospital and the remaining terms the supply prices expected to prevail during the budget period. We also may extract the coefficients representing the standard resource requirements and form the matrix

$$\mathbf{R} = \begin{bmatrix} 2.0 & 0.0 & 0.0 & 0.0 \\ 0.0 & 1.5 & 3.0 & 1.0 \\ 0.0 & 0.0 & 0.0 & 1.0 \\ 0.0 & 0.0 & 1.0 & 1.0 \\ \hline 2.0 & .5 & 0.0 & 0.0 \\ 0.0 & 3.0 & 6.0 & 0.0 \\ 0.0 & 2.0 & 0.0 & 2.5 \\ 0.0 & 0.0 & 0.0 & 4.0 \end{bmatrix} = \begin{bmatrix} \mathbf{R}_1 \\ \hline \mathbf{R}_2 \end{bmatrix}$$

**Table 17-3**  Standard Resource Requirement Per Unit of Service, by Type
of Service and by Type of Resource

| | Component of Care | | | | |
| Resource | Laboratory Tests $(S_1)$ | Operative Procedures $(S_2)$ | Days of Care $(N_1)$ | Days of Care $(N_2)$ | Standard Factor Price |
|---|---|---|---|---|---|
| Labor | | | | | |
| $SMH_1$ | 2.0 | 0.0 | 0.0 | 0.0 | $10.00 |
| $SMH_2$ | 0.0 | 1.5 | 3.0 | 1.0 | 3.00 |
| $SMH_3$ | 0.0 | 0.0 | 0.0 | 1.0 | 6.00 |
| $SMH_4$ | 0.0 | 0.0 | 1.0 | 1.0 | 4.00 |
| Supplies | | | | | |
| $SSR_1$ | 2.0 | .5 | 0.0 | 0.0 | 4.00 |
| $SSR_2$ | 0.0 | 3.0 | 6.0 | 0.0 | 1.00 |
| $SSR_3$ | 0.0 | 2.0 | 0.0 | 2.5 | 2.00 |
| $SSR_4$ | 0.0 | 0.0 | 0.0 | 4.0 | 1.50 |

where the entries above the dotted line correspond to standard staff hours, by
type of service and type of labor, while the coefficients below the dotted line
represent the standard supply requirements per unit of service. Consequently,
the standard unit cost of each component of care is given by

$$\mathbf{u}' = \mathbf{f}_s'\mathbf{R} = [\$28.00 \quad \$13.50 \mid \$19.00 \quad \$24.00]$$

Thus, the standard unit costs of laboratory examinations and operative procedures are $28.00 and $13.50, respectively. Similarly, the standard unit costs of
providing a day of care in nursing departments $D_1$ and $D_2$ are $19.00 and $24.00,
respectively.

These estimates are combined with the projections as to the volume of each
service to determine the total anticipated costs of program activity. Recalling
that budgeted program costs, BPC, are given by the product of standard unit
costs and the expected volume of care, we find that

$$BPC_g = \mathbf{u}'\mathbf{e}(\mathbf{v}_g) \tag{17.1}$$

yields the desired cost estimate. In this case, we let

$$\mathbf{e}(\mathbf{v}_g) = \begin{bmatrix} \mathbf{e}(\mathbf{s}_g) \\ ------ \\ \mathbf{e}(\mathbf{n}_g) \end{bmatrix}$$

where the elements of $\mathbf{e}(\mathbf{v}_g)$ were calculated earlier. Returning to our example,
we find that

$$BPC_g = [\$28.00 \quad \$13.50 \;\vdots\; \$19.00 \quad \$24.00] \begin{bmatrix} 5,700 \\ 400 \\ \hline 36,500 \\ 11,200 \end{bmatrix}$$

$$= \$1,127,300.00$$

Consider next the *actual* costs of program activity. In this case, we assume that the entries in Table 17-4 represent the actual distribution of the patient population in terms of diagnosis and service requirements. Further, assume that the actual volume of each service which was provided to the average patient who was hospitalized with a given diagnosis and required the service is represented by the set of coefficients appearing in Table 17-5. Using the approach introduced earlier, we find that

$$\mathbf{v}_g = \begin{bmatrix} 9,594 \\ 792 \\ \hline 55,560 \\ 25,080 \end{bmatrix}$$

where the elements of $\mathbf{v}_g$ represent the actual volume of laboratory examinations and operative procedures as well as the number of days of care in nursing departments $D_1$ and $D_2$ provided to the patient population of the program area.

To calculate the actual program costs it is necessary to determine the actual unit costs of each component of care. Assume that the coefficients in Table 17-

**Table 17-4** Actual Distribution of Patients, by Diagnosis and Service Requirements

| Component of Service | Diagnostic Condition | |
|---|---|---|
| | $M_1$ | $M_2$ |
| Ancillary services | | |
| $S_1$ | 840 | 1,440 |
| $S_2$ | 0 | 720 |
| Stay-specific services | | |
| $D_1$ | 3,000 | 3,840 |
| $D_2$ | 240 | 2,880 |

**Table 17-5** Actual Use of Service Per Patient

| Condition | Laboratory Tests $(S_1)$ | Operative Procedures $(S_2)$ | Days of Care $(D_1)$ | Days of Care $(D_2)$ |
|---|---|---|---|---|
| $M_1$ | 2.85 | 0 | 7.0 | 6.1 |
| $M_2$ | 5.0 | 1.1 | 9.0 | 8.2 |

6 represent the actual use of resources per unit of service. The actual factor prices are presented in the last column of the table.

Similar to our earlier work, we may form the row vector

$$\mathbf{f}'_a = [\$11.00 \quad \$3.50 \quad \$6.50 \quad \$4.00 \quad \vdots \quad \$10.50 \quad \$1.50 \quad \$2.60 \quad \$2.00]$$

where the first four elements correspond to the actual wage structure of the hospital and the remaining terms pertain to the actual prices of consumable supplies $R_1$, $R_2$, $R_3$, and $R_4$. We also extract the actual resource requirements per unit of service in Table 17-6 and form the matrix

$$\mathbf{R}^* = \begin{bmatrix} 2.5 & 0.0 & 0.0 & 0.0 \\ 0.0 & 1.6 & 3.5 & 1.5 \\ 0.0 & 0.0 & 0.0 & 2.0 \\ 0.0 & 0.0 & 1.5 & 0.0 \\ \hline 3.0 & .7 & 0.0 & 0.0 \\ 0.0 & 3.5 & 6.2 & 0.0 \\ 0.0 & 2.5 & 0.0 & 3.0 \\ 0.0 & 0.0 & 0.0 & 4.0 \end{bmatrix} = \begin{bmatrix} \mathbf{R}^*_1 \\ \hline \mathbf{R}^*_2 \end{bmatrix}$$

As a result, the actual unit cost of each service is given by

$$\mathbf{a}' = \mathbf{f}'_a \mathbf{R}^* \qquad\qquad (17.2)$$

$$= [\$59.00 \quad \$24.70 \quad \vdots \quad \$27.55 \quad \$34.05]$$

**Table 17-6** Actual Use of Resources Per Unit of Service, by Type of Service and Resource

| | Service | | | | |
|---|---|---|---|---|---|
| Resource | Laboratory Tests ($S_1$) | Operative Procedures ($S_2$) | Days of Care ($D_1$) | Days of Care ($D_2$) | Actual Factor Price |
| Labor | | | | | |
| $AMH_1$ | 2.5 | 0 | 0 | 0 | $11.00 |
| $AMH_2$ | 0 | 1.6 | 3.5 | 1.5 | 3.50 |
| $AMH_3$ | 0 | 0 | 0 | 2.0 | 6.50 |
| $AMH_4$ | 0 | 0 | 1.5 | 0 | 4.00 |
| Supplies | | | | | |
| $ARR_1$ | 3.0 | .7 | 0 | 0 | 10.50 |
| $ARR_2$ | 0 | 3.5 | 6.2 | 0 | 1.50 |
| $ARR_3$ | 0 | 2.5 | 0 | 3.0 | 2.60 |
| $ARR_4$ | 0 | 0 | 0 | 4.0 | 2.00 |

These findings indicate that the actual unit costs of providing laboratory examinations are $59.00; operative procedures, $24.70; a day of care in nursing department $D_1$, $27.55; and a day of care in nursing department $D_2$, $34.05.

Combining the actual unit costs and the actual quantity and composition of care to determine actual program costs (APC), we find that

$$\text{APC}_g = \mathbf{a}' \mathbf{v}_g \qquad (17.3)$$

$$= [\$59.00 \quad \$24.70 \quad \vdots \quad \$27.55 \quad \$34.05] \begin{bmatrix} 9,594 \\ 792 \\ \text{---------} \\ 55,560 \\ 25,080 \end{bmatrix}$$

$$= \$2,970,260.40$$

At this point in the analysis, we may calculate the variance in program costs by

$$\text{VAR}(C_g) = \text{APC}_g - \text{BPC}_g \qquad (17.4)$$

In terms of our example, we find that

$$VAR(C_g) = \$2{,}970{,}260.40 - \$1{,}127{,}300.00$$

$$= \boxed{\$1{,}842{,}960.40}$$

represents the total variance in the costs of program $g$. The objective of the following discussion is to partition the total variance calculated in this section into components that are attributable to differences between the actual and expected: (1) size and distribution of patients in terms of diagnosis and service requirements, (2) mix of services per patient, (3) use of resources per unit of service, and (4) factor prices.

## 17.4 DIAGNOSTIC MIX VARIANCE

The portion of the total variance in program costs attributable to differences between actual and expected distribution of patients in terms of diagnosis and service requirements may be found by

$$
\begin{array}{c}
\text{Diagnostic} \\
\text{Mix} \\
\text{Variance}
\end{array}
=
\left[
\begin{array}{c}
\text{Actual} \\
\text{Mix of} \\
\text{Patients}
\end{array}
-
\begin{array}{c}
\text{Expected} \\
\text{Mix of} \\
\text{Patients}
\end{array}
\right]
\times
\left[
\begin{array}{c}
\text{Standard} \\
\text{Mix of} \\
\text{Services}
\end{array}
\right]
\times
\left[
\begin{array}{c}
\text{Standard} \\
\text{Unit} \\
\text{Costs}
\end{array}
\right]
$$

In this formulation, it is important to note that, when we multiply differences between the actual and expected mix of patients by the standard mix of services, we obtain the difference between the actual and expected volume of service that is attributable to the treatment of a different group of patients than was expected at the time the budget was formulated. When we multiply this quantity by standard unit costs, we obtain the portion of the total variance in program costs attributable to the difference between the actual and expected distribution of the patient population of the program area.

Consider first the actual distribution of the patient population of the program area (Table 17-4). We may extract the data to form the matrix

$$
\mathbf{P}^* =
\left[
\begin{array}{cc}
840 & 1{,}440 \\
0 & 720 \\
\hline
3{,}000 & 3{,}840 \\
240 & 2{,}880
\end{array}
\right]
$$

Also recall that

$$P = \begin{bmatrix} 1{,}000 & 800 \\ 0 & 400 \\ \hline 3{,}000 & 2{,}000 \\ 700 & 1{,}200 \end{bmatrix}$$

represents the expected distribution of the patient population in terms of diagnosis and service requirements. As a consequence, we find

$$P^* - P = \begin{bmatrix} 840 & 1{,}440 \\ 0 & 720 \\ \hline 3{,}000 & 3{,}840 \\ 240 & 2{,}880 \end{bmatrix} - \begin{bmatrix} 1{,}000 & 800 \\ 0 & 400 \\ \hline 3{,}000 & 2{,}000 \\ 700 & 1{,}200 \end{bmatrix}$$

$$= \begin{bmatrix} -160 & 640 \\ 0 & 320 \\ \hline 0 & 1{,}840 \\ -460 & 1{,}680 \end{bmatrix}$$

represents the difference between the actual and expected mix of patients.

We now may obtain the product of each row of the matrix $P^* - P$ and a column vector consisting of appropriate coefficients selected from Table 17-2. For example, we might employ the coefficients in the first column of the table to form the vector

$$\begin{bmatrix} 2.5 \\ 4.0 \end{bmatrix}$$

which when multiplied by the first row of $P^* - P$ yields

$$\begin{bmatrix} -160 & 640 \end{bmatrix} \begin{bmatrix} 2.5 \\ 4.0 \end{bmatrix}$$

or 2,160 units. Thus, in relation to budgetary expectations, an additional 2,160 units of laboratory service were required to diagnose and monitor the conditions actually presented. Replicating the procedure for the other components of care, we find that

$$[0 \quad 320] \begin{bmatrix} 0.0 \\ 1.0 \end{bmatrix} = 320 \text{ units}$$

$$[0 \quad 1{,}840] \begin{bmatrix} 6.5 \\ 8.5 \end{bmatrix} = 15{,}640 \text{ days}$$

$$[-460 \quad 1{,}680] \begin{bmatrix} 5.2 \\ 6.3 \end{bmatrix} = 8{,}192 \text{ days}$$

represent differences between the actual and expected volumes of care attributable to disparities between the actual and expected diagnostic distribution. We may summarize our results by letting

$$\mathbf{v}_{dx} = \begin{bmatrix} 2{,}160 \\ 320 \\ 15{,}640 \\ 8{,}192 \end{bmatrix}$$

When we multiply $\mathbf{v}_{dx}$ by the standard costs per unit of service we obtain the portion of the total variance in program expenses attributable to the diagnostic mix of the program population. Recalling that

$$\mathbf{u}' = [\$28.00 \quad \$13.50 \quad \$19.00 \quad \$24.00]$$

represents the set of standard unit costs, the variance in program costs attributable to diagnostic mix is given by

$$\text{Var}(\mathbf{C}_{dx}) = \mathbf{u}'\mathbf{v}_{dx} \tag{17.5}$$

$$= [\$28.00 \quad \$13.50 \quad \$19.00 \quad \$24.00] \begin{bmatrix} 2,160 \\ 320 \\ 15,640 \\ 8,192 \end{bmatrix}$$

$$= \boxed{\$558,568.00}$$

These findings imply that approximately 30 percent (i.e., $558,568.00/ $1,842,960.40) of the total variance in program costs is attributable to differences between the actual and expected mix of patients.

## 17.5 SERVICE MIX VARIANCE

We may determine the portion of the total variance in program costs attributable to differences between the actual and standard mix of services per patient by

$$\begin{matrix} \text{Service} \\ \text{Mix} \\ \text{Variance} \end{matrix} = \begin{bmatrix} \text{Actual} \\ \text{Mix of} \\ \text{Patients} \end{bmatrix} \times \begin{bmatrix} \text{Actual} & \text{Standard} \\ \text{Mix of} & - & \text{Mix of} \\ \text{Services} & \text{Services} \end{bmatrix} \times \begin{bmatrix} \text{Standard} \\ \text{Unit} \\ \text{Costs} \end{bmatrix}$$

In this case, when we multiply the actual mix of patients by the difference between the actual and expected mix of services, we obtain the difference in the quantity and composition of service that is attributable to disparities between the actual and standard rates of use. Multiplying this quantity by standard unit costs results in the portion of the difference between actual and budgeted program costs that is attributable to the service mix variance.

Referring to Table 17-2, we may extract the coefficients representing the standard mix of services and form the matrix

$$\mathbf{S} = \begin{bmatrix} 2.5 & 0.0 & 6.5 & 5.2 \\ 4.0 & 1.0 & 8.5 & 6.3 \end{bmatrix}$$

Similarly, the data in Table 17-5 provide the basis for the formation of

$$\mathbf{S}^* = \begin{bmatrix} 2.85 & 0.0 & 7.0 & 6.1 \\ 5.0 & 1.1 & 9.0 & 8.2 \end{bmatrix}$$

where the first row of $S^*$ represents the per capita use of service by patients presenting condition $M_1$. Observe that

$$S^* - S = \begin{bmatrix} .35 & .00 & .50 & .90 \\ 1.00 & .10 & .50 & 1.90 \end{bmatrix}$$

represents the difference between the actual and standard mix of service per patient. Recalling that

$$P^* = \begin{bmatrix} 840 & 1,440 \\ \hline 0 & 720 \\ \hline 3,000 & 3,840 \\ \hline 240 & 2,880 \end{bmatrix}$$

we may obtain the product of each row in $P^*$ and the corresponding column of $S^* - S$ as follows

$$[840 \quad 1,440] \begin{bmatrix} .35 \\ 1.00 \end{bmatrix} = 1,734 \text{ units}$$

$$[0 \quad 720] \begin{bmatrix} .00 \\ .10 \end{bmatrix} = 72 \text{ units}$$

$$[3,000 \quad 3,840] \begin{bmatrix} .50 \\ .50 \end{bmatrix} = 3,420 \text{ days}$$

$$[240 \quad 2,880] \begin{bmatrix} .90 \\ 1.90 \end{bmatrix} = 5,688 \text{ days}$$

These calculations indicate that the difference between the actual and standard mix of services resulted in the provision of an additional 1,734 units of laboratory service, 72 units of operative care, 3,420 days of care in nursing department $D_1$, and 5,688 days of care in nursing department $D_2$. At this point, it is convenient to summarize our findings by letting

$$\mathbf{v}_{sv} = \begin{bmatrix} 1,734 \\ 72 \\ 3,420 \\ 5,688 \end{bmatrix}$$

Using this notation, we find that the variance in program costs attributable to differences between the actual and standard mix of services is given by

$$VAR(\mathbf{C}_{sv}) = \mathbf{u}'\mathbf{v}_{sv} \qquad (17.6)$$

Returning to our example, we find

$$VAR(\mathbf{C}_{sv}) = [\$28.00 \quad \$13.50 \quad \$19.00 \quad \$24.00] \begin{bmatrix} 1,734 \\ 72 \\ 3,420 \\ 5,688 \end{bmatrix}$$

$$= \boxed{\$251,016.00}$$

As a result, we conclude that just under 14 percent (i.e., \$251,016.00/ \$1,842,960.40) of the total variance in program costs is attributable to disparities between the actual and standard mixes of service.

## 17.6 LABOR EFFICIENCY VARIANCE

The labor efficiency variance is related to differences between the actual and standard amount of labor per unit of service. More specifically, the portion of the total variance in program costs that is attributable to the relative efficiency with which labor is used may be obtained by

$$\begin{matrix} \text{Labor} \\ \text{Efficiency} \\ \text{Variance} \end{matrix} = \begin{bmatrix} \text{Actual} \\ \text{Volume} \\ \text{of Service} \end{bmatrix} \times \begin{bmatrix} \text{Actual} & & \text{Standard} \\ \text{Staff Hours} & - & \text{Staff Hours} \\ \text{Per Service} & & \text{Per Service} \end{bmatrix} \times \begin{bmatrix} \text{Standard} \\ \text{Wage} \\ \text{Rate} \end{bmatrix}$$

In this case, the product of the actual volume of service and the difference between the actual and standard work hours per service yields the disparity between the actual and expected number of hours attributable to the relative efficiency with which personnel are employed in providing service. Multiplying this quantity by the standard wage rate yields the portion of the total variance in program costs attributable to differences between the actual and expected hours of labor per unit of service.

Recall that the matrix $\mathbf{R}$ was partitioned to reflect standard labor and supply requirements. Also recall that

$$\mathbf{R}_1 = \begin{bmatrix} 2.0 & 0.0 & 0.0 & 0.0 \\ 0.0 & 1.5 & 3.0 & 1.0 \\ 0.0 & 0.0 & 0.0 & 1.0 \\ 0.0 & 0.0 & 1.0 & 1.0 \end{bmatrix}$$

represents the standard labor hours per unit of service. Similarly, the matrix $\mathbf{R}^*$ was partitioned to reflect the actual personnel per unit of service. As can be verified, the actual work hours per service were summarized by

$$\mathbf{R}_1^* = \begin{bmatrix} 2.5 & 0.0 & 0.0 & 0.0 \\ 0.0 & 1.6 & 3.5 & 1.5 \\ 0.0 & 0.0 & 0.0 & 2.0 \\ 0.0 & 0.0 & 1.5 & 0.0 \end{bmatrix}$$

In this example, we find that the difference between the actual and standard hours per unit of service is given by

$$\mathbf{R}_1^* - \mathbf{R}_1 = \begin{bmatrix} .5 & 0.0 & 0.0 & 0.0 \\ 0.0 & .1 & .5 & .5 \\ 0.0 & 0.0 & 0.0 & 1.0 \\ 0.0 & 0.0 & .5 & -1.0 \end{bmatrix}$$

Referring to Table 17-3, observe that the set of standard wages may be summarized in the form

$$\mathbf{w}_s = \begin{bmatrix} \$10.00 \\ 3.00 \\ 6.00 \\ 4.00 \end{bmatrix}$$

while

$$\mathbf{v}'_g = [9{,}594 \quad 792 \quad 55{,}560 \quad 25{,}080]$$

represents the actual volume of each component of care. Consequently, the labor efficiency variance of the program area is given by

$$\text{VAR}(\mathbf{C}_\ell) = \mathbf{v}'_g(\mathbf{R}^*_1 - \mathbf{R}_1)'\mathbf{w}_s \qquad (17.7)$$

Returning to our example, the transpose of $(\mathbf{R}^*_1 - \mathbf{R}_1)$ is given by

$$(\mathbf{R}^*_1 - \mathbf{R}_1)' = \begin{bmatrix} .5 & 0 & 0 & 0 \\ 0 & .1 & 0 & 0 \\ 0 & .5 & 0 & .5 \\ 0 & .5 & 1.0 & -1.0 \end{bmatrix}$$

from which we find that

$$\text{VAR}(\mathbf{C}_\ell) =$$

$$[9{,}594 \quad 792 \quad 55{,}560 \quad 25{,}080] \begin{bmatrix} .5 & 0 & 0 & 0 \\ 0 & .1 & 0 & 0 \\ 0 & .5 & 0 & .5 \\ 0 & .5 & 1.0 & -1.0 \end{bmatrix} \begin{bmatrix} \$10.00 \\ 3.00 \\ 6.00 \\ 4.00 \end{bmatrix}$$

$$= [4{,}797 \quad 40{,}399.2 \quad 25{,}080 \quad 2{,}700] \begin{bmatrix} \$10.00 \\ 3.00 \\ 6.00 \\ 4.00 \end{bmatrix}$$

$$= \boxed{\$330{,}447.60}$$

On the basis of these findings we conclude that approximately 18 percent (i.e., $330,447.60/$1,842,960.40) of the total variance in program costs is attributable to the efficiency with which labor was used in providing service.

## 17.7 SUPPLY EFFICIENCY VARIANCE

The portion of the total variance in program costs attributable to the difference between the actual and expected use of consumable supplies per unit of service may be found by

$$\begin{matrix} \text{Supply} \\ \text{Efficiency} = \\ \text{Variance} \end{matrix} \begin{bmatrix} \text{Actual} \\ \text{Volume} \\ \text{of} \\ \text{Service} \end{bmatrix} \times \begin{bmatrix} \text{Actual} & \text{Standard} \\ \text{Supply} & \text{Supply} \\ \text{Requirement} - \text{Requirement} \\ \text{Per Service} & \text{Per Service} \end{bmatrix} \times \begin{bmatrix} \text{Standard} \\ \text{Supply} \\ \text{Price} \end{bmatrix}$$

We use $\mathbf{R}_2^*$ and $\mathbf{R}_2$ of matrices $\mathbf{R}^*$ and $\mathbf{R}$ respectively to calculate the difference between the actual and expected supply requirements per unit of service as follows:

$$\mathbf{R}_2^* - \mathbf{R}_2 = \begin{bmatrix} 3.0 & .7 & 0 & 0 \\ 0 & 3.5 & 6.2 & 0 \\ 0 & 2.5 & 0 & 3.0 \\ 0 & 0 & 0 & 4.0 \end{bmatrix} - \begin{bmatrix} 2.0 & .5 & 0 & 0 \\ 0 & 3.0 & 6.0 & 0 \\ 0 & 2.0 & 0 & 2.5 \\ 0 & 0 & 0 & 4.0 \end{bmatrix}$$

$$= \begin{bmatrix} 1.0 & .2 & 0 & 0 \\ 0 & .5 & .2 & 0 \\ 0 & .5 & 0 & .5 \\ 0 & 0 & 0 & 0 \end{bmatrix}$$

Further, the standard supply prices in the last column of Table 17-3 may be used to form the vector

$$
\mathbf{p}_s =
\begin{bmatrix}
\$4.00 \\
1.00 \\
2.00 \\
1.50
\end{bmatrix}
$$

We may now find the portion of the total variance in program costs attributable to differences between the actual and expected use of supplies per unit of service by

$$
\mathrm{VAR}(\mathbf{C}_r) = \mathbf{v}_g'(\mathbf{R}_2^* - \mathbf{R}_2)'\mathbf{p}_s \tag{17.8}
$$

where, in terms of our example, the transpose of $(\mathbf{R}_2^* - \mathbf{R}_2)$ is

$$
(\mathbf{R}_2^* - \mathbf{R}_2)' =
\begin{bmatrix}
1.0 & 0 & 0 & 0 \\
.2 & .5 & .5 & 0 \\
0 & .2 & 0 & 0 \\
0 & 0 & .5 & 0
\end{bmatrix}
$$

Consequently, we find

$$
\mathrm{VAR}(\mathbf{C}_r) =
$$

$$
[9{,}594 \quad 792 \quad 55{,}560 \quad 25{,}080]
\begin{bmatrix}
1.0 & 0 & 0 & 0 \\
.2 & .5 & .5 & 0 \\
0 & .2 & 0 & 0 \\
0 & 0 & .5 & 0
\end{bmatrix}
\begin{bmatrix}
\$4.00 \\
1.00 \\
2.00 \\
1.50
\end{bmatrix}
$$

$$= [9,752.4 \quad 11,508 \quad 12,936 \quad 0] \begin{bmatrix} \$4,00 \\ 1.00 \\ 2.00 \\ 1.50 \end{bmatrix}$$

$$= \boxed{\$79,389.60}$$

These calculations suggest that approximately 4 percent of the total variance in program costs is attributable to the difference between the actual and expected supply requirements per unit of service.

## 17.8 WAGE VARIANCE

Similar to the methods above, we may find the portion of the total variance in program costs attributable to differences between the actual and standard wage rate by

$$\begin{matrix} \text{Wage} \\ \text{Variance} \end{matrix} = \begin{bmatrix} \text{Actual} \\ \text{Volume of} \\ \text{Service} \end{bmatrix} \times \begin{bmatrix} \text{Actual Labor} \\ \text{Requirements} \\ \text{Per Service} \end{bmatrix} \times \begin{bmatrix} \text{Actual} & \text{Standard} \\ \text{Wage} & - & \text{Wage} \\ \text{Rate} & \text{Rate} \end{bmatrix}$$

It will be noted that the product of the actual volume of service and the actual labor requirements per unit of service yields the total number of personnel hours employed in providing service. When this quantity is multiplied by the difference between the actual and standard wage rates, we obtain the portion of the total variance in program costs attributable to the disparity between the actual and expected wage structure of the hospital.

Referring to our example, recall that

$$\mathbf{w}_s = \begin{bmatrix} \$10.00 \\ 3.00 \\ 6.00 \\ 4.00 \end{bmatrix}$$

represents the expected wage structure of the institution. On the other hand, actual wage rates in Table 17-6 may be used to form the column vector

$$\mathbf{w}_a = \begin{bmatrix} \$11.00 \\ 3.50 \\ 6.50 \\ 4.00 \end{bmatrix}$$

Consequently, differences between the actual and expected wage structure of the hospital is given by

$$\mathbf{w}_d = \mathbf{w}_a - \mathbf{w}_s = \begin{bmatrix} \$11.00 \\ 3.50 \\ 6.50 \\ 4.00 \end{bmatrix} - \begin{bmatrix} \$10.00 \\ 3.00 \\ 6.00 \\ 4.00 \end{bmatrix} = \begin{bmatrix} \$1.00 \\ .50 \\ .50 \\ .00 \end{bmatrix}$$

Similarly, the actual number of hours, by type of labor, used in providing service is obtained by

$$\mathbf{l}_a = \mathbf{R}_1^* \mathbf{v}_g$$

$$= \begin{bmatrix} 2.5 & 0 & 0 & 0 \\ 0 & 1.6 & 3.5 & 1.5 \\ 0 & 0 & 0 & 2.0 \\ 0 & 0 & 1.5 & 0 \end{bmatrix} \begin{bmatrix} 9,594 \\ 792 \\ 55,560 \\ 25,080 \end{bmatrix}$$

$$= \begin{bmatrix} 23,985.0 \\ 233,347.2 \\ 50,160.0 \\ 83,340.0 \end{bmatrix}$$

Hence, the portion of the total variance in program costs attributable to differences between the actual and expected wage structure of the institution is given by

$$\boxed{\text{VAR}(\mathbf{C}_w) = \mathbf{l}_a' \mathbf{w}_d \qquad\qquad (17.9)}$$

$$= [23{,}985.0 \quad 233{,}347.20 \quad 50{,}160.0 \quad 83{,}340.0] \begin{bmatrix} \$1.00 \\ .50 \\ .50 \\ .00 \end{bmatrix}$$

$$= \boxed{\$165{,}738.60}$$

## 17.9 SUPPLY PRICE VARIANCE

The portion of the total variance in program costs attributable to differences between actual and expected supply prices is given by

$$\begin{bmatrix} \text{Supply} \\ \text{Price} \\ \text{Variance} \end{bmatrix} = \begin{bmatrix} \text{Actual} \\ \text{Volume of} \\ \text{Service} \end{bmatrix} \times \begin{bmatrix} \text{Actual Supply} \\ \text{Requirements} \\ \text{Per Service} \end{bmatrix} \times \begin{bmatrix} \text{Actual} & \text{Standard} \\ \text{Supply} - & \text{Supply} \\ \text{Price} & \text{Price} \end{bmatrix}$$

The total quantity of supplies used to provide service is the product of the actual volume of service and the actual supply requirements per unit of service. Multiplying this result by the last term in the equation yields the portion of the total variance in program costs attributable to disparities between the actual and standard cost per unit of consumable supply.

As can be verified, differences between actual and expected supply prices are given by

$$\mathbf{p}_d = \mathbf{p}_a - \mathbf{p}_s$$

where, in terms of our example

$$\mathbf{p}_a = \begin{bmatrix} \$10.50 \\ 1.50 \\ 2.60 \\ 2.00 \end{bmatrix} ; \quad \mathbf{p}_s = \begin{bmatrix} \$4.00 \\ 1.00 \\ 2.00 \\ 1.50 \end{bmatrix}$$

and

$$\mathbf{p}_d = \begin{bmatrix} \$6.50 \\ .50 \\ .60 \\ .50 \end{bmatrix}$$

The actual quantity of supplies by type of supply item is given by

$$\mathbf{r}_a = \mathbf{R}_2^* \mathbf{v}_g$$

$$= \begin{bmatrix} 3.0 & .7 & 0 & 0 \\ 0 & 3.5 & 6.2 & 0 \\ 0 & 2.5 & 0 & 3.0 \\ 0 & 0 & 0 & 4.0 \end{bmatrix} \begin{bmatrix} 9,594 \\ 792 \\ 55,560 \\ 25,080 \end{bmatrix} = \begin{bmatrix} 29,336.4 \\ 347,244.0 \\ 77,220.0 \\ 100,320.0 \end{bmatrix}$$

Consequently, we find

$$\text{VAR}(\mathbf{C}_p) = \mathbf{r}_a' \mathbf{p}_d \qquad\qquad (17.10)$$

yields the portion of the total variance in program costs attributable to differences between actual and expected supply prices. In terms of our example, $\text{VAR}(\mathbf{C}_p)$ is given by

$$\text{VAR}(\mathbf{C}_p) = [29,336.4 \quad 347,244.0 \quad 77,220.0 \quad 100,320.0] \begin{bmatrix} \$6.50 \\ .50 \\ .60 \\ .50 \end{bmatrix}$$

$$= \boxed{\$460,800.60}$$

These findings suggest that approximately 25 percent of the total variance in program costs is attributable to differences between actual and expected supply prices.

## 17.10 MANAGEMENT REPORTS

We may summarize our findings concerning the hypothetical program as follows

$$
\begin{aligned}
\text{VAR}(\mathbf{C}_{dx}) &= \$558{,}568.00 \\
\text{VAR}(\mathbf{C}_{sv}) &= 251{,}016.00 \\
\text{VAR}(\mathbf{C}_{\ell}) &= 330{,}447.60 \\
\text{VAR}(\mathbf{C}_{r}) &= 76{,}389.60 \\
\text{VAR}(\mathbf{C}_{w}) &= 165{,}738.60 \\
\text{VAR}(\mathbf{C}_{p}) &= \underline{460{,}800.60} \\
\text{VAR}(\mathbf{C}_{g}) &= 1{,}842{,}960.40
\end{aligned}
$$

Given that the size and diagnostic distribution of the program population and the quantity and composition of services provided to each patient are determined by the physician, these calculations suggest that $558,568.00 + $251,016.00 or $809,584.00 (approximately 44 percent) of the total cost variance is the responsibility of physicians associated with the program area. Control over these components of the cost variance must be exerted through the utilization review committee that has the responsibility of ascertaining the extent to which individual physicians have contributed to excessive costs by overprescribing care for their patients. Obviously, such a determination is accomplished best by a review of the care prescribed by individual physicians in specific cases.

As seen earlier, line management exerts direct control over the quantity and composition of real resources that are used in providing ancillary services and nursing care. In this case, the portion of the total cost variance attributable to line managers is given by the sum of $\text{VAR}(\mathbf{C}_{\ell})$ and $\text{VAR}(\mathbf{C}_{r})$. In terms of our example, $406,837.20, or approximately 22 percent of the total variance in program costs, is the responsibility of line management. This suggests that the use of real resources in support of the program area should be evaluated and, where appropriate, management should develop and implement courses of action designed to redress imbalances between their actual and expected use.

Consider next the two price variances that were computed above. With respect to $\text{VAR}(\mathbf{C}_{p})$, the primary responsibility for controlling the prices paid for consumable supplies usually is assigned to the purchasing department or a centralized purchasing agent. In terms of our example, the price variance associated with consumable supplies is $460,800.60 (25 percent of the total), which suggests that: (1) standard supply prices were systematically underestimated, (2) supplies were not acquired at the most advantageous prices, or (3) a combination of these two factors. Concerning the first of these elements, a systematic underestimate of standard factor prices indicates that the forecasting techniques used in developing the program budget must be improved. Differences between expected and actual factor prices must be minimized when the hospital is reimbursed prospectively or determines its fee schedule on a prospective basis. As to the second factor, a failure to obtain required stock at the most advantageous price requires a thorough examination of the process by which supplies are purchased. This will provide the basis for designing and implementing remedial policies or courses of action.

Regarding the wage variance, the results of the calculations suggest that the portion of the variance in program costs attributable to differences between actual and expected wage rates, $VAR(C_w)$, amounts to $165,738.60 (approximately 9 percent of the total). As in the case of the supply price variance, the wage variance may be a result of (1) a failure to adhere to established wage policies, (2) economic factors over which management exerts little control, or (3) a combination of these two. In the event that this variance is attributable to a discrepancy between the wages that actually were paid and the wage policy or the collective agreement of the hospital, a thorough examination of the personnel department should provide the basis for implementation of corrective action. On the other hand, the second factor suggests that the difference between actual and expected wages might be reduced by giving explicit recognition, in the model by which standard factor prices are estimated, to the economic elements over which management exerts little control. As before, minimizing the difference between actual and standard wage rates is of particular importance to the hospital that is reimbursed on a prospective basis or develops a prospective fee schedule that may not be altered during the future period.

Once the cost variance and the contribution of each of the factors to the difference between current and expected costs have been computed for each program area, the information can be summarized in a report similar to Table 17-7. Such a report provides senior management with the total variance in the costs of each program area as well as the portion of each variance that is attributable to differences between the actual and expected: (1) distribution of program patients by diagnosis and service requirements, (2) mix of services per patient, (3) mix of resources per unit of service, and (4) factor prices. As seen above, the individuals responsible for each of these variances may be identified by management and, where appropriate, should then develop and implement corrective actions or policies to redress the imbalance.

---

**ADDITIONAL READINGS***

American Hospital Association. *Managerial Cost Accounting for Hospitals*. Chicago, 1980.

Dirksen, C. J. "Determining How and Why Your Costs Are Changing," *Hospital Financial Management,* 14, December 1978.

Holder, W. W. and J. Williams. "Better Cost Control With Flexible Budgets and Variance Analysis," *Hospital Financial Management,* 30(1):12, Jan. 1976.

---

* These readings would also be helpful as additional resources for Chapters 16 and 18.

**Table 17-7** Analysis of the Variance in Program Costs for the Period

| Program Area ($P_a$) | Variance Due to Diagnostic Mix | Variance Due to Service Mix | Labor Efficiency Variance | Supply Efficiency Variance | Wage Variance | Supply Price Variance | Total Variance |
|---|---|---|---|---|---|---|---|
| $P_1$ | | | | | | | |
| $P_2$ | | | | | | | |
| $P_3$ | | | | | | | |
| ⋯ | | | | | | | |
| $P_g$ | \$558,568.00 | \$251,016.00 | \$330,447.60 | \$76,389.60 | \$165,738.60 | \$460,800.60 | \$1,842,960.40 |
| ⋯ | | | | | | | |
| $P_v$ | | | | | | | |
| Total | | | | | | | |

# Chapter 18

# Controlling the Responsibility Center

## Objectives

After completing this chapter, you should be able to:

1. Determine the total variance in the costs of the responsibility center.
2. Partition the total variance in the costs of the responsibility center into portions that are attributable to the:
   a. volume variance.
   b. efficiency variance.
   c. price variance.
   d. interactive variance.
3. Prepare summary reports for the various levels of managerial responsibility.

This chapter shifts the focus of discussion from the program area to the responsibility center. Similar to the analysis of the program area, the objectives of this chapter are to determine the total variance in cost and to divide exceptions to the budget into four components: (1) a volume variance, (2) an efficiency variance, (3) a factor price variance, and (4) an interactive variance. Symbolically, the approach used in this chapter may be represented in the general form

$$VAR(Cost) = VAR(Vol) + VAR(Eff) + VAR(Price) + VAR(Inter)$$

where

| | |
|---|---|
| VAR(Cost) | represents the total variance in cost; |
| VAR(Vol) | represents the volume variance; |
| VAR(Eff) | represents the variance in cost attributable to the relative efficiency with which labor and supplies are used; |

VAR(Price)    represents the variance in cost due to differences between actual and expected factor prices; and

VAR(Inter)    corresponds to the interactive term.

To simplify the analysis, assume that the department and the responsibility center are synonymous.

## 18.1 THE TOTAL COST VARIANCE

As in the case of the program area, the total cost variance of the responsibility center is given by

$$\frac{\text{Total Cost}}{\text{Variance}} = \frac{\text{Actual Costs of the}}{\text{Responsibility Center}} - \frac{\text{Budgeted Costs of the}}{\text{Responsibility Center}}$$

Similar to our earlier discussion, we shall find that

$$\frac{\text{Budgeted Costs}}{\text{of the Center}} = \left[\begin{array}{c}\text{Anticipated}\\\text{Volume of Service}\end{array}\right] \times \left[\begin{array}{c}\text{Standard}\\\text{Unit Costs}\end{array}\right]$$

while the

$$\frac{\text{Actual Costs}}{\text{of the Center}} = \left[\begin{array}{c}\text{Actual}\\\text{Volume of Service}\end{array}\right] \times \left[\begin{array}{c}\text{Actual}\\\text{Unit Costs}\end{array}\right]$$

For illustration, assume that the laboratory department employs labor of types $L_1, L_2,$ and $L_3$ as well as consumable supplies of types $R_1, R_2,$ and $R_3$ in providing services $S_1, S_2,$ and $S_3$. Also suppose that the data in Table 18-1 represent the actual and expected volumes of laboratory service $S_1, S_2,$ and $S_3$ while the coefficients in Tables 18-2 and 18-3 represent the actual and standard resource requirements per unit of service. The actual and expected factor prices are presented in the last column of these tables.

**Table 18-1** Expected and Actual Work Load of Laboratory Department

| Service | Expected Volume of Service $E(S_k)$ (1) | Actual Volume of Service $V_k^*$ (2) | Difference Between Actual & Expected Volume of Service (3) |
|---|---|---|---|
| $S_1$ | 52,000 | 59,220 | 7,220 |
| $S_2$ | 66,000 | 75,600 | 9,600 |
| $S_3$ | 85,000 | 102,375 | 17,375 |

**Table 18-2** Standard Resource Requirements by Type of Service and Resource

| Resource | Service | | | Standard Factor Price |
|---|---|---|---|---|
| | $S_1$ (1) | $S_2$ (2) | $S_3$ (3) | (4) |
| Labor | | | | |
| $L_1$ | 1.0 | 3.0 | 0.0 | $3.00 |
| $L_2$ | 2.0 | 0.0 | 4.0 | 4.00 |
| $L_3$ | 0.0 | .5 | 1.5 | 8.00 |
| Supplies | | | | |
| $R_1$ | 4.0 | 0.0 | 0.0 | 1.00 |
| $R_2$ | 0.0 | 2.0 | 0.0 | 3.00 |
| $R_3$ | 0.0 | 1.0 | 4.0 | 5.00 |

As before, we may form the row vector

$$\mathbf{f}'_s = [\$3.00 \quad \$4.00 \quad \$8.00 \quad \vdots \quad \$1.00 \quad \$3.00 \quad \$5.00]$$

where each element corresponds to one of the standard factor prices. Similarly, we use the resource coefficients in Table 18-2 to form the matrix

$$\mathbf{R}_s = \begin{bmatrix} 1.0 & 3.0 & 0.0 \\ 2.0 & 0.0 & 4.0 \\ 0.0 & .5 & 1.5 \\ \hline 4.0 & 0.0 & 0.0 \\ 0.0 & 2.0 & 0.0 \\ 0.0 & 1.0 & 4.0 \end{bmatrix}$$

where the elements of matrix $\mathbf{R}_s$ correspond to the set of standard work hours and supply requirements per unit of service. Accordingly, standard unit costs are found by

$$\mathbf{u}' = \mathbf{f}'_s \mathbf{R}_s$$

**Table 18-3** Actual Resource Requirements by Type of Resource and Service

| Resource | Service $S_1$ (1) | $S_2$ (2) | $S_3$ (3) | Actual Factor Price (4) |
|---|---|---|---|---|
| Labor | | | | |
| $L_1$ | 1.2 | 3.1 | 0.0 | $4.00 |
| $L_2$ | 2.1 | 0.0 | 4.3 | 4.50 |
| $L_3$ | 0.0 | .7 | 1.7 | 8.50 |
| | | | | |
| Supplies | | | | |
| $R_1$ | 4.3 | 0.0 | 0.0 | 2.00 |
| $R_2$ | 0.0 | 2.1 | 0.0 | 3.50 |
| $R_3$ | 0.0 | 1.3 | 4.2 | 6.20 |

$$= [\$3.00 \quad \$4.00 \quad \$8.00 \mid \$1.00 \quad \$3.00 \quad \$5.00] \begin{bmatrix} 1.0 & 3.0 & 0.0 \\ 2.0 & 0.0 & 4.0 \\ 0.0 & .5 & 1.5 \\ \hline 4.0 & 0.0 & 0.0 \\ 0.0 & 2.0 & 0.0 \\ 0.0 & 1.0 & 4.0 \end{bmatrix}$$

$$= [\$15.00 \quad \$24.00 \quad \$48.00]$$

Letting

$$\mathbf{v}_s = \begin{bmatrix} 52,000 \\ 66,000 \\ 85,000 \end{bmatrix}$$

where each element corresponds to an expected volume of service, budgeted departmental costs are given by

$$\boxed{BDC = \mathbf{u}'\mathbf{v}_s}$$

$$= [\$15.00 \quad \$24.00 \quad \$48.00] \begin{bmatrix} 52,000 \\ 66,000 \\ 85,000 \end{bmatrix}$$

$$= \boxed{\$6,444,000}$$

By analogy, the actual departmental costs are obtained by

$$\boxed{ADC = \mathbf{a'v}_a}$$

$$= [\$22.85 \quad \$33.76 \quad \$59.84] \begin{bmatrix} 59,220 \\ 75,600 \\ 102,375 \end{bmatrix}$$

$$= \boxed{\$10,031,553.00}$$

In this case, the elements of $\mathbf{a'}$ represent the actual unit costs of providing ancillary services $S_1$, $S_2$, and $S_3$ while the elements of $\mathbf{v}_a$ correspond to the actual volume of service provided by the department. On the basis of these calculations, the total variance in departmental costs is given by

$$ADC - BDC = \$10,031,553.00 - \$6,444,000.00$$

$$= \boxed{\$3,587,553.00}$$

The objective of the following discussion is to divide the total variance into the components mentioned earlier.

## 18.2 VOLUME VARIANCE

The portion of the total variance in departmental costs attributable to the difference between the actual and expected rates of providing service is given by

$$\begin{matrix} \text{Volume} \\ \text{Variance} \end{matrix} = \begin{bmatrix} \text{Actual} & \text{Expected} \\ \text{Volume of} - \text{Volume of} \\ \text{Service} & \text{Service} \end{bmatrix} \times \begin{bmatrix} \text{Standard} \\ \text{Unit Costs} \end{bmatrix}$$

Referring to our example, we find that the deviation between expected and actual rates of operation is given by

$$\mathbf{v}_a - \mathbf{v}_s = \begin{bmatrix} 59{,}220 \\ 75{,}600 \\ 102{,}375 \end{bmatrix} - \begin{bmatrix} 52{,}000 \\ 66{,}000 \\ 85{,}000 \end{bmatrix} = \begin{bmatrix} 7{,}220 \\ 9{,}600 \\ 17{,}375 \end{bmatrix}$$

Consequently, the variance attributable to differences in the volume of care is obtained by

$$\text{VAR(Vol)} = \mathbf{u}'[\mathbf{v}_a - \mathbf{v}_s] \qquad (18.1)$$

$$= [\$15.00 \quad \$24.00 \quad \$48.00] \begin{bmatrix} 7{,}220 \\ 9{,}600 \\ 17{,}375 \end{bmatrix}$$

$$= \boxed{\$1{,}172{,}700}$$

From the perspective of internal control and preparing reports that depict the results of operational activity, it also is desirable to calculate the volume variance by type of service. In this case, we employ the elements of the vector $(\mathbf{v}_a - \mathbf{v}_s)$ and form the diagonal matrix

$$\mathbf{S}_d = \begin{bmatrix} 7{,}220 & 0 & 0 \\ 0 & 9{,}600 & 0 \\ 0 & 0 & 17{,}375 \end{bmatrix}$$

Using the matrix $\mathbf{S}_d$, the volume variance, by type of service, is obtained by

$$\text{VAR(Vol}_k) = \mathbf{u}'\mathbf{S}_d \qquad (18.2.1)$$

where the subscript $k$ indicates that a volume variance is calculated for each service. Returning to our example, an application of Equation 18.2 yields

$$\text{VAR}(\text{Vol}_k) = [\$15.00 \quad \$24.00 \quad \$48.00] \begin{bmatrix} 7,220 & 0 & 0 \\ 0 & 9,600 & 0 \\ 0 & 0 & 17,375 \end{bmatrix}$$

$$= [\$108,300 \quad \$230,400 \quad \$834,000]$$

The portion of the volume variance attributable to service $S_1$, $S_2$, and $S_3$ thus is $\$108,300$, $\$230,400$, and $\$834,000$. The sum of the elements in the resulting row vector is $\$1,172,700$, which represents the total variance in cost attributable to differences between the actual and expected work load of the department.

It also is desirable to calculate the influence of the difference between the actual and expected volume of a given service on the cost of each resource used by the department. Letting the subscript $r$ refer to the resources used in providing each service, the volume variance associated with each resource used for service $k$ is given by

$$\text{VAR}(\text{Vol}_{rk}) = \mathbf{S}_d\,\mathbf{R}_s'\,\mathbf{F}_s \qquad (18.2.2)$$

where $\mathbf{F}_s$ is a diagonal matrix representing the set of standard factor prices. Returning to our example, we find that

$$\mathbf{F}_s = \begin{bmatrix} \$3.00 & 0 & 0 & 0 & 0 & 0 \\ 0 & \$4.00 & 0 & 0 & 0 & 0 \\ 0 & 0 & \$8.00 & 0 & 0 & 0 \\ 0 & 0 & 0 & \$1.00 & 0 & 0 \\ 0 & 0 & 0 & 0 & \$3.00 & 0 \\ 0 & 0 & 0 & 0 & 0 & \$5.00 \end{bmatrix}$$

and, as can be verified

$$\text{VAR}(\text{Vol}_{rk}) = \begin{bmatrix} \$21,660 & \$57,760 & \$0 & \$28,880 & \$0 & \$0 \\ 86,400 & 0 & 38,400 & 0 & 57,600 & 48,000 \\ 0 & 278,000 & 208,500 & 0 & 0 & 347,500 \end{bmatrix}$$

In summary, the first row of $\mathbf{VAR(Vol}_{rk})$ represents the influence of the difference between the actual and expected volume of care on the use of each resource used in providing service $S_1$. The volume variance associated with the use of resources $L_1$, $L_2$, $L_3$, $R_1$, $R_2$, and $R_3$ in providing service $S_1$ amounted to $21,660, $57,760, $0, $28,800, $0 and $0, respectively. The findings of this section are summarized in Table 18-4.

## 18.3 EFFICIENCY VARIANCE

Similar to the discussion in Chapter 17, the efficiency variance is the portion of the total exception to the budget attributable to differences between the actual and expected use of resources. In this case, the efficiency variance is given by

$$
\begin{bmatrix} \text{Efficiency} \\ \text{Variance} \end{bmatrix} = \begin{bmatrix} \text{Actual} \\ \text{Volume} \\ \text{of} \\ \text{Service} \end{bmatrix} \times \begin{bmatrix} \text{Actual} \\ \text{Resource} \\ \text{Requirements} \\ \text{Per Service} \end{bmatrix} - \begin{bmatrix} \text{Standard} \\ \text{Resource} \\ \text{Requirements} \\ \text{Per Service} \end{bmatrix} \times \begin{bmatrix} \text{Standard} \\ \text{Factor} \\ \text{Price} \end{bmatrix}
$$

Referring to our example, we extract the resource coefficients in Table 18-3, and form the matrix

## Table 18-4 Summary of Volume Variance Calculations

| Resource | Ancillary Service $S_1$ | $S_2$ | $S_3$ | Total |
|---|---|---|---|---|
| Labor | | | | |
| $L_1$ | $21,660.00[1] | $86,400.00[1] | $    0.00[1] | $108,060.00 |
| $L_2$ | 57,760.00[1] | 0.00[1] | 278,000.00[1] | 335,760.00 |
| $L_3$ | 0.00[1] | 38,400.00[1] | 208,500.00[1] | 246,900.00 |
| | | | | |
| Supplies | | | | |
| $R_1$ | 28,880.00[1] | 0.00[1] | 0.00[1] | 28,880.00 |
| $R_2$ | 0.00[1] | 57,600.00[1] | 0.00[1] | 57,600.00 |
| $R_3$ | 0.00[1] | 48,000.00[1] | 347,500.00[1] | 395,500.00 |
| Total | 108,300.00[2] | 230,400.00[2] | 834,000.00[2] | 1,172,700.00[3] |

[1] Value appears in $\mathbf{VAR(Vol}_{rk}) = S_d R'_s F_s$
[2] Value appears in $\mathbf{VAR(Vol}_k) = u'S_d$
[3] Value given by $\text{VAR(Vol)} = u'[v_a - v_s]$

$$\mathbf{R}_a = \begin{bmatrix} 1.2 & 3.1 & 0.0 \\ 2.1 & 0.0 & 4.3 \\ 0.0 & .7 & 1.7 \\ \hline 4.3 & 0.0 & 0.0 \\ 0.0 & 2.1 & 0.0 \\ 0.0 & 1.3 & 4.2 \end{bmatrix}$$

Consequently, the difference between the actual and expected use of resources per unit of service is given by

$$\mathbf{R}_a - \mathbf{R}_s = \begin{bmatrix} 1.2 & 3.1 & 0.0 \\ 2.1 & 0.0 & 4.3 \\ 0.0 & .7 & 1.7 \\ 4.3 & 0.0 & 0.0 \\ 0.0 & 2.1 & 0.0 \\ 0.0 & 1.3 & 4.2 \end{bmatrix} - \begin{bmatrix} 1.0 & 3.0 & 0.0 \\ 2.0 & 0.0 & 4.0 \\ 0.0 & .5 & 1.5 \\ 4.0 & 0.0 & 0.0 \\ 0.0 & 2.0 & 0.0 \\ 0.0 & 1.0 & 4.0 \end{bmatrix}$$

$$= \begin{bmatrix} .2 & .1 & 0 \\ .1 & 0 & .3 \\ 0 & .2 & .2 \\ .3 & 0 & 0 \\ 0 & .1 & 0 \\ 0 & .3 & .2 \end{bmatrix}$$

Now, since

$$\mathbf{v}_a' = [59{,}220 \quad 75{,}600 \quad 102{,}375]$$

while

$$\mathbf{f}_s' = [\$3.00 \quad \$4.00 \quad \$8.00 \quad \$1.00 \quad \$3.00 \quad \$5.00]$$

the portion of the cost variance attributable to the difference between the actual and expected use of resources is obtained by

$$\mathrm{VAR(Eff)} = \mathbf{v}_a'(\mathbf{R}_a - \mathbf{R}_s)'\mathbf{f}_s \qquad\qquad (18.3.1)$$

$$= [59{,}220 \quad 75{,}600 \quad 102{,}375] \begin{bmatrix} .2 & .1 & 0 & .3 & 0 & 0 \\ .1 & 0 & .2 & 0 & .1 & .3 \\ 0 & .3 & .2 & 0 & 0 & .2 \end{bmatrix}$$

$$\times \begin{bmatrix} \$3.00 \\ 4.00 \\ 8.00 \\ 1.00 \\ 3.00 \\ 5.00 \end{bmatrix}$$

$$= [19{,}404 \quad 36{,}634.5 \quad 35{,}595 \quad 17{,}766 \quad 7{,}560 \quad 43{,}155]$$

$$\times \begin{bmatrix} \$3.00 \\ 4.00 \\ 8.00 \\ 1.00 \\ 3.00 \\ 5.00 \end{bmatrix}$$

$$= \$745{,}731$$

These calculations mean that approximately 21 percent of the total cost variance (i.e., \$745,731/\$3,587,553) is attributable to the relative efficiency with which management employed labor and consumable supplies in providing services.

From the perspective of monitoring, evaluating, and controlling the responsibility center, it also is of value to calculate the efficiency variances associated with each of the resources used. In this case, the product $v_a' (R_a - R_s)'$ yields the row vector

$$[19{,}404 \quad 36{,}634.5 \quad 35{,}595 \ \vdots \ 17{,}766 \quad 7{,}560 \quad 43{,}155]$$

where the first three elements represent differences between the actual and expected use of labor of type $L_1, L_2$, and $L_3$ and the last three elements correspond to the differences between the actual and expected use of consumable supplies $R_1, R_2$, and $R_3$. We may use the elements of the row vector to form the diagonal matrix

$$\mathbf{Q}_r = \begin{bmatrix} 19{,}404 & 0 & 0 & 0 & 0 & 0 \\ 0 & 36{,}634.5 & 0 & 0 & 0 & 0 \\ 0 & 0 & 35{,}595 & 0 & 0 & 0 \\ 0 & 0 & 0 & 17{,}766 & 0 & 0 \\ 0 & 0 & 0 & 0 & 7{,}560 & 0 \\ 0 & 0 & 0 & 0 & 0 & 43{,}155 \end{bmatrix}$$

which, in turn, may be used to calculate the portion of the total efficiency variance attributable to each of the resources. Letting the subscript $r$ indicate that the efficiency variance is calculated for each of the resources, we use matrix $\mathbf{Q}_r$ to obtain

$$\mathbf{VAR(Eff}_r) = \mathbf{Q}_r \mathbf{f}_s \tag{18.3.2}$$

$$= \begin{bmatrix} \$58{,}212 \\ 146{,}538 \\ 284{,}760 \\ \hdashline 17{,}766 \\ 22{,}680 \\ 215{,}775 \end{bmatrix}$$

Thus, in department $D_3$, the efficiency variance for labor of type $L_1, L_2$, and $L_3$ amounts to \$58,212, \$146,538, and \$284,760, respectively, for a total of \$489,510. The efficiency variance for consumable supplies $R_1, R_2$, and $R_3$ is \$17,766, \$22,680, and \$215,775, respectively, totaling \$256,221.

Consider next the efficiency variance, $VAR(Eff_{rk})$ that is associated with each resource used in providing each of the services. In this case, the value of $VAR(Eff_{rk})$ is given by

$$VAR(Eff_{rk}) = V_a(R_a - R_s)'F_s \qquad (18.3.3)$$

where $V_a$ is a diagonal matrix representing the actual mix of services provided during the period. Returning to our example, notice that

$$V_a = \begin{bmatrix} 59{,}220 & 0 & 0 \\ 0 & 75{,}600 & 0 \\ 0 & 0 & 102{,}375 \end{bmatrix}$$

while the transpose of $(R_a - R_s)$ is given by

$$(R_a - R_s)' = \begin{bmatrix} .2 & .1 & 0 & .3 & 0 & 0 \\ .1 & 0 & .2 & 0 & .1 & .3 \\ 0 & .3 & .2 & 0 & 0 & .2 \end{bmatrix}$$

As a result, it can be verified that

$$VAR(Eff_{rk}) = \begin{bmatrix} \$35{,}532 & \$23{,}688 & \$0 & \$17{,}766 & \$0 & \$0 \\ 22{,}680 & 0 & 120{,}960 & 0 & 22{,}680 & 113{,}400 \\ 0 & 122{,}850 & 163{,}800 & 0 & 0 & 102{,}375 \end{bmatrix}$$

Focusing on the first row of $VAR(Eff_{rk})$, these findings indicate that the efficiency variance in using resources $L_1, L_2, L_3, R_1, R_2$, and $R_3$ in providing service $S_1$ amounted to \$35,532, \$23,688, \$0, \$17,766, \$0, and \$0 respectively. Recognizing that the second and third rows of $VAR(Eff_{rk})$ pertain to services $S_2$ and $S_3$, respectively, we summarize the findings of this section in Table 18-5.

**Table 18-5** Summary of Efficiency Variance

| Resource | S₁ | S₂ | S₃ | Total |
|---|---|---|---|---|
|  | $S_1$ | $S_2$ | $S_3$ | *Total* |
| Labor |  |  |  |  |
| $L_1$ | $35,532[1] | $22,680[1] | $0[1] | $58,212[2] |
| $L_2$ | 23,688[1] | 0[1] | 122,850[1] | 146,538[2] |
| $L_3$ | 0[1] | 120,960[1] | 163,800[1] | 284,760[2] |
| Subtotal | 59,220 | 143,640 | 286,650 | 489,510 |
| Supplies |  |  |  |  |
| $R_1$ | 17,766[1] | 0[1] | 0[1] | 17,766[2] |
| $R_2$ | 0[1] | 22,680[1] | 0[1] | 22,680[2] |
| $R_3$ | 0[1] | 113,400[1] | 102,375[1] | 215,775[2] |
| Subtotal | 17,766 | 136,080 | 102,375 | 256,221 |
| Total | 76,986 | 279,720 | 389,025 | 745,731[3] |

[1] Value given by $VAR(Eff_{rk}) = \mathbf{v}_a(\mathbf{R}_a - \mathbf{R}_s)'\mathbf{F}_s$
[2] Value given by $VAR(Eff_r) = \mathbf{Q}_r\mathbf{f}_s$
[3] Value given by $VAR(Eff) = \mathbf{v}_a'(\mathbf{R}_a - \mathbf{R}_s)'\mathbf{f}_s$

## 18.4 PRICE VARIANCE

The portion of the departmental cost variance attributable to differences between actual and expected factor prices may be calculated by

$$
\begin{bmatrix} \text{Price} \\ \text{Variance} \end{bmatrix} = \begin{bmatrix} \text{Expected} \\ \text{Volume of} \\ \text{Service} \end{bmatrix} \times \begin{bmatrix} \text{Standard} \\ \text{Resource} \\ \text{Requirements} \\ \text{Per Service} \end{bmatrix} \times \begin{bmatrix} \text{Actual} & \text{Standard} \\ \text{Factor} - & \text{Factor} \\ \text{Price} & \text{Price} \end{bmatrix}
$$

The product of the first two terms yields the total standard resource requirements; when multiplied by the last term, this yields the portion of the cost variance attributable to differences between actual and expected prices.

Referring to our example, we let

$$
\mathbf{f}_a = \begin{bmatrix} \$4.00 \\ 4.50 \\ 8.50 \\ 2.00 \\ 3.50 \\ 6.20 \end{bmatrix} \quad \text{and} \quad \mathbf{f}_s = \begin{bmatrix} \$3.00 \\ 4.00 \\ 8.00 \\ 1.00 \\ 3.00 \\ 5.00 \end{bmatrix}
$$

so that

$$\mathbf{f}_a - \mathbf{f}_s = \begin{bmatrix} \$1.00 \\ .50 \\ .50 \\ 1.00 \\ .50 \\ 1.20 \end{bmatrix}$$

represents the difference between actual and standard factor prices.

Making use of the column vector $(\mathbf{f}_a - \mathbf{f}_s)$, we find that the portion of the departmental cost variance attributable to differences between actual and expected factor prices is given by

$$\text{VAR(Price)} = \mathbf{v}_s' \mathbf{R}_s' (\mathbf{f}_a - \mathbf{f}_s) \qquad (18.4)$$

In terms of our example, an application of Equation 18.4 yields

$$= [52{,}000 \quad 66{,}000 \quad 85{,}000] \begin{bmatrix} 1.0 & 2.0 & 0.0 & 4.0 & 0.0 & 0.0 \\ 3.0 & 0.0 & .5 & 0.0 & 2.0 & 1.0 \\ 0.0 & 4.0 & 1.5 & 0.0 & 0.0 & 4.0 \end{bmatrix} \begin{bmatrix} \$1.00 \\ .50 \\ .50 \\ 1.00 \\ .50 \\ 1.20 \end{bmatrix}$$

$$= [250{,}000 \quad 444{,}000 \quad 160{,}500 \quad 208{,}000 \quad 132{,}000 \quad 406{,}000] \begin{bmatrix} \$1.00 \\ .50 \\ .50 \\ 1.00 \\ .50 \\ 1.20 \end{bmatrix}$$

$$= \boxed{\$1,313,450}$$

The price variance for each of the services also may be calculated by

$$\mathbf{VAR(Price}_k) = \mathbf{V}_s\mathbf{R}_s'(\mathbf{f}_a - \mathbf{f}_s) \qquad (18.5)$$

where $\mathbf{V}_s$ is a diagonal matrix representing the standard volume of service. Returning to our example, we find that

$$\mathbf{V}_s = \begin{bmatrix} 52,000 & 0 & 0 \\ 0 & 66,000 & 0 \\ 0 & 0 & 85,000 \end{bmatrix}$$

Thus, it can be verified that an application of Equation 18.5 to our hypothetical data yields

$$\mathbf{VAR(Price}_k) = \begin{bmatrix} \$312,000 \\ 359,700 \\ 641,750 \end{bmatrix}$$

These findings indicate that the price variance associated with service $S_1$, $S_2$, and $S_3$ amounts to $312,000, $359,700, and $641,750 respectively. The sum of the elements in $\mathbf{VAR(Price}_k)$ is equal to $1,313,450, which is the price variance for departmental activity.

We also may calculate the price variance $\mathbf{VAR(Price}_{rk})$ for each resource in providing a given service by

$$\mathbf{VAR(Price}_{rk}) = \mathbf{V}_s\mathbf{R}_s'\mathbf{F}_d \qquad (18.6)$$

where $\mathbf{F}_d$ is a diagonal matrix representing differences between actual and expected factor prices. Returning to our example, the diagonal matrix $\mathbf{F}_d$ is given by

$$\mathbf{F}_d = \begin{bmatrix} \$1.00 & 0 & 0 & 0 & 0 & 0 \\ 0 & \$.50 & 0 & 0 & 0 & 0 \\ 0 & 0 & \$.50 & 0 & 0 & 0 \\ 0 & 0 & 0 & \$1.00 & 0 & 0 \\ 0 & 0 & 0 & 0 & \$.50 & 0 \\ 0 & 0 & 0 & 0 & 0 & \$1.20 \end{bmatrix}$$

and, as can be verified, an application of Equation 18.6 yields

**VAR(Price$_{rk}$)** =

$$\begin{bmatrix} \$52,000 & \$52,000 & \$0 & \$208,000 & \$0 & \$0 \\ 198,000 & 0 & 16,500 & 0 & 66,000 & 79,200 \\ 0 & 170,000 & 63,750 & 0 & 0 & 408,000 \end{bmatrix}$$

As before, the elements in rows of **VAR(Price$_{rk}$)** represent the price variances for each resource used in providing one of the services. At this point, the reader should understand the process by which each entry summarized in Table 18-6 was obtained.

**Table 18-6** Summary of the Price Variances

| Resource | $S_1$ | $S_2$ | $S_3$ | Total |
|---|---|---|---|---|
| | | Service | | |
| Labor | | | | |
| $L_1$ | $52,000 | $198,000 | $0 | $250,000 |
| $L_2$ | 52,000 | 0 | 170,000 | 222,000 |
| $L_3$ | 0 | 16,500 | 63,750 | 80,250 |
| Supplies | | | | |
| $R_1$ | 208,000 | 0 | 0 | 208,000 |
| $R_2$ | 0 | 66,000 | 0 | 66,000 |
| $R_3$ | 0 | 79,200 | 408,000 | 487,200 |
| Total | 312,000 | 359,700 | 641,750 | 1,313,450 |

## 18.5 THE INTERACTIVE VARIANCE

Thus far this analysis has ignored the interaction between factor prices and the use of real resources. This section considers the joint effect of differences between the actual and expected use of resources as well as the effect of differences between actual and expected factor prices on the total cost variance of the department. The interactive variance is defined by

$$
\begin{matrix} \text{Interactive} \\ \text{Variance} \end{matrix} = \begin{bmatrix} \text{Actual} & \text{Expected} \\ \text{Use of} & - & \text{Use of} \\ \text{Resources} & \text{Resources} \end{bmatrix} \times \begin{bmatrix} \text{Actual} & \text{Standard} \\ \text{Factor} & - & \text{Factor} \\ \text{Price} & \text{Price} \end{bmatrix}
$$

In this formulation, the actual use of resources is given by

$$
\begin{bmatrix} \text{Actual} \\ \text{Use of} \\ \text{Resources} \end{bmatrix} = \begin{bmatrix} \text{Actual} \\ \text{Volume of} \\ \text{Service} \end{bmatrix} \times \begin{bmatrix} \text{Actual Resource} \\ \text{Requirements} \\ \text{Per Service} \end{bmatrix}
$$

while the expected use of resources may be obtained by

$$
\begin{bmatrix} \text{Expected} \\ \text{Use of} \\ \text{Resources} \end{bmatrix} = \begin{bmatrix} \text{Expected} \\ \text{Volume of} \\ \text{Service} \end{bmatrix} \times \begin{bmatrix} \text{Standard Resource} \\ \text{Requirements} \\ \text{Per Service} \end{bmatrix}
$$

Returning to our example and using the notation developed earlier, we find that the expected use of resources, $r_s$, may be obtained as follows

$$
r_s = R_s v_s
$$

$$
= \begin{bmatrix} 1.0 & 3.0 & 0.0 \\ 2.0 & 0.0 & 4.0 \\ 0.0 & .5 & 1.5 \\ 4.0 & 0.0 & 0.0 \\ 0.0 & 2.0 & 0.0 \\ 0.0 & 1.0 & 4.0 \end{bmatrix} \begin{bmatrix} 52,000 \\ 66,000 \\ 85,000 \end{bmatrix} = \begin{bmatrix} 250,000 \\ 444,000 \\ 160,500 \\ 208,000 \\ 132,000 \\ 406,000 \end{bmatrix}
$$

Similarly, the actual use of resources, as represented by the column vector $r_a$, is given by

$$\mathbf{r}_a = \mathbf{R}_a \mathbf{v}_a$$

$$= \begin{bmatrix} 1.2 & 3.1 & 0.0 \\ 2.1 & 0.0 & 4.3 \\ 0.0 & .7 & 1.7 \\ 4.3 & 0.0 & 0.0 \\ 0.0 & 2.1 & 0.0 \\ 0.0 & 1.3 & 4.2 \end{bmatrix} \begin{bmatrix} 59,220 \\ 75,600 \\ 102,375 \end{bmatrix} = \begin{bmatrix} 305,424.0 \\ 564,574.5 \\ 226,957.5 \\ 254,646.0 \\ 158,760.0 \\ 528,255.0 \end{bmatrix}$$

Consequently, the difference between the actual and expected use of resources is given by

$$\mathbf{r}_a - \mathbf{r}_s = \begin{bmatrix} 55,424.0 \\ 120,574.5 \\ 66,457.5 \\ 46,646.0 \\ 26,760.0 \\ 122,255.0 \end{bmatrix}$$

On the basis of these results, we find that

$$\text{VAR (Inter)} = (\mathbf{r}_a - \mathbf{r}_s)'(\mathbf{f}_a - \mathbf{f}_s) \qquad (18.7.1)$$

$$= [55,424.0 \quad 120,574.5 \quad 66,457.5 \quad 46,646.0 \quad 26,760.0 \quad 122,255.0]$$

$$\times \begin{bmatrix} \$1.00 \\ .50 \\ .50 \\ 1.00 \\ .50 \\ 1.20 \end{bmatrix}$$

$$= \boxed{\$355,672}$$

represents the portion of the departmental cost variance attributable to the interactive effect.

Consider next the interactive variance, $\mathbf{VAR(Inter}_{rk})$, which is associated with each resource used in providing service $k$. Using the notation developed earlier, the interactive variance, by type of resource and service, is given by

$$\boxed{\mathbf{VAR(Inter}_{rk}) = (\mathbf{V}_a \mathbf{R}_a' - \mathbf{V}_s \mathbf{R}_s')\mathbf{F}_d \qquad \textbf{(18.7.2)}}$$

$$= \mathbf{V}_a \mathbf{R}_a' \mathbf{F}_d - \mathbf{V}_s \mathbf{R}_s' \mathbf{F}_d$$

Returning to our example, it should be verified that

$$\mathbf{VAR(Inter}_{rk}) = \begin{bmatrix} \$19,064.00 & \$10,181.00 & \$0.00 \\ 36,360.00 & 0.00 & 9,960.00 \\ 0.00 & 50,106.25 & 23,268.75 \end{bmatrix}$$

$$\begin{bmatrix} \$46,646.00 & \$0.00 & \$0.00 \\ 0.00 & 13,380.00 & 38,736.00 \\ 0.00 & 0.00 & 107,970.00 \end{bmatrix}$$

As before, the elements in the rows of $\mathbf{VAR(Inter}_{rk})$ represent the interactive variance for the use of each resource in providing one of the three services. At this point, the reader should understand the process by which each of the entries summarized in Table 18-7 was obtained.

## 18.6 MANAGEMENT REPORTS

A set of reports that might be prepared for line management is summarized in Tables 18-8, 18-9, and 18-10. When the information in these tables is reported on a timely and accurate basis, the factors over which line managers exert direct control are separated clearly from those over which there is little or no control. In this case, the line manager is provided with information that depicts:

1. the total cost variance for each service provided in the unit (i.e., the sum of the values in the last row or last column of the illustration);

**Table 18-7** Summary of Interactive Variances

| Resource | Service $S_1$ | $S_2$ | $S_3$ | Total |
|---|---|---|---|---|
| $L_1$ | $19,064.00 | $36,360.00 | $0.00 | $55,424.00 |
| $L_2$ | 10,181.00 | 0.00 | 50,106.25 | 60,287.25 |
| $L_3$ | 0.00 | 9,960.00 | 23,268.75 | 33,228.75 |
| $R_1$ | 46,646.00 | 0.00 | 0.00 | 46,646.00 |
| $R_2$ | 0.00 | 13,380.00 | 0.00 | 13,380.00 |
| $R_3$ | 0.00 | 38,736.00 | 107,970.00 | 146,706.00 |
| Total | 75,891.00 | 98,436.00 | 181,345.00 | 355,672.00 |

**Table 18-8** Analysis of Cost Variance for Ancillary Service $S_1$, for the Period Ending _____

| Resource | Efficiency Variance (1) | Price Variance (2) | Volume Variance (3) | Interactive Variance (4) | Total Variance (5) |
|---|---|---|---|---|---|
| $L_1$ | $35,532 | $52,000 | $21,660 | $19,064 | $128,256 |
| $L_2$ | 23,688 | 52,000 | 57,760 | 10,181 | 143,629 |
| $L_3$ | 0 | 0 | 0 | 0 | 0 |
| $R_1$ | 17,766 | 208,000 | 28,880 | 46,646 | 301,292 |
| $R_2$ | 0 | 0 | 0 | 0 | 0 |
| $R_3$ | 0 | 0 | 0 | 0 | 0 |
| Total | 76,986 | 312,000 | 108,300 | 75,891 | 573,177 |

**Table 18-9** Analysis of Cost Variance for Ancillary Service $S_2$ for the Period Ending _____

| Resource | Efficiency Variance (1) | Price Variance (2) | Volume Variance (3) | Interactive Variance (4) | Total Variance (5) |
|---|---|---|---|---|---|
| $L_1$ | $22,680 | $198,000 | $86,400 | $36,360 | $343,440 |
| $L_2$ | 0 | 0 | 0 | 0 | 0 |
| $L_3$ | 120,960 | 16,500 | 38,400 | 9,960 | 185,820 |
| $R_1$ | 0 | 0 | 0 | 0 | 0 |
| $R_2$ | 22,680 | 66,000 | 57,600 | 13,380 | 159,660 |
| $R_3$ | 113,400 | 79,200 | 48,000 | 38,736 | 279,336 |
| Total | 279,720 | 359,700 | 230,400 | 98,436 | 968,256 |

**Table 18-10** Analysis of Cost Variance for Ancillary Service $S_3$ for the Period Ending _____

| Resource | Efficiency Variance (1) | Price Variance (2) | Volume Variance (3) | Interactive Variance (4) | Total Variance (5) |
|---|---|---|---|---|---|
| $L_1$ | $0 | $0 | $0 | $0.00 | $0.00 |
| $L_2$ | 122,850 | 170,000 | 278,000 | 50,106.25 | 620,956.25 |
| $L_3$ | 163,800 | 63,750 | 208,500 | 23,268.75 | 459,318.75 |
| $R_1$ | 0 | 0 | 0 | 0.00 | 0.00 |
| $R_2$ | 0 | 0 | 0 | 0.00 | 0.00 |
| $R_3$ | 102,375 | 408,000 | 347,500 | 107,970.00 | 965,845.00 |
| Total | 389,025 | 641,750 | 834,000 | 181,345.00 | 2,046,120.00 |

2. the cost variance for each resource used in providing each of the departmentally specific services (i.e., the row totals which appear in the last column);
3. the volume variance, efficiency variance, price variance, and interactive variance for each service (i.e., the column totals in the last row); and
4. the distribution of each component of the total variance by type of resource and service (i.e, the individual entries in the tables, excluding the row and column totals).

The values in column (1) are of fundamental importance since the efficiency variance usually results from factors over which the line manager exerts direct control. To assist line management in identifying areas requiring remedial action, the individual entries of column (1) can be expressed as a percentage of the sum of the efficiency variance for the unit. In Tables 18-8, 18-9, and 18-10,

$$\$76,986 + \$279,720 + \$389,025 = \$745,731$$

represents the total efficiency variance for the laboratory department. Expressing each entry in column (1) as a percentage of the total efficiency variance for the department results in the summary information presented in Table 18-11. This illustrates that line management should reexamine the process by which laboratory services $S_2$ and $S_3$ are provided. These data also indicate that management should carefully assess the use of resources $L_2$, $L_3$, and $R_3$ in providing these services and should examine alternate methods of improving the efficiency with which these resources are used.

Consider next the values in column (2) of Tables 18-8, 18-9, and 18-10. Recall that the personnel department is responsible for ensuring that the actual

**Table 18-11** Summary Analysis of Departmental Efficiency Variance by Type of Service and Resource for the Period Ending _____

| Resource | Service $S_1$ | $S_2$ | $S_3$ | Total |
|---|---|---|---|---|
| $L_1$ | 4.8 | 3.0 | 0.0 | 7.8 |
| $L_2$ | 3.2 | 0.0 | 16.5* | 19.7* |
| $L_3$ | 0.0 | 16.2* | 22.0* | 38.2* |
| $R_1$ | 2.4 | 0.0 | 0.0 | 2.4 |
| $R_2$ | 0.0 | 3.0 | 0.0 | 3.0 |
| $R_3$ | 0.0 | 15.2* | 13.7* | 28.9* |
| Total | 10.4 | 37.4* | 52.2* | 100.0 |

* Indicates relatively large differences between actual and expected performances.

remuneration paid to employees corresponds to the established wage and salary structure. The first three entries in column (2) of these tables indicate a need to review the performance of the personnel department or the process by which the expected wage structure is formulated.

Similarly, the price variances in the use of consumable supplies normally are the responsibility of the purchasing department or a central purchasing agent. The last three values in column (2) of Tables 18-8, 18-9, and 18-10 may indicate that supplies have not been acquired at the most favorable prices, which implies that the performance of the purchasing unit requires improvement. Alternatively, these data may suggest that all factors that influence expectations concerning factor prices have not been given adequate consideration by management. In such a situation, these data may indicate the need to improve the technique of estimating factor prices.

As mentioned, the volume variances in column (3) of Tables 18-8, 18-9, and 18-10 reflect the decisions of physicians to whom the hospital has extended privileges. In this case, the volume variances may be attributable to the management of more severe cases than was expected originally. On the other hand, an unfavorable (favorable) volume variance also may be attributable to the overuse (underuse) of service. In either case, control over volume variances should be exercised by the professional staff through the utilization review committee.

A final comment concerning this analysis is worthy of note. The interactive component of the cost variance indicates the need for coordinated action by a well-informed management team. As should be obvious from the earlier discussion, improvement by line management in the use of real resources reduces the efficiency variance while improvement by the purchasing or personnel departments reduces the price variance. In such a situation, the effects of the improved performance are *not* limited to the efficiency and price variances. Rather, these staff improvements are reflected by a reduction in the portion of the total cost variance that is attributable to interactive effects. For example, a better performance by the purchasing or personnel departments reduces the values in $(\mathbf{f}_a - \mathbf{f}_s)$ while an improvement by line management reduces the values in $(\mathbf{r}_a - \mathbf{r}_s)$. Thus, in addition to reducing the efficiency and price variance, staff improvements also reduce the interactive variance. Reductions in the variance attributable to interactive effects provide an additional incentive to improve performance.

When developing reports for higher levels of management it is necessary to summarize the detailed information that normally is required by line managers. Consider first a summary report that might be prepared for the manager of a division in which the laboratory department examined in the previous section is a component. The division manager should be provided with a report containing the data in Table 18-12 or in Table 18-13. The first of these tables summarizes the departmental variances by type of resource, the second by type of service. When similar reports are prepared for the other departments, division managers are provided with a summary of the operational performance for each department for which they are responsible.

In Table 18-13, the value in row (1) and column (1) is simply the sum of the values in row (1) and column (1) of Tables 18-8, 18-9, and 18-10. In this case, it can be verified that

$$\$58,212 = \$35,532 + \$22,680 + \$0$$

The other entries in this table are obtained in similar fashion. The data in the last row of Tables 18-8, 18-9, and 18-10 are extracted to form the body of Table 18-13 while the row and column totals of this table represent the total variance by type of service and by source of variance, respectively.

The information reported to division managers, in turn, should be summarized in reports prepared for senior management. It is convenient to divide the operations of the hospital into units that provide ancillary services, nursing care, and indirect patient services. Table 18-14 is an example of a report that summarizes the cost variances by division and by department. Entries that pertain to the laboratory department are obtained from the bottom row of Table 18-12 or Table 18-13 (they are identical). When such a report is provided on a timely and accurate basis, senior management not only can evaluate the hospital's overall performance but also can assess the extent to which imbalances have been reduced by improvements in the performance of line managers, division managers, and the heads of the purchasing and personnel departments.

**Table 18-12** Analysis of Cost Variance by Type of Resource Employed in the Laboratory Department for the Period Ending _____

| Resource | Departmental Efficiency Variance (1) | Departmental Price Variance (2) | Departmental Volume Variance (3) | Departmental Interactive Variance (4) | Total Departmental Variance (5) |
|---|---|---|---|---|---|
| $L_1$ | $58,212 | $250,000 | $108,060 | $55,424.00 | $471,696.00 |
| $L_2$ | 146,538 | 222,000 | 335,760 | 60,287.25 | 764,585.25 |
| $L_3$ | 284,760 | 80,250 | 246,900 | 33,228.75 | 645,138.75 |
| $R_1$ | 17,766 | 208,000 | 28,880 | 46,646.00 | 301,292.00 |
| $R_2$ | 22,680 | 66,000 | 57,600 | 13,380.00 | 159,660.00 |
| $R_3$ | 215,775 | 487,200 | 395,500 | 146,706.00 | 1,245,181.00 |
| Total | 745,731 | 1,313,450 | 1,172,700 | 355,672.00 | 3,587,553.00 |

**Table 18-13** Analysis of Cost Variance by Type of Service in the Laboratory Department for the Period Ending _____

| Ancillary Service | Total Efficiency Variance | Total Price Variance | Total Volume Variance | Total Interactive Variance | Total |
|---|---|---|---|---|---|
| $S_1$ | $76,986 | $312,000 | $108,300 | $75,891 | $573,177 |
| $S_2$ | 279,720 | 359,700 | 230,400 | 98,436 | 968,256 |
| $S_3$ | 389,025 | 641,750 | 834,000 | 181,345 | 2,046,120 |
| Total | 745,731 | 1,313,450 | 1,172,700 | 355,672 | 3,587,553 |

## 18.7 PRODUCTIVITY REPORTS

Since the operational manager exerts direct control only over the use of real resources in providing departmental services, the hospital's reporting system should be capable of presenting information that depicts differences between planned and current use of labor services and consumable supplies as expressed in physical terms. In particular, a set of ratios depicting differences between those two rates is of considerable value when attempting to identify problem areas requiring managerial attention and action designed to realign the actual use of resources with the planned rate of using these factor inputs. Letting $AMH_{kj}$ represent the use of labor $j$ in providing a unit of service $k$ and $SMH_{kj}$ represent the standard hours of type $j$ labor required to provide a unit of service $k$, the set of ratios given by

$$L_{kj}^* = \frac{AMH_{kj}}{SMH_{kj}} \gtreqless 1 \qquad (18.8)$$

**Table 18-14** Summary of Cost Variances by Division and Department for the Period Ending _____

| Division & Department | Efficiency Variance | Price Variance | Volume Variance | Interactive Variance | Total |
|---|---|---|---|---|---|
| *Ancillary services* | | | | | |
| Laboratory | $745,731 | $1,313,450 | $1,172,700 | $355,672 | $3,587,553 |
| Radiology | | | | | |
| Inhalation therapy | | | | | |
| . | | | | | |
| . | | | | | |
| *Nursing services* | | | | | |
| Medical | | | | | |
| Surgical | | | | | |
| Orthopedics | | | | | |
| . | | | | | |
| . | | | | | |
| *Indirect patient care* | | | | | |
| Medical records | | | | | |
| Dietary | | | | | |
| Laundry | | | | | |
| . | | | | | |
| . | | | | | |
| Total | | | | | |

reflects the extent to which the rate of using labor of type $j$ in producing service $k$ departs from the expectations of management. Returning to our example, the set of ratios depicting relative rates of using each type of labor in providing services $S_1$, $S_2$, and $S_3$ is presented here. As can be seen from the ratios in this table, the rate at which labor is used currently in producing each of the services in the department exceeds the planned rate. These data suggest that the most pronounced differences involve the use of labor category $L_3$ in providing services $S_2$ and $S_3$ and labor category $L_1$ in providing service $S_1$.

| | Type of Labor | | |
|---|---|---|---|
| Service | $L_1$ | $L_2$ | $L_3$ |
| $S_1$ | 1.20* | 1.05 | 0.00 |
| $S_2$ | 1.03 | 0.00 | 1.40* |
| $S_3$ | 0.00 | 1.08 | 1.13* |

* Indicates relatively large differences between actual and expected performance.

Management also should review systematically the use of consumable supplies in providing the services of the responsibility center. Letting $ASR_{kq}$ represent the actual use of consumable supply $q$ in providing a unit of service $k$ and $SSR_{kq}$

correspond to the standard quantity of supply item $q$ that management expects
to employ in providing a unit of service $k$, the set of ratios given by

$$R^*_{kq} = \frac{ASR_{kq}}{SSR_{kq}} \qquad (18.9)$$

reflects the difference between the current and planned rate of using inventory
by type of consumable supply and service. Returning to our example, the set
of ratios presented by $R^*_{kq}$ suggest that even though the current use of consumable
supplies exceeds the planned rate in all cases, the most pronounced difference
involves supply item $R_3$ in providing service $S_2$. These data also suggest that
the use of resources in this department is not as efficient as originally planned.

| Service | Type of Supply | | |
| | $R_1$ | $R_2$ | $R_3$ |
| --- | --- | --- | --- |
| $S_1$ | 1.08 | 0.00 | 0.00 |
| $S_2$ | 0.00 | 1.05 | 1.30* |
| $S_3$ | 0.00 | 0.00 | 1.05 |

* Indicates relatively large differences between actual and expected performance.

The ratios $L^*_{kj}$ and $R^*_{kq}$ provide information of considerable value to the process
of monitoring, controlling, and evaluating the performance of the responsibility
center. The primary advantages of productivity reporting are that

1. the information pertains to factors over which management exerts direct
   control;
2. ratios computed for all productive units in the hospital provide an index
   of performance that facilitates the comparison of one responsibility center
   with another;
3. ratios pertaining to a single responsibility center indicate disparities between planned and current rates of resource use by type of resource and
   by type of service, which is of assistance in the identification of problem
   areas and the steps required to realign actual and desired performance; and
4. data required for the construction of the indexes also may be subjected to
   statistical analysis.

The values of the computed ratios coupled with a statistical examination of
observed differences between the planned and actual use of each resource can
be helpful in performance analysis. For example, assume that the ratios $L^*_{kj}$ and
$R^*_{kq}$ pertain to a given responsibility center and that these ratios all are greater
than one. Further, suppose that several of the differences are found to be statistically significant. This suggests that, in general, the responsibility center is

not managed as efficiently as planned and that, in specific areas, it is quite likely that the difference between planned and current use cannot be attributed to chance. In such a situation, management should examine the reasons for the disparity. Further, when appropriate, it is necessary to formulate and initiate a plan of action designed to redress the imbalance. However, even though all aspects of the responsibility center should be investigated in detail, the areas with statistically significant differences between planned and current use of resources should be the object of more intensive examination.

# Chapter 19

# Short-Term Forecasting

## Objectives

After reading this chapter, you should be able to:

1. Describe the importance of projections concerning the use or provision of service in developing working capital plans.
2. Describe time series analysis as a technique for developing projections of use.
3. Describe causal models and regression as methods of projecting use.
4. Describe simulation as a forecasting technique.

## 19.1 INTRODUCTION

That the development of both long-term and short-term plans is of vital importance to the management of working capital and controlling operational activity has been emphasized throughout this text. Many of the decision models and resulting optimal solutions depend on the accuracy of the forecasts developed by management. For example, we found that the economic order quantity and the reorder point depend, in part, on forecasting inventory usage, which in turn relies on projections as to the use or provision of hospital services. Similarly, cash disbursements depend on the quantity and composition of the labor force, which also is influenced by the provision and use of hospital services. In fact, many of the formal decision models discussed relied on forecasts of the use or provision of care.

At the risk of oversimplifying, the importance of projections as to the use of service might be documented by observing that

Revenues = f(use);
Accounts receivable = f(revenues) = f(use);
Cash receipts = f(realization of accounts receivable) = f(revenues) = f(use);
Cash balances = f(cash receipts) = f(realization of accounts receivable) = f(revenues) = f(use);
Investment in marketable securities = f(cash balances) = f(cash receipts) = f(realization of accounts receivable) = f(revenues) = f(use).

Similarly, it might be argued that the hospital's demand for factor inputs such as labor, capital, and consumable supplies depends to a significant extent on the quantity and composition of service provided. In this case, we might posit that

Resource demand = f(provision of service);
Expenses = f(resource demand) = f(provision of service);
Liabilities = f(resource demand) = f(provision of service);
Cash outflows = f(expenses, liabilities) = f(resource demand) = f(provision of service);
Cash balances = f(cash outflows) = f(liabilities, expenses) = f(resource demand) = f(provision of service).

As these functional relationships indicate, the focal point for developing working capital plans and controlling operational activity involves projections concerning the use or provision of service. On the basis of such projections, these functional relations suggest that management may develop fairly reliable assumptions concerning future revenues, expenses, liabilities, accounts receivable, inventories, and investment in marketable securities. Thus, service estimates exert a significant impact on projections concerning the hospital's current assets and liabilities.

Historically, forecasts concerning future service have been based on a planning process that does not give explicit recognition to the underlying patterns or variables that influence the demand for care. However, there now exist a wide variety of forecasting techniques that may be used to derive predictions as to the use or provision of service. Many of these techniques have resulted in increased accuracy and explicit statements of the uncertainties that accompany any projection. For the purposes of working capital management and controlling the performance of the institution, short-term forecasts are most appropriate and frequently are required. As a result, the following discussion reviews methods by which short-term forecasts concerning the future use, provision, and costs of services might be developed.

## 19.2 FORECASTING TECHNIQUES

Three forecasting techniques are relevant to the problem of developing service projections—time series analysis, regression, and simulation.

### 19.2.1 Time Series Analysis—Regression Analysis

Many methods of short-term projections of use may be derived from time series data. Forecasts based on time series data consist of establishing a trend in a set of historical information and extrapolating the trend into the future. Such an approach assumes that the factors reflected in the historical pattern will remain constant and that the relationship observed historically will recur during the planning period. Such an assumption is perhaps more valid in the short run than in the long run.

When time series data are used, historical information is arranged sequentially to provide the basis for establishing a pattern or relationship over time. It frequently is necessary to use a specific functional relation in order to establish a pattern or trend from which extrapolations may be used as a forecast. Although it is not possible to discuss all of the functions that may be used to depict the behavior of a variable over time, some of the more common forms are described here.

Exponential curves are used frequently when examining variables, such as population growth or the use of outpatient services, that increase at a more or less constant rate over time. The usual form of the exponential curve is

$$y = a^x \tag{19.1}$$

where $y$ represents the variable whose value we wish to estimate. Equation 19.1 causes the variable $y$ to increase at a constant rate and, as a result, this expression represents geometric progression.

Occasionally the secular trend exhibited by a set of data may be approximated by a linear equation of the form

$$y = a + bx \tag{19.2}$$

where $y$ is the dependent variable (e.g., use) and $x$ is a single predictor variable (e.g., time). In Equation 19.2, the term $a$ represents the $y$ intercept (i.e., the value of $y$ when $x = 0$) while the term $b$ is the slope of the line (i.e., the change in $y$ associated with a unit change in $x$). Given the values of $a$ and $b$, the value of $y$ may be estimated by substituting a known or assumed value of $x$ into the linear relationship.

If we modify Equation 19.2 slightly, we may obtain the equation

$$y = a + bx + cx^2 \tag{19.3}$$

which is referred to as a second order polynomial. Second and higher order polynomials are of considerable value when estimating the relationship between costs and output or rates of operation. Such a study uses total costs as the dependent variable $y$ and output or the rate of operation as the independent variable $x$. As can be seen in any standard econometrics text, Equation 19.3 results in a "U"-shaped average cost curve and a linear marginal cost function for values of $x$ that are greater than or equal to zero. Concerning this latter point, the third order polynomial of the form

$$y = a + bx - cx^2 + dx^3 \qquad (19.4)$$

also results in a "U"-shaped average cost curve as well as a "U"-shaped marginal cost curve. Higher order polynomials of the form

$$y = a + bx + cx^2 + dx^3 + ex^4 + \cdots \qquad (19.5)$$

also may be used when establishing the relationship on which the forecast will be based.

When examining the secular movement in a set of data or establishing the relation between two variables, the first step is to plot the relevant data on graph paper. This provides a visual image of the pattern of movement or relationship that must be approximated by one of the special functions. Once management has decided to employ one of the functions, it may use regression analysis to estimate the coefficients of the equation and to assess the extent to which a specific functional relation accommodates a set of data.

In addition to special curves to reflect the movement of use or cost of service over time, management also may use moving averages and exponential smoothing techniques. Since these methods were discussed earlier, they are not considered here.

## 19.2.2 Causal Models—Regression Analysis

Occasionally, it is possible to develop a causal model in which a dependent variable (the variable to be projected) is related to a set of independent variables that exert an impact on the factor or phenomenon of interest. Such a model expresses a causal relation between the dependent variable and the set of independent variables in mathematical terms. For example, the use of service might be expressed in terms of the incidence of a disease or injury, case complexity, and case severity, as well as other factors that determine the extent to which care is utilized. We might describe such a model by

$$\text{Use} = aI + bC + cS \qquad (19.6)$$

where

| $I$ | represents the incidence of disease or injury; |
|---|---|
| $C$ | represents a composite index of the complexity of the cases managed; |
| $S$ | is a composite index of the severity of the cases managed; and |

$a, b, c$   are weights attached to $I$, $C$, and $S$, respectively.

On the basis of historical data, we might quantify Equation 19.6 and assess the model as a predictive device. In this case, multiple regression techniques usually are required.

Once the predictive capabilities of the model have been verified, the projection concerning the dependent variable may be derived by using historical values assumed by the independent variables or by using forecasts based on them. Thus, in many situations, the accuracy of projections concerning the factor of interest depends on the precision with which the set of independent variables has been estimated.

In addition to providing a mechanism by which multiple predictor variables might be incorporated in the analysis, causal models permit management to perform tests of significance and to develop confidence intervals that express the probable variation in expected outcomes. Moreover, models that incorporate several predictor variables allow management to examine the sensitivity of the dependent variable to the assumptions that define the environment of the hospital during the planning period as well as the operational decisions that must be contemplated. In this regard, causal or multiple predictor models are preferred to the time series methods. As mentioned, the use of time series methods assumes that the factors that gave rise to the historical relationship will remain constant when projecting data by extrapolation. Unfortunately, such an assumption may not be valid and the observed relationship may prove to be useless when developing forecasts.

Although causal models have many advantages, they also have disadvantages that should be considered before implementing such an approach. Causal models (1) are more costly and require more data than other approaches; and (2) normally are quite sophisticated and may require special training to interpret the results.

## 19.2.3 Simulation

Finally, there are situations in which management wishes to examine a process that involves several variables and is so complicated that it cannot be expressed in equation form. In such a situation, management should resort to simulation techniques. These require a considerable amount of data reflecting various outcomes, their probabilities of occurrence, and a specification of the process in which the relationships among the variables is identified clearly. Random numbers then may be used to simulate the process and to obtain the resulting outcomes as well as the probability of their occurrence.

All of the techniques described in this chapter are applicable to the problem of developing projections concerning the use, provision, or costs of hospital care. The major advantages of the time series methods are that they are relatively inexpensive to operate and fairly easy to develop. Causal models may be used in developing longer term projections and in expressing the variability associated with possible outcomes as well as the impact of differing assumptions concerning the operating environment of the hospital. On the other hand, causal models can be quite expensive to construct and operate on a day-to-day basis.

As might be surmised, the selection of the technique that is most appropriate in a given situation depends on the needs of management as well as the data requirements, costs, and predictive capabilities of the approaches considered. The relative weights assigned to these considerations, of course, will vary from situation to situation and from hospital to hospital. However, the application of an appropriate technique can improve the accuracy of the financial plans of the institution and thereby enhance the likelihood of achieving operational goals.

---

**REFERENCE**

Wheelwright, S. C. and Makridakis, S. *Forecasting Methods for Management*, Second Edition. New York: John Wiley & Sons, 1977.

# Index

## A

ABC inventory classification system, 230-232
Ability to pay, 117, 118
Absorbing states, 137, 140, 143
Accelerated depreciation techniques, 17
Accountants, 187
Accounting
  defined, 10
  systems of, 261
Accounting department, 235
Accounts payable, 70, 96, 99, 112
Accounts receivable, 5, 11, 69, 70, 79, 80, 81, 92, 93
  *See also* Number of days' charges in receivables (NODCIR)
  age composition of, 122, 123, 124
  average age of, 122
  and cash inflows, 7
  characteristics of, 112-113
  control of, 116-124
  costs of, 113-115
  defined, 112
  evaluation of management of, 120-124
  forecasting of, 480
  management of, 25, 116-124
  mathematical expectation of, 126
  number vs. value of, 124
  rate of conversion to cash, 8
  reduction in cycle of, 76, 79, 111
Accounts receivable turnover ratio (ART), 121
Accrued salaries and wages payable, 70
Acquisition costs. *See* Order costs
Actual costs, 10, 431
Actual unit costs, 432, 433
Adequate inventory, 9
Administration role in credit and collection departments, 120
Admission phase of accounts receivable, 118
Age composition of accounts receivable, 122, 123, 124
Allowable costs
  for Blue Cross, 15-18

in Canada, 38-40
for Medicare, 25
Allowances, 17, 18
Ambulance service, 15
Ambulatory care, 42
American Hospital Association, 282
Ancillary services, 15, 20, 27, 28,
   360, 365, 384, 386
Annual interest rates, 102, 103, 107
Annual usage, 231, 232
APL´(A Programming Language),
   284
Apportionment
   direct, 263-267
   double distribution, 274-279
   methods of, 262-284
   step-down, 267-274
AR. See Accounts receivable
ART. See Accounts receivable
   turnover ratio
Assets
   components of, 99
   current, 227
   inventory, 228
   and liabilities, 71
   lien on, 189
   long-term. See Long-term assets
   nonmoney, 153
   quick, 227
Assignment, 22
Audits, 156, 161
   fees for, 164
Average age of outstanding
   accounts, 122
Averaging historical data, 403


B

Bad debts, 22, 25, 91, 92, 93, 114,
   120, 121, 131, 140, 145
   expense of, 17
   probability of, 125
Balance sheet, 88-97, 98
Bank deposits, 158
Bank perspective, 169, 170

Bank receipts, 159
Bank statement reconciliation, 164
Basic cash contribution (BCC), 42, 43
Batching process, 403
BCC. See Basic cash contribution
Benefit period under Medicare, 23
Benefit structure
   for Blue Cross, 14-15
   in Canada, 34-37
   for commercial insurance
      companies, 20-21
   for Medicare, 23-24
Bequests, 39
Blood and blood products, 15
Blue Cross, 14-19, 26, 285
   allowable costs, 15-18
   benefit package, 14-15
   payment methods, 18-19
Bonding of employees, 155, 164
Bonds, 153, 189-190
   evaluation of, 191-195
   market price of, 192
Borrowing, 100, 166, 167, 173
   cash, 99, 107, 171
   short-term, 8, 170, 173, 175, 176
Break-even analysis, 82-88, 90, 108
Break-even point, 84, 85, 88
Budgeting, 10
   approaches to, 306-309
   importance of, 285-286
   and management functions,
      286-289
   program, 291-296, 371
   responsibility, 290-291, 405
   techniques of, 289-306
   zero-base, 296, 306, 317
Budgets, 9
   capital, 287, 318, 322, 349-350
   cash, 8, 287, 318, 322, 350-354
   cash disbursement, 353-354
   cash receipts, 350-353
   components of, 321-323
   comprehensive, 307
   expense, 287, 318, 322, 331-339
   financial, 410-416
   fixed, 307-309

flexible, 307-309
global, 289-290
line item, 290
operational, 171, 322, 375, 376,
    377-392, 406-410
partial, 307
preparation of, 311-319
responsibility, 290-291, 405
revenue, 258, 287, 318, 322,
    339-349
salary, 331-337
supply expense, 337-339
systematic development of, 312
wage, 331-337
Buffer stock, 9, 228, 229, 246, 247,
    248, 249, 251
Buildings, 39
Built-in equipment, 39

**C**

Canada
    contractual allowances in, 341
    cost containment in, 257
    financing mechanisms in, 33-48
    global budgeting system in, 289
    noninstitutional sources of
        payments in, 132
    prospective reimbursement in,
        11, 19
    provinical plan in, 34, 44-45, 285
    sources of payment in, 112, 113,
        132
Canadian Hospital Accounting
    Manual, 261
Canadian Hospital Association, 261
Capital, 70
    forecasting of, 480
Capital assets, 39
Capital budget, 287, 318, 322,
    349-350
Capital costs, 9, 17
Capital equipment, 5
    costs of, 16
Carrying costs, 237-239, 241, 242,
    245, 247

Cash, 5, 70, 71, 72, 81
    availability of, 7
    composition of, 154
    control of, 155-165
    costs of holding, 94, 166, 185
    defined, 154
    idle, 8, 94, 155, 166, 187
    importance of, 154-155
    management of, 7, 8, 11, 155-165
    misappropriation of, 155, 156, 158,
        159
    motives for holding, 165, 166
    on hand, 94
    ownership of, 155
    precautionary demands for, 165,
        166
    separation of functions of handling
        and accounting, 156, 158, 164
    shortages of, 8, 175
    speculative demand for, 165, 166
    surpluses of, 131, 175
    surprise checks on, 156, 164
    transaction demand for, 165, 166
Cash asset management, 25
Cash balance, 7, 69, 94
    under certainty conditions, 170-172
    decision on, 165-167
    and expected costs, 179
    forecasting of, 480
    and long-costs, 179
    minimum, 169-170
    optimum, 178-185
    and short-costs, 176
    under uncertainty conditions,
        172-185
Cash borrowing, 99, 107, 171
Cash budget, 8, 287, 318, 322,
    350-354
Cash buffer, 165
Cash disbursements, 7, 74, 81, 89,
    159-161, 167, 168
    budget for, 353-354
    control of, 160
    summary of, 354
Cash flows, 72-81, 90, 105, 111,
    169, 170, 171, 172

estimation of, 127
merging sets of, 169
nature of, 167-169
negative net, 175
net, 173, 174, 175, 176, 180,
    181, 182, 183
by planning period, 129
timing and magnitude of, 125
Cash forecasting, 8
Cashier's facilities, 156
Cash inflows, 7, 81, 99, 122, 168,
    171, 180, 181, 323, 353
expected, 203
in prospective reimbursement,
    76-80
in retrospective reimbursement,
    73-76
Cash outflows, 73, 74, 76, 81, 99,
    167, 171, 179, 180
Cash receipts, 7, 8, 72, 73, 74,
    76, 81, 111, 124, 156-159, 167,
    168
budget for, 350-353
estimation of, 125-148
forecasting of, 480
by mail, 57
magnitude of, 137
nonrandom, 353
over-the-counter, 158, 159
present value of future, 203
random, 180
summary of, 354
timing of, 137
Cash registers, 156
Cash reserves, 170
Catastrophic insurance, 20, 21
Causal models, 482-483
CDs. See Certificates of deposit
Census reports, 362, 364
Central supply, 234
Certificates of deposit (CDs), 188-189
Chapel receipts, 39
Charity care, 17, 18, 25, 91, 92,
    93, 118, 120, 121
Chart of accounts, 260
Check handling, 157, 160, 161

Chief financial officer, 120, 172,
    188, 224
CI. See Cash inflows
CO. See Cash outflows
Coinsurance charges, 14, 17, 18, 21,
    24, 25, 26, 34, 131
Collateral trust bonds, 189
Collection
costs of, 114
procedures for, 38
Collection agency, 114
Collection department, 114, 115, 120,
    124
Collective bargaining, 259
Column vector, 51
Combination method of Medicare
    payment, 27-29
Commercial insurance companies,
    14, 19-22
Common stock, 190, 191
equity in, 197
Components of hospital care, 373-375
Compound interest, 192
Comprehensive budgets, 307
Comprehensive insurance coverage,
    20
Computer applications, 284
Consumable supplies. See Supplies
Contractual allowances, 91, 92, 93,
    341
Contractual obligations, 167, 168
Contributed services, 39
Control, 287-288
of accounts receivable, 116-124
of cash, 155-165
of cash disbursements, 160
internal. See Internal controls
of inventory, 232-236
of operational activity, 287, 424
of program area, 423
of responsibility center, 451
Controllable costs, 424
Coordination, 288
Corporate bonds, 189-190
Corporate stocks, 190-191
Cost analysis, 9, 10, 257-284

alternate methods of, 283-284
prerequisites for, 260-262
Cost based charges, 29
Cost-benefit analysis, 297, 302-306
Cost centers, 29, 258, 359
  classification of, 260
Cost containment, 3-4, 19, 257
Cost-effectiveness analysis, 297, 298-302
Cost finding. *See* Cost analysis
Cost-plus basis, 14, 15
Costs
  *See also* Expenses
  accounts receivable, 113-115
  actual, 10, 431, 432, 433
  ancillary services, 27, 28
  capital, 9, 17
  capital equipment, 16
  carrying, 237-239, 241, 242, 245, 247
  charity, 17, 25
  collection, 114
  controllable, 424
  credit, 102, 114
  credit extension, 116
  delinquency, 114-115, 116, 120
  direct, 419-420
  educational activity, 15, 25
  employment, 39
  equipment, 398-401, 416-418
  expected, 10, 179, 184
  external indirect, 341
  fixed. *See* Fixed costs
  historical, 16
  of holding cash, 94, 166, 185
  hospital care, 19, 40
  indirect, 420-421
  inventory, 236-241
  labor, 392-393, 394-397
  long-. *See* Long-costs
  marginal, 249, 250
  medical care, 3
  net opeating, 80
  occupancy, 39
  operating, 9, 80, 81, 228
  opportunity, 8, 80, 81, 107,
      113-114, 116, 120, 122, 166, 171,
      187, 209, 210, 228, 237, 238, 239
  order, 236-237, 239, 240, 241, 242,
      245, 247
  overhead, 416-418, 420-421
  production, 341
  program activity, 431
  projection of, 201
  of providing support services, 9
  purchased services, 39
  replacement, 16
  research, 15, 25, 40
  revenue-generating center
      operations, 341
  routine services, 27
  short-. *See* Short-costs
  storage, 237, 238
  supply, 39, 84, 337, 392-393,
      397-398
  total. *See* Total costs
  transaction, 215
  uncontrollable, 424
  unit, 232, 432, 433
  variable, *See* Variable costs
  working capital, 97, 111
Cost variances, 365-366, 367
  defined, 424
  total, 426, 427-434, 451,
      452-455, 469
Coupon bonds, 189, 190
Courtesy discounts, 91, 92, 93, 121
Credit, 152
  costs of, 102, 114
  extension of, 101, 115, 116
  liberalizing of, 115
  open line of, 166
Credit department, 120, 124
Credit rating, 8, 104, 155, 166,
      170, 173
Current assets, 5, 7, 70, 71, 72,
      80, 98, 227
  estimation of, 90-95
Current market value of stocks, 203
Current ratios, 198
Cutoff, 195
Cycle stock, 246

**D**

Data base, 229
Data collection, 402-404
Days of supply expenses financed
  by accounts payable
  (DOSEFAP), 96
Debentures, 189
Debt principal, 39
Decision matrix, 231
Declining balance method, 17
Deductible clauses, 14, 17, 18, 21,
  24, 25, 26, 131
Delinquency costs, 114-115, 116, 120
Demand for health care, 4, 99, 228,
  240, 241, 246, 247, 248, 252
  nature of, 307
Departmental method of Medicare
  payment, 26-27
Depreciation charges, 16, 17, 25, 39,
  40, 84, 89, 90
Derivative functions of money, 152
Determinant, 59-65
Diagnostic mix, 377-381, 428,
  434-437
Direct apportionment, 263-267, 282
Direct costs, 419-420
  equipment, 398-401
  operational, 9
Direct patient services, 342-344
Discharge phase of accounts
  receivable, 119
Discounted present value (DPV), 194
Discounting, 194
Discount period, 103
Discount rate, 205
Discounts, 17, 18, 120
Dispensing of inventories, 232
Dividends, 190
  projection of, 201-202
DOSEFAP. See Days of supply
  expenses financed by accounts
  payable
Double distribution apportionment,
  274-279, 282
DPV. See Discounted present value

**E**

Earnings per share (EPS) ratio, 199
Economic order quantity (EOQ), 9,
  243, 246-252
Educational activities, 15, 25
Efficiency variance, 451, 458-466
Emergency treatment, 15, 20, 23
Employment costs, 39
Endorsement of checks, 157
Endowments, 39, 222
End-of-year adjustments, 45
EOQ. See Economic order quantity
EPS. See Earnings per share
Equipment, 5, 39, 40, 70, 84, 94
  acquisition of, 353
  cost of, 16, 398-401, 416-418
Equipment trust bonds, 189
Equity, 99, 100
  common stock, 197
Estate mortgage bonds, 189
Estimation
  of cash flow, 127
  of cash receipts, 125-148
  of current assets, 90-95
  of liabilities, 96-97
  of long-term assets, 95-96
  of probability of requiring health
    care, 132
  procedures for, 136-148
  of resouce requirements, 387-392
  of work load, 323-331
Evaluation
  of accounts receivable
    management, 120-124
  of bonds, 191-195
  of cash control system, 161-165
Excluded costs, 15
Expected cash inflow, 203
Expected costs, 10, 184
  and cash balance, 179
Expected diagnostic mix, 377-381
Expected expenses, 81
Expected long-cost function, 176-178
Expected revenues, 81, 258
Expected short-cost function, 173-176

Expense budget, 9, 10, 287, 318, 322, 331-339
Expenses
 *See also* Costs
 bad debt, 17
 expected, 81
 forecasting of, 480
 operating, 230
 reporting of, 366-368
 supply, 228
Expert opinions, 403
Exponential smoothing, 328-330
Extended health care, 42
Extension of credit, 101, 115, 116
External auditors, 161, 164
External debt, 16
External indirect costs, 341

**F**

Factor inputs, 5
Factor price variance, 451
Federal contribution in Canada, 41-44
Federal-Provincial Fiscal Arrangements and Established Programs Financing Act, 33, 34, 41
Fee schedule, 258
Financial budget, 410-416
Financial forecasting, 131
Financial information, 262
Financial management, 10
Financial manager, 81
Financial planning, 81
Financial statements, 81-97
Financing
 in Canada, 40-45
 of health care, 10-11, 18, 21-22, 24-25
 mechanisms of, 5, 40-45
 of temporary working capital, 104-106
 of working capital, 97-107, 99-106
 of working capital assets, 5
Fiscal services division, 172

Fixed assets, 70, 71, 80
Fixed budgets, 307-309
Fixed costs, 83, 84, 108
 reduction of, 87
Flexible budgets, 307-309
Forecasting
 short-term, 479
 in stock evaluation, 200-206
 techniques of, 480-484
Foregone returns, 80
Free care. *See* Charity
Full cost pricing, 421-422
Functions of management, 286-289
Functions of money, 151-154
Funding. *See* Financing
Furniture, 40

**G**

Generalized purchasing power, 152
General service centers, 258, 263, 267
Geometric mean, 323-328
Gifts, 39
Global budget, 289-290
Goals, 288, 373
 *See also* Objectives
 of responsibility centers, 323
"Goods in process," 228
Government bonds, 189-190
Government treasury bills, 188
Gross interest rate, 113

**H**

Health care
 components of, 373-375
 costs of, 3, 19
 demand for, 4, 99, 228, 240, 241, 246, 247, 248, 252, 307
 estimation of probability of requiring, 132
 financing of, 10-11
Health and Human Services Department, 282
Historical analysis of stocks, 196-199
Historical costs, 16

Historical data, 403
Holiday relief, 334
Home care, 42
Home health agencies, 24
Hospital Financial Management
    Association, 282
Hospital Insurance and Diagnostic
    Services Act, 33, 34, 41
Hospital services, defined, 41

I

Identity matrix, 145
Idle cash, 8, 94, 155, 166, 187
Imprest funds, 160
Income statements, 82-88, 89, 90
Income tax reduction, 44
Incremental approach to budgeting,
    307
Indemnity benefits, 21
Indirect costs, 9, 420-421
Inflation, 4, 8, 16, 17, 26, 153, 155
Information systems, 120, 229,
    261-262, 402-404
Inpatient benefits, 34, 35-36
Inpatient services, 20, 33, 38
Institutional sources of payment, 112,
    125-131
Insurance companies, 14, 19-22
Insurance premiums, 84
Interactive variance, 451, 467-469,
    472
Interest charges, 8, 39
    on past due accounts, 115
Interest-earning securities, 111
Interest income, 7, 153
Interest rates, 102, 103, 107
    on bonds, 189, 192
    gross, 113
    nominal, 192
    risk-free, 203
Internal audits, 156, 161
Internal controls, 155, 162-164,
    357-360
    and working capital management,
    5-7

Internal rates of return, 8, 195,
    203-204
Intrinsic value of investments, 8,
    204-205
Inventory, 5, 7, 9, 70, 80
    See also Supplies
    control of, 232-236
    costs of, 236-241
    cycles of, 237
    importance of, 228-229
    lifesaving qualities of, 232
    management of. See Inventory
        management
    perishability component of, 239
    physical, 235
    protection of, 238
Inventory asset, 228
Inventory holdings, 69, 228
Inventory management, 9
    in certainty, 241-245
    defined, 229
    functions of, 229-230
    in uncertainty, 245-254
Inventory-purchase ratio, 93
Inventory turnover ratio, 199
Inverse of a matrix, 59-65
Investment analyst, 187, 224
Investments, 8, 69, 154
    alternatives, 188-191
    forecasting of, 480
    income from, 39
    possibilities in, 131
    single, 206-221
    strategy for, 223-224
IOUs, 154

J

Job rotation, 164

L

Labor, 5, 71, 73
    See also Salaries; Wages
    cost of, 392-393, 394-397
    forecasting of, 480

hours of per unit of service, 361
Labor efficiency variance, 439-442
Land, 5
  improvements in, 39, 70
Lawyers for collection, 114
Lead time, 237, 245, 247, 248, 251
Least cost solution, 254
Leveling payments, 43-44
Liabilities, 5, 7, 71, 98
  estimation of, 96-97
  forecasting of, 480
  long-term, 98, 99
  recording of, 159
  short-term, 99
  validation of, 161
Liens on assets, 189
Lifesaving qualities of inventory, 232
"Life-time" reserve under Medicare, 23
Line item budgeting, 290
Liquid assets, 70
Liquidity
  of portfolios, 222-223, 224
  ratios of, 198-199
Locked cashier's facilities, 156
Long-costs, 166, 170, 172, 173, 183
    239, 241, 242, 245, 252, 253
  and cash balance, 179
  expected, 176-178
Long-term assets, 70, 95-96, 98
Long-term borrowing, 100
Long-term debt, 7, 104, 105
Long-term financing, 5
Long-term indebtedness, 84
Long-term liabilities, 98, 99

**M**

Mail receipts, 157
Major medical, 20, 21
Management
  functions of, 286-289
  objectives of, 4
Management information system, 120
Management model on investments, 206-221

Management reports, 448-450, 469-474
Marginal costs, 249, 250
Marketability of portfolios, 222-223
Marketable securities, 5, 7, 8, 69, 104, 107, 165, 170
  forecasting of, 480
  management of, 187-224
  sale of, 166, 167, 171, 173, 215, 216
  short-term, 70
Markov chains, 132-136, 140
Maternity benefits, 20
Mathematical expectation model
  for accounts receivable, 126
  for reorder point, 252-254
Matrix
  decision, 231
  defined, 50
  determinant and inverse of, 59-65
  identity, 145
  inverse of, 59-65
  partitioned, 146
  square, 59
  transitional probability, 133, 140
Matrix addition, 52
Matrix algebra, 49-65, 128, 262, 276, 284, 371
Matrix multiplication, 53-59
Matrix subtraction, 52-53
Maturity of securities, 225
Medicaid, 14, 22, 29-30
Medical care costs, 3
Medical records, 402
Medical technology, 4, 16
Medicare, 14, 22-29, 286
  receipt of payments from, 26-29
Medium of exchange, 152, 154, 165
Merchandising function, 348-349
Minimum cash balance, 169-170
Minimum working capital need (MWCN), 74
Misappropriation of cash by employees, 155, 156, 158, 159
Monetary costs of insufficient inventories, 240

Money
functions of, 151-154
ratio of to nonmonetary assets, 153
time value of, 203
Monthly summary statement, 426
Moody's Investors Service, 191
Mortgages, 153
Motivation for holding cash, 165, 166
Movable equipment, 40
Moving average, 323-328
Mutually exclusive states, 132, 137
MWCN. See Minimum working
capital need

N

Negative net cash flows, 175
Net cash flows, 90, 171, 173, 174,
175, 176, 180, 181, 182, 183
Net costs, 25, 80
Net expense, 16, 25
Net income, 5, 81, 90
Net interest charges, 25
Net interest rates, 113
Net loss, 5, 81, 90
Net operating costs, 80
Net patient service revenue, 121
Net period, 103
Net working capital, defined, 70
New forecasst of use, 328
NODCIR. See Number of days'
charges in receivables
Nominal rate of interest, 192
Nonabsorbing states. See Transitional
states
Nonfinancial information, 261, 262
Noninstitutional sources of payment,
112, 113, 131-148
Nonmonetary costs of insufficient
inventories, 240
Nonmoney assets, 153
Nonmovable equipment, 40
Nonoperating revenues, 38, 80
Nonplan revenues, 89, 91, 92
Nonrandom cash flows, 169, 170
Nonrandom cash inflows, 168, 180

Nonrandom cash outflows, 179, 180
Nonrandom cash receipts, 73, 76, 353
Number of days' charges in
receivables (NODCIR), 91, 92,
94, 121, 122
Nurse therapists, 24
Nursing facilities, 23, 25, 38
NWC. See Net Working capital

O

Objectives, 371
See also Goals
of institution, 229
of management, 4
of responsibility centers, 323
Obstetrical benefits, 20
OC. See Opportunity costs or
Order costs
Occupancy costs, 39
Offset revenues, 39, 40
On-call duty requirements, 334
Open line of credit, 166
Operating cash flow, 90
Operating costs, 9, 81, 228
Operating expenses, 230
Operating loss, 89
Operating stock, 246, 247
Operational activity, 5
control of, 259-260, 287, 424
planning of, 258-259
recording and reporting of, 357
reports on, 426
Operational budget, 9, 10, 171, 322,
375, 376, 377-392, 406-410
Opportunity costs, 8, 80, 81, 107,
113-114, 116, 120, 122, 166, 171,
187, 209, 210, 228, 237, 238,
239
Optimal reorder point, 248
Optimization problems, 302-303
Optimum cash balance, 94, 178-185
Optimum order quantity, 243, 247,
248
Optimum reorder point, 241, 252
Order costs, 236-237, 239, 240, 241

242, 245, 247
Order quantity, 243
Order size, 241, 247, 248
Organizational structures, 283
Organization chart, 260
Organizing, 288-289
Outpatient benefits, 15, 20, 23, 34, 36
Outpatient services, 33, 36-37
Output, defined, 7
Over-the-counter cash receipts, 158, 159
Overhead costs, 398-401, 416-418, 420-421
Overstocked costs. *See* Long-costs

**P**

Partial budgets, 307
Participating preferred stocks, 190
Partitioned matrix, 146
Passive transactions, 167
Patient accounts manager, 120
Patient day forecast, 323
Patient population size and mix, 377, 424, 428, 429
Patient profile, 360
Patient records, 402
Patient service centers, 258, 267
Payment methods, 22
  Blue Cross, 18-19
  in Canada, 44-45
Payoffs, 206
Payroll checks, 161
PCB. *See* Per capita base
PCR. *See* Per capita rate
Per capita base (PCB), 42
Per capita rate (PCR), 42, 43
Performance reports, 426
Performance standards, 9
Periodic adjustments, 45
Periodic Interim Payments (PIP), 26, 167, 286
Periodic inventory system, 235
Perishability component of inventory, 239
Perpetual inventory system, 229, 235

Personal payment plans for patients, 117, 118
Personnel management, 259
Petty cash funds, 164
Pharmaceutical stocks, 239
Physical inventory, 235
Physical plant, 39, 70, 84
Physician role in cost containment, 19
Physician services, 41
PIP. *See* Periodic Interim Payments
Planned staffing patterns, 259
Planning, 131, 286-287
Planning period, 129, 171
Plan revenues, 89, 91
Plant budget. *See* Capital budget
Portfolios, 221-224
Possession costs. *See* Storage costs
Postage stamps, 154
Postdated checks, 154
Post-discharge phase of accounts receivable, 120
Postsecondary education, 42
Preadmission phase of accounts receivable, 116-118
Precautionary demand for cash, 165, 166
Preferred stock, 190, 191
Premium pay hours, 334
Prenumbered checks, 160
Prepayment, 7, 26
Present value analysis, 8, 195, 202-203
Price information, 402
Price variances, 463-466, 472
Pricing, 421-422
Primary functions of money, 151
Prime symbol, 51
Probability models, 8, 9
  on distribution of patients, 428
  on health, 133
  Markov chains, 132-136, 140
Production costs, 341
Production function, 71
Production phase of accounts receivable, 118-119

Productivity reports, 425, 474-477
Professional investment analyst, 187,
	224
Profitability forecasting, 200, 201
Profitability ratios, 196-198
Program areas, 372-373
	control of, 423
	direct equipment costs of,
		398-401
	labor costs of, 398-401
	overhead of, 398-401
	service requirements of, 381-387
	supply costs of, 392-393
Program budgeting, 291-296, 371
Projected balance sheet, 95, 98
Projected fee schedule, 258
Projected income statement, 89
Projection
	of costs, 201
	of dividends, 201-202
	of profits, 201
	of sales, 200-201
	of working capital needs, 81
Promissory notes, 153
Prospective reimbursement, 11, 13,
	19, 33, 72, 80, 81, 88, 91, 111,
	115, 167, 168
	cash inflows in, 76-80
Protection of inventory, 238
Provincial plan in Canada, 34, 44-45,
	285
Purchasing, 232
Purchasing agent, 234
Purchasing department, 234
Purchasing power, 152, 153

Q

Quick assets, 227
Quick ratios, 198

R

Random cash flows, 169, 170
Random cash inflows, 168, 181
Random cash receipts, 73, 76, 180

Random variables, 72
Rate of return, 203-204
Rate setting, 419-422
Ratio analysis, 88-97, 196
Reasonable cost basis, 25
Receivables. See Accounts receivable
Receiving department, 232, 234
Recovery, 38, 121
Registered bonds, 189
Regression analysis, 330-331,
	481-483
Rental payments, 84
Reorder point, 234, 241, 246-252,
	247, 248, 249, 251, 252
Replacement costs, 16
Reporting systems, 229, 287, 425-426
Reports, 448-450, 469-474
	statistical, 360-366
Requisitioning, 232
Research costs, 15, 25, 40
Residential care, 42
Resource requirements, 387-392, 426,
	430
	forecasting of, 480
Responsibility budgeting, 290-291,
	405
Responsibility centers, 287, 288, 290,
	323, 359, 373
	control of, 451
	equipment cost in, 416-418
	financial budget of, 410-416
	operational budget of, 406-410
	overhead of, 416-418
Retrospective reimbursement, 5, 11,
	13, 72, 79, 81, 89, 90, 93, 111,
	115
	cash inflows in, 73-76
Return on assets ratio, 197
Return on investment, 222
Revenue budget, 9, 258, 287, 318,
	322, 339-349
Revenue-generating activities,
	29, 121, 122, 263, 341
Revenues
	expected, 10, 81, 258
	net patient service, 121

nonoperating, 38, 80
nonplan, 89, 91, 92
offset, 39, 40
plan, 89, 91
reporting of, 366-368
sources of, 14, 34-38
total, 4, 85, 86, 87, 88, 89
and volume of patient care, 83
Risk
attitude toward, 170, 222, 223
reduction of, 221-222, 223
and return, 191, 222
of stocks, 191
and uncertainty, 205-206
Risk capital, 223
Risk-free interest rate, 203
Risk premium, 205
Row vectors, 51, 129, 130, 131

**S**

Safety stock. *See* Buffer stock
Salaries, 70, 73, 74, 84, 94, 353
*See also* Labor; Wages
budget for, 331-337
structure of, 425
of top management, 84
Sales projections, 200-201
Savings accounts, 154
Scalar multiplication, 53
Secured bonds, 189
Securities. *See* Marketable securities
Self-liquidating nature of working
capital needs, 99
Separation of cash handling and
accounting functions, 156, 158,
164
Serial bonds, 189
Service mix variance, 437-439
Short-costs, 166, 169, 170, 172, 182,
183, 239, 240-241, 242, 245,
246, 247, 252, 253
expected, 173-176
Short-term borrowing, 8, 100, 167,
170, 173, 175, 176
Short-term debt, 7, 104, 105, 152

Short-term financing, 5, 106-107
Short-term forecasting, 479
Short-term liabilities, 99
Short-term loans, 173
Short-term marketable securities, 70
Short-term obligations, 70
SHUR. *See* System for Hospital
Uniform Reporting
Signing of checks, 160, 161
Simulation, 483-484
Single distribution apportionment.
*See* Step-down apportionment
Single security strategy, 206-221
Sinking fund bonds, 189
Skilled nursing facilities, 23, 25
Social Security Act, 22, 29
Social Security Administration, 25
Sources of revenue, 14, 34-38
Speculative demand for cash, 165,
166
Square matrices, 59
Staffing patterns, 259, 360
Standard of deferred payments,
152-153
Standard factor prices, 393-394
Standardized direct patient services,
342-344
Standard mix of services, 429
Standard & Poor's Corporation, 191
Standards of performance, 9
State funds, 30
Statistical reports, 360-366
Stay-specific services, 15, 344-347,
360, 374, 384, 386
Step-down apportionment, 267-274,
282
Stock-out, 240
costs of. *See* Short-costs
Stocks, 190-191
analysis of, 202-206
selection of, 195-206
Storage
costs of, 237, 238
problems of, 232
Store of value, 153-154, 165
Straight-line depreciation, 17

Summary analysis, 121
Sum-of-years-digit, 17
Supplies, 5, 7, 9, 71, 73, 74,
    94, 228, 238, 353, 403
    See also Inventory
    costs of, 39, 84, 337, 392-393,
        397-398
    forecsting of, 480
Supply efficiency variance, 442-444
Supply expenses, 228
    budget for, 337-339
Supply of hospital services, 4
Supply price variance, 446-447
Support centers, 258
Surgical benefits, 20
Surprise checks on cash, 156, 164
System for Hospital Uniform
    Reporting (SHUR), 261

T

T bills. See Treasury bills
Teaching and research program costs,
    15, 25
Technology, 4, 16
Temporary investments, 154
Temporary working capital, 99,
    104-106
Term deposits, 154
Third party payers, 37, 117, 118,
    125
    defined, 14
Time-and-motion studies, 404
Time series analysis, 481-482
Time value of money, 203
Timing of receipts, 19
Title XVIII of Social Security
    Act, 22, 23, 24, 30
Title XIX of Social Security Act,
    22, 29
Total assets, 80
Total cost curves, 84, 85
Total cost function, 242
Total costs, 4, 83, 87, 247, 248
    and volume of patient care, 84,
        85, 86, 88, 89

Total cost variance, 427-434, 452-455,
    469
Total entity approach to budgeting,
    306
Total revenue curve, 84
Total revenues, 4, 85, 86, 87, 88, 89
Total variance, 426, 451
Trade credit, 100-104, 106, 107, 113
    advantages of, 115-116
Transaction costs, 215
Transaction demand for cash,
    165, 166
Transient states, 140
Transitional probability matrix, 133,
    140
Transitional states, 137, 143, 146
Transpose, 51
Trapping states. See Absorbing states
Treasury (T) bills, 188

U

Uncollectable receivables, 131, 137,
    138, 351
Uncontrollable costs, 424
Uncontrollable transactions, 167
Unit costs, 232, 432, 433
Unit of value function of money, 152
Universal approach to budgeting, 306
Unsecured bonds. See Debentures

V

Vacation relief, 334
Vacuum approach to budgeting, 306
Variable costs, 84, 87, 108
    reduction in, 88
Variance
    cost. See Cost variances
    diagnostic mix, 434-437
    efficiency, 451, 458-466
    factor price, 451
    interactive, 451, 467-469, 472
    labor efficiency, 439-442
    price, 463-466, 472
    supply efficiency, 442-444

supply price, 446-447
total, 451
total cost, 469
volume, 451, 455-458, 471, 472
wage, 444-446
Vaults, 156
Vector-matrix products, 54
Vectors, 51, 53, 129, 130, 131
Volume of patient care, 83, 84, 85, 86, 88, 89, 90
Volume variance, 451, 455-458, 471, 472
Voluntary prepayment plan, 26
Voucher, 161

**W**

Wages, 70, 73, 74, 84, 94, 353
*See also* Labor; Salaries
budget for, 331-337
information on, 402
structure of, 425
Wage variance, 444-446
WC. *See* Working capital
Working capital
*See also* Working capital needs
costs of, 97, 111
defined, 69

financing of, 97-107
management of. *See* Working capital management
nature of, 98-99
temporary, 99
Working capital management
defined, 5
importance of, 70-72
and internal control, 5-7
value of, 7-10
Working capital needs, 72-97, 97
and financial statements, 81-97
financing of, 99-104
projection of, 81
Work load, 452
estimation of, 323-331
Workmen's compensation, 14
Workmen's Compensation Board, 37
Work sampling, 404

**Y**

Y transpose, 51

**Z**

Zero-base budgeting, 296-306, 317

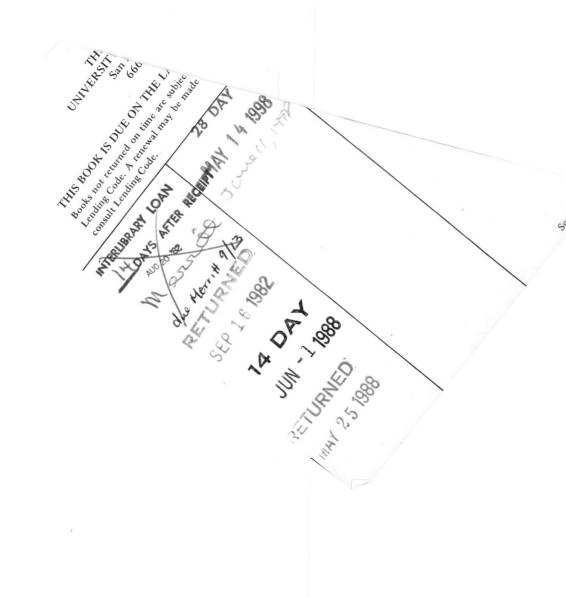